Vision and Aging

Second Edition

Vision and Aging

Second Edition

Edited by

Alfred A. Rosenbloom, Jr., M.A., O.D., D.O.S.
Director, Low Vision Services
The Chicago Lighthouse for People Who Are Blind or
  Visually Impaired
Past President and Dean Emeritus
Illinois College of Optometry
Chicago, Illinois
Chair, Geriatric Optometry Committee
American Optometric Association

Meredith W. Morgan, O.D., Ph.D.
Professor and Dean Emeritus
University of California, Berkeley
School of Optometry
Berkeley, California
Visiting Professor, School of Optometry
The Medical Center, University of Alabama
Birmingham, Alabama
Visiting Professor, School of Optometry
University of Waterloo
Waterloo, Ontario, Canada

With 19 Contributing Authors

Butterworth–Heinemann
Boston   London   Oxford   Singapore   Sydney   Toronto   Wellington

Every effort has been made to ensure that the drug dosage schedules within this text are accurate and conform to standards accepted at time of publication. However, as treatment recommendations vary in the light of continuing research and clinical experience, the reader is advised to verify drug dosage schedules herein with information found on product information sheets. This is especially true in cases of new or infrequently used drugs.

 Recognizing the importance of preserving what has been written, it is the policy of Butterworth–Heinemann to have the books it publishes printed on acid-free paper, and we exert our best efforts to that end.

Library of Congress Cataloging-in-Publication Data
Vision and Aging / edited by Alfred A. Rosenbloom, Jr., Meredith W. Morgan; with 19
  contributing authors. — 2nd ed.
    p. cm.
  Includes bibliographical references and index.
  ISBN 0-7506-9311-8 (acid-free paper)
    1. Geriatric ophthalmology.   2. Vision disorders in old age.   3. Eye — Diseases and
      defects — Age factors.   I. Rosenbloom, Alfred A.   II. Morgan, Meredith W.
  RE48.2.A5V57   1992
  618.97'77 — dc20   92-37391
                                                                                    CIP

British Library Cataloguing–in–Publication Data.
A catalogue record for this book is available from the British Library.

Butterworth–Heinemann
80 Montvale Avenue
Stoneham, MA 02180

10 9 8 7 6 5 4 3 2 1

Printed in the United States of America

Contents

Foreword

Eye care specialists find themselves in the enviable position of having the skills to contribute significantly to the quality of life of most older people. Nowhere are the principles of excellence in geriatrics so well illustrated as in the provision of quality primary eye and vision care with its emphasis on prevention, early detection, comprehensive assessment, and functional improvement. Excellence in the practice is distinguished by breadth and depth of knowledge, interdisciplinary cooperation, community outreach, and extension of service to nontraditional settings.

The editors deserve commendation for organizing a text that is so timely, authoritative, and relevant to comprehensive vision care of older people. Building on the excellent first edition, this new edition, *Vision and Aging,* provides updated information in areas of special importance to optometrists. It emphasizes the importance of early detection of eye problems and prevention of blindness, probably the greatest fear of older people. Although directed primarily to optometrists, the text does not neglect the importance of interdisciplinary team care of older patients. The management approaches described in this text are significant in fostering a sense of independence and in enhancing enjoyment of favorite activities. There is also excellent practical advice concerning assessment and care of older patients in both home and institutional settings. Despite the advances in eye and vision care, there is often a failure to recognize that aging does not result in inevitable loss of vision and independence. This book helps to dispel that myth. As a medical colleague specializing in geriatric patient care, I encourage optometrists and ophthalmologists to reach out to the community and let people know that life can be satisfying and fulfilling. A baby's smile, a rainbow, a home run that clears two fences, city lights at sunset, and a garden's first seedlings are visual pleasures that can make life worth living at any age!

Warmest Aloha,

Patricia Lanoie Blanchette, M.D., M.P.H.
Associate Professor of Medicine and Public Health
Chief, Division of Geriatric Medicine
Director, Pacific Islands Geriatric Education Center
John A. Burns School of Medicine
University of Hawaii

Preface to the First Edition

The purpose of this book is to bring into focus the vast variety of concepts concerning vision and aging. By so doing, vision care practitioners will be able to relate these concepts to the larger goal of providing vision care as a part of comprehensive health service to older persons. In various respects this text is an updating and expansion of optometry's first and only volume on aging — *Vision of the Aging Patient*, edited by Monroe J. Hirsch and Ralph E. Wick. Over 25 years have passed since its publication; moreover, it has been out of print for at least a decade. In the meantime, the number of aging individuals both healthy and unhealthy, vigorous and infirm has increased dramatically so that today every eighth person in the United States is over 65 years of age. Nearly every individual in this diverse group needs optometric care. Optometrists must be prepared to offer this needed care as informed and sympathetic health care practitioners.

Several guiding principles which serve as a framework for this text deserve comment. Aging is *not* a disease — even though there are physiological, psychological, sociological and visual changes with time. Diversity rather than homogeneity becomes the norm with increasing age. Physiological indicators, for example, show a greater range of differences in persons over 65 than in any other age group. As a consequence, norms as performance guidelines cannot be accurately established with any certainty.

Chronological age is a convenient but imprecise indicator of physical, mental and emotional status. For general reference and purposes of discussion only, the editors have defined the aged as being at least 65 years of age. Persons in the age bracket 65 to 74 are sometimes referred to as the *young-old* in contrast to persons in the age range from 75 to 84 who are referred to as the *old*. Those persons over 85 are referred to as the *old-old* and they are more likely to have some significant health care problems due to degenerative or disease conditions.

Because of the unique characteristics of aging, its diversity and complexity, this book is necessarily the work of many individuals. Each of the 27 contributors has undertaken to discuss the aspect of vision and aging with which he or she is most conversant. These authors include optometrists, physicians, psychologists, sociologists and other health professionals. Many participating authors are also educator-scientists who have made important contributions to the advancement of knowledge through research and teaching.

This text is not intended to be a specific topic text, such as refraction techniques and analyses, disease recognition and/or treatment. For example, the chapter on disease and pathology does not include illustrations of the conditions discussed since these are available in many specific texts as identified in the chapter's reference list. This particular chapter is, however, as others, an overview of those specific ocular conditions which are most prevalent in the elderly and which should be kept in mind when serving an older population. This text, then, is directed to the complex vision care of a specific category of patients.

The editors were guided by the overriding goal of imparting knowledge and understanding fundamental to comprehensive and primary vision care of elderly persons rather than imparting skill in testing methodology. In the selection of topics to be discussed and the type of information to be provided, the editors had in mind a primary readership of vision care colleagues, both practitioners and students. What would these readers want and need to know? How much prior knowledge could be assumed? The editors have, for example, assumed that the reader already has skill and knowledge in the various techniques of routine vision and eye examination procedures.

Limitations of space prohibited the inclusion of everything we wished to include; consequently, some topics have been treated only briefly or omitted entirely. So, too, many authors and colleagues who have made important contributions to the field of vision and aging are missing from this book. In some instances, the editors have recognized some of these important contributors through appropriate bibliographic references.

In order to provide the older patient with comprehensive primary care, the optometrist must be aware of not only the ocular and vision conditions of the elderly patient but also must be knowledgeable about those services within the community which improve the quality of life for elderly persons.

The collaborating authors have not met to discuss their special contributions. In a larger sense the prevailing theme of aging is the single concept to which each author adds a unique contribution. The necessary unity in planning and presentation has been the task of the editors. Having read and re-read the various chapters, the editors feel particular pride in and appreciation for the writers who so generously and painstakingly have given of themselves by sharing with us their knowledge and by helping us to understand and appreciate the concepts that each has discussed.

The editors also wish to acknowledge the valued editorial assistance of the copy editor, Mary C. Berry. She provided valuable assistance with details of the editorial process and with the solution of problems of contemporary English usage and style.

Science, it has been said, lives in the details which are universally valid. *Vision and Aging: General and Clinical Perspectives* is not a text whose only purpose is recounting past and present knowledge. Rather its overriding intent is to bring into perspective the continuing quest of practitioners and scientists seeking a more perfect understanding not only of patient care but also of other human services for all aging individuals. The editors hope that every reader of this book may someday find the material personally beneficial.

Meredith W. Morgan
Alfred A. Rosenbloom, Jr.

Preface to the Second Edition

As co-editors we have come to the conclusion that a second edition of *Vision and Aging: General and Clinical Perspectives* is needed at this time for at least four very important reasons. First, there has been a significant increase in our knowledge concerning vision and aging. Second, the scope of optometry has continued to expand and the emphasis of the profession has become increasingly that of a primary health care provider. Today every school and college of optometry includes in its curriculum a course in geriatric optometry; there are also an increased number of residencies in this emerging specialty. Third, the number of persons in the world requiring vision care who are over 65 years of age continues to grow at an ever expanding rate; indeed, one of the fastest growing categories of potential vision-care patients is that of persons over the age of 85 — the so-called old-old of the population. In the United States this population is growing at a rate four times faster than any other segment of the population. Fourth, the first edition is out of print.

Significant knowledge concerning the vision care of the elderly patient has expanded. This, along with a continued growth of new knowledge in optometry, has created a dilemma for both the editors and the publishers: How can all of the pertinent information on vision and aging be included in a single text of reasonable size and cost? The answer is, of course, that it cannot. The editors have reluctantly agreed with the publishers that selected chapters in the first edition discussing psychology, sociology, and socio-economic aspects of aging should be omitted. The editors believe that these are important aspects of the vision care of the elderly and essential for a complete understanding of elder care. As a consequence, selected chapters have been revised to include essential knowledge in these areas. As a further acknowledgment of the importance of these aspects, the chapter authors have included pertinent references to the gerontological literature. Most of the other chapters that have been retained have been rewritten to bring them up to date.

The editors wish to emphasize that they have continued to be guided by the objectives and point of view expressed in the preface to the first edition. As a book on primary care optometry within the field of geriatrics, this is not a text concerned with specific treatment of selected conditions. Rather, it is a text about understanding both older individuals and their vision problems as an entity. It is essential that optometrists recognize that a particular visual condition cannot be separated from the individual and that, likewise, the individual cannot be separated from his or her visual conditions. The important concept is that the patient receive comprehensive optometric care and, where appropriate, within an inter-disciplinary framework. Our ultimate goal is to improve the quality of life for the individual, fostering goal-directed activities and an independent life style. A new chapter entitled "Optometric Primary Care in Geriatrics" by Lesley L. Walls, O.D., M.D., and Earl P. Schmitt, O.D., emphasizes the importance of this concept.

The most important guiding principle in the preparation of this second edition has been to bring together in a single volume the relevant clinical concepts and information useful for the effective vision care of the elderly patient. Without the invaluable scientific and clinical insights of the contributing authors, the central purpose of this text could not have been achieved. It is our expectation that these concepts will continue to be clinically sound even when new techniques of vision care are developed in the future.

Alfred A. Rosenbloom, Jr.
Meredith W. Morgan

Contributing Authors

Ian L. Bailey, O.D., M.S., F.B.D.A. (H.D.)
Professor Optometry and Vision Sciences
Director, Low Vision
School of Optometry
University of California, Berkeley
Berkeley, California

Edward S. Bennett, O.D., M.S.Ed.
Associate Professor of Optometry
University of Missouri, St. Louis
School of Optometry
Adjunct Assistant Professor of Ophthalmology
St. Louis University School of Medicine
St. Louis, Missouri

David M. Cockburn, D.Sc., M.Sc.
Senior Academic Associate in Optometry
University of Melbourne
Victoria, Australia

Samuel M. Genensky, Ph.D
Founder and Chairman of the Executive Committee, Board of Directors
Center for the Partially Sighted
Santa Monica, California

Siret Desiree Jaanus, Ph.D
Professor Emeritus
Southern California College of Optometry
Fullerton, California
Visiting Professor of Pharmacology
Pennsylvania College of Optometry
Philadelphia, Pennsylvania

Gary L. Mancil, O.D.
Research Health Scientist
Rehabilitation Research and Development Center
Veterans Administration Medical Center
Decatur, Georgia

David D. Michaels, M.S., O.D., M.D.
Professor of Ophthalmology
University of California, Los Angeles
Los Angeles, California
Chairman, Department of Ophthalmology
San Pedro and Peninsula Hospital
San Pedro, California

David Pickwell, M.Sc., F.B.C.O., F.B.O.A. (H.D.), D.Orth.
Professor and Head of Optometry
University of Bradford
Bradford, Yorkshire
United Kingdom

Albert L. Pierce
Formerly of School of Optometry
University of Alabama
Birmingham, Alabama

J. Randall Pitman, O.D.
Primary Care Optometric Practitioner
Boise, Idaho

Melvin J. Remba, M.Opt., O.D.
Chief of Clinic
Department of Optometry
Cedars-Sinai Medical Center
Los Angeles, California

Earl P. Schmitt, O.D., M.S., Ed.D., D.O.S.
Professor of Optometry
Northeastern State University
Tahlequah, Oklahoma

Christina M. Sorenson, O.D.
Gary Hall Eye Surgery Institute
Phoenix, Arizona

Suresh Viswanathan, B.Opt.
Graduate Student in Clinical Optometry
College of Optometry
Pacific University
Forest Grove, Oregon

Lesley L. Walls, O.D., M.D.
Dean, College of Optometry
Pacific University
Forest Grove, Oregon

Barry A. Weissman, O.D., Ph.D.
Professor of Ophthalmology
Chief, Contact Lens Service
Jules Stein Eye Institute and Department of Ophthalmology
University of California School of Medicine
Los Angeles, California

Bruce C. Wick, O.D., Ph.D.
Associate Professor of Optometry
University of Houston
Houston, Texas

Robert L. Yolton, O.D., Ph.D.
Professor of Optometry
Pacific University
Forest Grove, Oregon

Steven H. Zarit, Ph.D.
Professor of Human Development
Assistant Director of the Gerontology Center
Pennsylvania State University
University Park, Pennsylvania

Introduction

A characteristic of mature industrialized societies is increased average longevity and increased average age of the population. The United States is now becoming such a society and will reach a steady state around 2030, when the distribution of the population by age will be rectangular; there will be equal proportions of people under age 19 and over age 55, as well as a substantial percentage over 75 (and even 85) years of age. With increased expectations of living into old age and with the anticipation of approaching the biologically determined upper limit of the human life-span (estimated at 110 to 120 years), the prevalence of age-related disorders will increase. Indeed, a byproduct of increased average longevity is an increased probability that a given individual will survive to the age of risk of certain diseases prevalent in both old age and, increasingly, old-old age.

Visual disorders are high on the list of such diseases, and impaired vision is one of the most common and disabling conditions of old age. Geriatricians and laypeople alike are increasingly concerned with issues of the quality—more than simply the quantity—of life as old age is achieved. To paraphrase John F. Kennedy, it is more the life in the years than simply the years of life that we must sustain as the population ages progressively. In this regard, no function appears more important than the retention of vision—not only for the maintenance of independence and function, but also for the fullest enjoyment of life.

The frontiers of knowledge relating to the aging process are also being extended through an intensified research effort. This effort has a dual purpose: (1) to understand the aging process ("primary aging") stripped of the associated time-determined concomitants of aging that, through interventions both prior to and during old age, may be retarded or prevented altogether ("secondary aging"); and (2) to determine the means whereby the disabilities associated with aging might be alleviated through treatment.

In both regards *Vision and Aging: General and Clinical Perspectives* is of major interest. It is becoming increasingly apparent that much of what we have accepted as inevitable in aging may indeed not be so. A fuller understanding of the nutritional, behavioral, and environmental determinants of time-related disease emphasizes that function can be preserved into very old age at levels not significantly less than those of middle age and young adulthood. For example, if atherosclerosis can be prevented, cardiovascular function can be maintained into the eighth and ninth decades. The same may prove to be true for the visual disorders of old age; cataract, glaucoma, and macular degeneration may possibly be preventable or even able to be delayed further through appropriate preventive strategies. At the same time, improved surgical, medical, and prosthetic treatment of the disorders highly prevalent in old age may preserve function and retard progression and disability. Finally, geriatric practitioners are becoming increasingly aware of the inextricable interrelationships among the biological, psychological, and social determinants of function and the quality of life in old age. The integration of information about, and sensitivity to, all three spheres of human feelings and endeavor mark the effective geriatric practitioner. Equally important is an awareness that attitudes that preserve the dignity and self-respect of aging patients, although important in caring for patients of all ages, are central to the appropriate care of elderly people.

Increased awareness of the emotional and physical needs of the growing proportion of elderly people, the changing patterns of normal versus abnormal aging in our maturing society, and the sophistication of scientific advances require widespread dissemination of the principles and practice of gerontology among health professionals. *Vision and Aging: General and Clinical Perspectives* is a text that practitioners addressing the visual needs of an aging population will find indispensable. The scope and depth of this text and the wide range of expertise characteristic of its contributors make this volume a significant contribution to the field of gerontology.

William R. Hazzard, M.D.
David J. Carver Professor of Medicine
Director, Center on Aging
Johns Hopkins Medical Institutions
Baltimore

1

Optometric Primary Care in Geriatrics

Earl P. Schmitt
Lesley L. Walls

OPTOMETRIC PRIMARY CARE: DEMOGRAPHICS

While age means are increasing slowly in nearly every nation of the world (Graying of Nations, 1986; Templeman, 1989; Aging America 1985–1986 ed.), longevity is a fairly recent phenomenon for humankind.

It has been during the 20th century that the life expectancy figures have changed the most remarkably, however, with dramatic demographic shifts taking place within the past 50 years (Graying of Nations, 1986). By 1982, there were an estimated 48.9 million adults in the 55 years and over age bracket, and they embraced 20% of the national census. Of these, 32,000 were centenarians (Taeuber 1983). Despite the susceptibility to illness, accidents, physiologic dysfunctions, and the general ravages of time, approximately 5,000 Americans in 1984 became 65 years of age each day. When allowances are made for losses from all sources, this resulted in a net daily increase of some 1,400 to 1,500 elderly individuals in the 65 years and older age bracket (Cadmus, 1989; Fowles, 1985). This trend still continues.

By 2020, the number of senior citizens in the United States will reach a total count of 52 million (Barrow, 1986; Owens, 1986). In 2030, the post-World War II "baby-boomers" will begin to enter the elderly category, increasing the number of older Americans to 65.6 million, which will represent 21.8% of the entire population. By 2080, people 65 years and older in the United States will comprise 24.5% of the country's residents.

The median age in America rose from 30.0 in 1980 to 32.9 in 1990. Twenty-six percent of the population today is under the age of 18 years, compared to 28% in the early 1980s (Geographical Mobility, 1988). At the same time, the most significant future growth among the elderly has occurred within the "old" cohort, those between the ages of 75 and 84 years, and in the "old-old" group, persons who are 85 years old and older (Altergott, 1986). In 1982, fewer than 5% of Americans were age 75 years or older. This percentage will double by

2030. During that time, the "old-old" will grow in numbers as well. In 1982, people who were age 85 years and older represented a mere 1% of the country's entire population. By 2050, this cohort will be 5% of the total, will number 16 million individuals, and will constitute the single, most rapidly expanding segment in the nation (Taeuber, 1983; Barrow, 1986). A large portion of this group will be female (Owens, 1986).

OPTOMETRIC PRIMARY CARE: ECONOMIC IMPLICATIONS

During the past 20 years, the number of optometrists actively practicing in the United States has been increasing, rising from 18,400 in 1970 to 24,300 in 1986. This growth represented an increase in the ratio of optometric practitioners from 8.9 to 10.1 for every 100,000 members of the general population. By 2020, it is projected that there will be 35,700 practicing optometrists in the nation. At that time, the number of ophthalmologists in America is anticipated to reach 21,850 (Soroka, 1991).

Although the supply of health professionals has expanded recently, the costs of providing health care has increased each year for the past several decades. For example, in 1950, the expenses for health services, including long-term care, amounted to 12.7 billion dollars, constituting 4.4% of the Gross National Product (GNP). By 1982, this expenditure had grown to 322.6 billion dollars, or 10.5% of the GNP. By the year 2000, approximately 12% of the GNP is expected to be spent on health-care costs (Technology and Aging in America, 1985).

Although the nation's population continues to age, relatively few elderly citizens require intensified health-care services. Addressing this point, one observer has reported that approximately eight of the ten Americans who today are age 65 years or older are healthy enough to live comparatively normal lives without needing ongoing medical assistance. This includes the five million individuals who are 80 years old or more (Bingaman, 1985). Generally speaking, senior citizens tend to have better health habits than do younger age groups. Senior citizens smoke less, are less apt to be overweight, enjoy better eating habits, and consume fewer alcoholic beverages than do their younger cohorts. Older persons exercise less regularly than do their younger counterparts, however (Aging America, 1989).

In 1984, older Americans consumed more than one-third of all the funds spent nationally on personal health care, even though this segment constituted only about 12% of the total population. By 2030, however, when the elderly will represent close to one-quarter of all Americans, two-thirds of health-care spending in the United States is expected to be used to meet the needs of senior citizens. It is feared that Social Security will be confronting a major financial crisis as early as the year 2000, resulting from Medicare, Medicaid, and other health-related entitlement programs facing a predicted annual expenditure liability of nearly one trillion dollars (Califano, 1986).

The costs of providing optometric vision services are escalating along with all other areas of health care. A recent poll (Winslow, 1991) determined that 70%

of office gross income was spent by practitioners on overhead items such as ophthalmic supplies, salaries and personnel costs, space and equipment, utilities, insurance, professional dues, subscriptions, and related issues.

The assumption of primary health-care responsibilities by optometrists inevitably will lead to changes in office income levels and the manner in which patients are scheduled. Now that greater equity in Medicare support has been established among the health-care disciplines, optometry can justify charging for services on the same basis as do other providers. Moreover, because Medicare remuneration will be tied to the procedures actually undertaken, patients can be rescheduled without sacrificing the income that might be realized from simply maintaining a larger clientele volume (Christensen, 1990).

At present, approximately one-third of the American population has some form of third-party vision care coverage, and this proportion is predicted to climb to two-thirds by the turn of the century. Currently, about 32% of the average optometrist's gross income is received from third-party reimbursement schemes, compared to 18% reported in 1985 to 1986. The profession has had to overcome resistance to reach this level of third-party parity, however (Soroka, 1991). However, many third-party plans do not match usual and customary office fees. At the same time, they require an immense amount of paper work that demands the attention and energies of numerous skilled and qualified office personnel. Such staff support, in turn, necessitates a significant practice investment, with salaries and benefits taking about 16% of the gross income from most optometric offices during 1990 (Winslow, 1991).

Optometric parity was realized by passage of the Budget Reconciliation Act of 1986. The law permits all eye health services provided by optometrists, as defined by state jurisdictions, to be reimbursed through Medicare at the same level as that paid to medical physicians (Klopfer et al., 1990). This has resulted in optometry starting to reclaim the elderly as patients. Consequently, by the year 2000, optometry is projected to be caring for half of the geriatric eye and vision patients who are eligible for Medicare support (A.O.A., 1990).

New Medicare rules became effective January 1, 1991 and were developed as a result of the Physician Payment Review Commission report that was presented to Congress in 1991 (Medicare Reform, 1991). The new fee schedule will be phased-in over a five-year period. A notable impact will be to provide more income for primary care practitioners in all fields of health care, not only optometry (Barresi, 1991). As the majority of services rendered by optometrists are considered to be at the primary care level, it follows that reimbursement for optometric practitioners should increase under the new guidelines (Medicare Reform, 1991).

Total Medicare expenditures are anticipated to increase about 15% annually during the five-year implementation period. The revised fee schedule is the first serious adjustment of the law since its initiation. Historically, Medicare paid health-care providers at a level that reflected regional or customary charges, whichever was less. The new three-part formula will consider the skill and professional expertise involved in delivering the care, office costs and overhead in maintaining the practice facilities in order to supply the services, and regional economic differences throughout the country. Each part of the formula will receive a sum of "work relative value units," which pertain to the professional services involved. The sum of these work units then will represent the "total relative value unit" for the service provided. This last figure, in turn, will be multiplied by a constant of $26.87 in order to arrive at the dollar figure that is paid to the practitioner, providing that the practitioner is willing to accept the Medicare formula as a total fee for services.

For offices not participating and not accepting in full the Medicare schedule for professional services, a reduction in claims of 5% from the published payment scale will be made (Hanlen, 1992). Such practitioners then will be prohibited from charging their patients more than 20% above the established Medicare fees. Regardless, the costs to the program will be significant. Medicare presently finances health care for 34 million elderly and disabled persons. In 1991, the federal outlay for such care was expected to reach 104 billion dollars, almost 31% of which was to have been for services alone. This 32 billion dollar service cost is predicted to rise to 50 billion dollars by 1996 (A.O.A., 1991).

To the extent that governmental participation in health-care funding is involved, Medicare budgeting will be affected (AOA, 1991). The administrative complexities of Medicaid has led the federal government to contract with private insurance companies to implement the processing of claims, handle billings, and arrange for payment details. Firms called "intermediaries" are responsible for claims filed under Part-A, while others termed "carriers" process applications concerning Part-B. Every state has its own intermediate and carrier organizations, and these companies must follow strictly the guidelines mandated by Congress, as well as the regulations set by the Health Care Financing Administration, the governmental agency that oversees all carrier and intermediary operations (Medicare Handbook, 1990).

Augmenting Medicare is Title XIX of the Social Security Act, also known as Medicaid. This, too, is a federal program, but it is administered locally by the various states in accordance with congressional regulations. The program became operational in January 1966 with the primary intent of expediting health-care services to the indigent. Both state and federal funds pay for Medicaid costs, with state participation ranging from one-half to around three-quarters of the total expenditures.

In 1980, Medicaid, on the average, represented 9% of any state's budget. In 1990, this rose to about 14%. In 1989, the 50 states spent a total of 26.3 billion dollars on their Medicaid programs. In fiscal year 1990, that figure advanced to 30.9 billion dollars, and by the end of 1991 the expected outlay will equal 34.2 billion dollars. The main reason given for the steady climb is that more citizens are needing health care as the population continues to age (Rising Medicare Costs, 1991).

Specific services often are restricted from Medicaid coverages, including eye and vision care, depending on regional stipulations. Most of Medicaid's benefits are paid for medical services, even though freedom-of-choice is guaranteed to recipients. In selected instances, Medicaid will pay for low vision appliances or, in some instances, contact lenses (Jolley, 1990).

While Medicaid is available to most citizens, eligibility will differ among the several state jurisdictions. For example, even if elderly persons have limited incomes but possess other assets such as savings accounts, they may be disqualified from Medicaid payments. At present, it is estimated that only about one-third of the elderly poor, that is, those who have an annual income that falls below the poverty level of $11,400 as defined by the United States government, actually receive Medicaid benefits (Lublen, 1989).

Nursing homes (See Chapter 14) represent one of the fastest growing segments of the national health-care industry. In 1960, Americans spent 500 million dollars on nursing home care for the elderly and infirm. In 1984, this figure had risen to 32 billion dollars, and by 1990, a total of 60 billion dollars had been paid for nursing home services. However, the number of spaces available in nursing homes and centers is not keeping pace with the growing demands. In 1986, there were 1.5 million beds in nursing home facilities. Between the years of 1975 to 1984, the population figure of old-old Americans, that is, those 85 years or older, increased by 4%, while the number of nursing care beds rose only by 3%. Among the elderly, the old-old are 15 times more likely to need institutionalization than those between the ages of 65 to 74 years.

Crooks (1989) reported that a majority of Americans are favorably inclined toward some form of government-sponsored health plan, while wanting to retain the right to choose both the provider and the service center. Consideration of a national health policy currently is a hot political topic. Resolution of this issue will consume the energies of public officials and representatives of professional organizations in the immediate future. Until these decisions are made, however, Medicare, Medicaid, and their related programs probably will remain the most viable options for health care for most older Americans. These are complex and often bureaucratically cumbersome systems. However, Medicare now reimburses optometry for most routine primary health-care services, which the profession can supply within jurisdictional mandates. Because it is a diagnosis-driven system, care and patience must be exercised by professional offices in filing claims and documenting services. But so far, optometry has established a good record concerning Medicare billings (Hanlen, 1991). Whether or not Medicare stands as a model for a larger, national health-care plan in the future remains to be seen.

OPTOMETRIC GERIATRIC PRIMARY CARE: OVERVIEW
Primary Aging

Primary aging refers to the anatomic and physiologic changes associated with the aging process, irrespective of any concomitant or coexisting disease mechanism. It is much more complicated than simply the loss of cells in various organs. It is well known, for example, that proper nutrition, reasonable exercise, and the maintenance of a proper mental outlook all have a positive effect on the process of aging.

In "normal" primary aging, every organ of the body loses function. This functional loss seldom becomes a problem until around age 65 years unless there are associated secondary age-related complications, which will be discussed in the next section. Most of the body organs reach a peak of efficiency and reserve at about age 20 and remain relatively stable then until around age 30 years. Thereafter, a steady and gradual decline is experienced in functional activity and ability. At about age 75 or 80 years, most physiologic structures have lost about 50% of their original functional capabilities. The good news is that most organs and organ systems have well over a 50% reserve, so adequate life-support activities remain but the reserve capacities dwindle. For instance, the liver and kidneys have a 90% reserve capacity when a person is 20 years old, so they should remain viable and perform adequately when a person reaches his or her seventies or eighties under normal conditions.

The main problem resulting from the primary aging process is that of a diminishing reserve potential in the bodily organs. This means that a serious disease or injury is tolerated less well, and that recovery time for most debilities and dysfunctions becomes longer and is less satisfactory in many cases, as a person grows older. The goal in health care, therefore, should be to minimize the primary aging changes and to control the factors that accelerate the entire aging process.

Secondary Aging

Secondary aging is defined as the aging process that has been accelerated because of otherwise controllable or preventable circumstances. These conditions arise from treatable diseases or disorders, social problems, psychological difficulties, and economic stresses. Chronic diseases have replaced acute illness as the leading cause of death in the elderly. Often an acute illness such as pneumonia is secondary only to the explicit, long-standing, terminal diseases or events from which the elderly person is dying. (See Chapter 2.)

The leading maladies associated with secondary aging include cardiovascular diseases, cancer, cerebrovascular disease, diabetes, rheumatic disorders, and so forth. (See Chapter 2.) In addition, it is well documented that smoking, poor nutrition, excessive use of alcohol, and a lack of proper exercise accelerate the aging process.

Preventive health care must be at the forefront of all health-care programs. This is especially true for the elderly. Screening programs to detect diseases associated with secondary aging are very important. Obviously, appropriate patient education and referrals into the health-care system are vital if screening programs are to be effective in getting better control of the diseases associated with secondary aging.

Bones, Muscles, and Joints

The incidence of osteoarthritis escalates with age. Other diseases in the rheumatic classification, such as temporal arteritis, also increase in frequency through time. Normal "wear and tear" begins to affect a substantial number of the elderly by their sixty-fifth year. (See Chapter 2.)

Cardiovascular

Cardiovascular diseases are the leading cause of mortality in the United States. Heart attack secondary to atherosclerosis is the single most common event leading to mortality as a result of cardiovascular complications. Virtually everyone above the age of infancy has some degree of atherosclerosis. As a condition, however, it has a long and insidious history and normally does not cause problems until late in life unless there are underlying complexities that accelerate the process, such as hypertension, elevated cholesterol levels, diabetes, and cigarette smoking. It is estimated that 40% of Americans over the age of 65 will die from some form of cardiac disease.

Diabetes

With advancing age comes a definite increase in the incidence of diabetes, that being almost exclusively of the form known as Type-2, previously known as "adult onset diabetes." Type-2 patients tend to be stable, ketosis-resistant, and obese in contrast to the Type-1 diabetic who is unstable, becomes ketotic easily, and usually is not obese at the time of diagnosis.

In the Type-2 diabetic that commonly is found among the geriatric population there is a delayed insulin release by the pancreas. Moreover, there is insulin resistance at the membrane receptor level, usually as a result of decreased numbers and functioning of insulin receptor sites. Obesity, decreased amounts of exercise, and a gradual reduction of muscle mass that accompanies the onset of old age all contribute to increasing susceptibility to Type-2 diabetes and worsening its consequences once contracted.

Auditory Considerations

Problems with hearing are extremely common in the geriatric population. Hearing losses severe enough to interfere with daily living activities, a condition termed presbycusis, occur in approximately 30% of individuals between the ages of 65 to 74 years, and in about 50% of persons 75 years of age and older. Hearing aids often will help and increase the quality of life for those affected.

The onset of hearing loss, particularly in the higher frequency ranges, begins soon after age 30 as a result of cochlear changes that occur in the inner ear. The three ossicles of the middle ear are connected by synovial joints that are susceptible to sclerosis that results from the normal aging process. Ear wax also becomes thicker for older people and dries more readily. This wax may become impacted in the ear canal, thus contributing to decreased hearing capabilities. Good ear hygiene and screening for hearing problems are to be recommended strongly for the elderly. Protection to prevent noise-induced damage from further deteriorating an already compromised auditory system is a valuable service to offer the aged, in an effort to preserve as much of the individual's hearing as possible.

One-third of all persons over the age of 65 years suffer from tinnitus. This is true whether or not there is an associated hearing loss. The incidence of vertigo also increases with age as a secondary result from the atherosclerotic reduction of blood supplies to the inner ear and the central nervous system.

There are several "tricks" one might use in an office setting to communicate with the hearing impaired. One is to roll a piece of paper into a funnel, place the small end at the patient's external ear canal, and then speak into the larger end. Another approach is to put a stethoscope into the patient's ears and talk into the bell. Caution is advised here, however, because tremendous concentration of the sound results from this arrangement, and it may be too loud for the patient's comfort. Various electronic devices and amplification units exist, and are recommended for optometric use.

PSYCHOLOGICAL CONSIDERATIONS

The deterioration of mental capabilities that sometimes is observed in association with aging can create serious psychological and emotional problems for older patients, as well as cause intense stress for the family members involved. It is estimated that 1.5 million Americans of all ages are suffering today from some type of severe, chronic dementia, and an equal number have a more mild form of ongoing and progressive intellectual or cognitive impairment. (See Chapters 2 and 15.) As the population both increases in number and gradually becomes older, predictions are that there may be 7.4 million Americans incapacitated by a dementia by 2040. In current financial terms, this translates into an annual national health-care expense of 40 billion dollars for long-term care alone (Billig and Reisberg, 1989).

Although older persons seem to process information more deliberately and are less inclined to make hasty decisions or snap judgments, actual decrements in cognitive abilities do not appear to be indigenous to the aging experience. Only when an individual is close to the end of life may significant losses from past performance levels in such areas as verbal information processing, psychomotor response times, and computational abilities be demonstrated. This decline in mental agility, known as "terminal drop," is a phenomenon recognized by gerontologists, but the cause is obscure (Botwinick, 1978).

The majority of older persons do not lose their abilities to reason so much as they demonstrate a less rapid response time to stimuli of all descriptions. This slowing of psychomotor and cognitive reactions probably is the most prominent characteristic that has been documented in gerontologic research. Human response times to all modalities generally have been found to decrease as age increases, even when no other health complications are present. Too often this natural process is misinterpreted as being a form of senility by insensitive observers as well as unknowing health-care practitioners. Age-related changes of structure within the central nervous system (CNS), including losses of neurones, a decrease in the number of neural synapses, and the gradual accumulation of waste products from cellular metabolism probably contribute to this overall loss of mental efficiency (Devereaux, et al., 1981).

While older age groups are at higher risk for certain kinds of psychological damage than are younger persons, for the most part, few senior citizens seem interested or willing to seek the services of mental health specialists. The primary health-care practitioner has been urged to be alert for the elderly patient who appears to be showing aberrant or otherwise unexplainable behavioral changes (Bruce and Leaf, 1989). Appropriate referrals could be helpful.

Too often, older people increasingly experience feelings of isolation. Loss of sensory facilities, in particular, decrease their contact with the environment and may induce feelings of loneliness and despondency. Enforced quiescence because of frailty also tends to isolate one from the rest of the world. Frustration, anger, and self-pity tend to compound the increasingly narrow world enforced upon too many elderly and infirm individuals by the aging process (Cason and Thompson, 1980).

Primary optometric care is capable of making a significant contribution by helping older people maintain meaningful visual contact with their environment. By establishing for them an optimum level of visual efficiency, optometrists contribute to elderly patients' abilities to function as efficiently as possible. In turn, their capability to achieve meaningful cognitive processing and psychological well-being is enhanced during their later years (Schmitt, 1990).

PRESCRIBING CONSIDERATIONS
Pharmacokinetics

Most medications are metabolized and excreted by either the liver or the kidneys. Because both organs undergo a dramatic decrease in total function through time, prescribing systemic pharmaceuticals for the elderly is much different than for standard adults. The distribution of medications into the body's compartments also changes with age. There is a decrease in muscle mass and an increase in total body fat over the years. There also is a decrease in serum protein with age, which results in less protein binding of medications in the blood serum. All of these factors increase the likelihood of pharmaceutical toxicity in the elderly. (See Chapter 5.)

The primary care practitioner can explore drug regimens and histories, evaluating the status of the patient during the office visit and communicating with the patient's medical provider as may be deemed necessary. Case history questions should be thorough, and, if need be, family members or care-givers should be queried regarding specific legend medications taken by the older adult. The prescription of benzodiazepines is but one example of a widespread, sometimes inappropriate, and occasionally hazardous use of pharmaceuticals for elderly patients (Garnett and Barr, 1984). Derivatives of benzodiazepines such as chlordiazepoxide (Librium, Roche Products, Manati, Puerto Rico) and diazepam (Valium, Roche Products) may be given to treat states of anxiety and depression, as well as to serve as a muscle relaxant or an anti-convulsant. These drugs are potentiated when combined with such substances as alcohol, barbiturates, and phenothiazines, such as chlorpromazine (Thorazine, Smith Kline Beecham Pharmaceuticals, Philadelphia, PA). These derivatives can induce drowsiness, dampen reflexes, exacerbate depression syndromes, cause lethargy, and generally cause psychological changes that can dull sensory processes. The optometrist who is unaware of these iatrogenic complications may have difficulties when dealing with an older patient who is taking such medications, which is a strong argument for obtaining an in-depth health history during the preliminary patient care interview (Bevan, 1969; Hussar, 1987).

SOCIAL ISSUES

While the elderly are the most rapidly growing cohort in American society, there is no consensus by the nation at large as to how they are to be perceived or cared for. Estimations of the economic resources held by older citizens vary, but Social Security benefits remain the single most important source of income for most elderly individuals. When dependent on these funds alone, many older citizens are placed at, or near, the poverty line (Siegel and Davidson, 1984). Most elderly and retired persons have other sources of income, however, which may include pension funds, income from rental properties, and returns from investments. Despite this ancillary support, nearly all older adults are eligible for some additional form of government assistance. The manner in which to provide for the health and welfare of elderly Americans through entitlement programs is a major topic of debate, both at state and national levels (Swisher, 1990).

Before 1935 there were never less than ten working-aged adults for every American over the age of 65 years. At the start of World War II, there were nine working adults for every senior citizen. Today, the differential is about four and one-half gainfully employed persons for every one that is retired. By the year 2030, it is predicted that this supporting ratio will barely equal two working adults to one elderly American (Cowan, 1977).

In addition, the work force will have two million fewer gainfully employed persons between the ages of 18 and 25 years by the year 2000, compared to 1989 figures, a fact which will have significant social impact on everything from local school board elections to government entitlement programs. A larger proportion of workers by then will be female and of minority groups. With the drop in a younger aged labor pool, older workers will be retained longer by necessity, with retirement options being delayed so that business can use the skills and experience of the mature employee. While older workers accounted for 20% of the work force in 1980, they will comprise nearly 33% of all industrial employees by the turn of the century. In return, marked changes in work-related benefits will be granted by the business world, including choices for flex-time working hours and health insurance packages that will change the insurance and hence the payment scales and the delivery of health care by providers (Crooks, 1989; Bowker, 1989).

At present, eligibility is gained for Social Security benefits at age 62, and there are a number of senior citizens who are ready to leave their jobs and retire (Denzer, 1990). If a number of retired, older citizens descend on a community because of attractive living conditions, the area's entire social structure can be altered (Heckheimer, 1989). But not all of those who qualify for retirement elect the option. McGoldrick (1989) summarizes the current research on retirement and its resulting effect on the health and longevity of those who leave the work force as a consequence of age. One survey found that 32% of those who stayed on the job past the time of minimum retirement age did so not for monetary reasons, but because they liked to work (Bird, 1989). Industry has found that older employees are reliable, often have greater company loyalty than their younger counterparts, and record fewer absentee days as well (Wright, 1991). This growing appreciation of older workers has helped erode many of the stereotypes that Americans have held regarding the elderly. The fears, distrusts, and prejudices that have been directed toward our more mature and aged adults slowly are melting as senior citizens continue to make economic and leadership contributions for longer times. Currently, approximately 59% of those between the ages of 65 and 69 years receive regular wages. Noteworthy also is the fact that a large number of older workers want to stay on the job (Grad, 1985)!

In spite of renewed interests by business and the elderly themselves in continued employment, not all older citizens can remain economically productive and independent. Frailty and cognitive debilities may require an older person to withdraw and be rendered care, either on a part-time or full-time basis. As the number of elderly people increases, so do the social needs for their housing and life-support services. While a vast majority of care-givers provide dedicated and loving attention, recently there have been an increasing number of disturbing reports concerning abuse and neglect of the elderly. One problem area involves guardianship, and the rights which may be forfeited by an older person when placed under the control of a court-appointed custodian. There are no uniform jurisdictions, and each state has its own laws governing how and when senior citizens may be declared to be legally incompetent. Restrictions may vary, but it is not unknown for older persons to lose their right to travel, handle money, or buy or sell property once placed under a guardianship decree (Broyles, 1987).

Abuse of the elderly, whether by an official guardian or by family members, unfortunately is not rare in American society. Elder abuse can assume many forms, including psychological, sexual, and the violation of personal and constitutional rights. Cases of negligence, neglect, and financial impoverishment have been recorded. Victims often are age 75 or older, and tend to be female. When perpetrated by family members, the abuser most likely will be the victim's son, followed by a daughter. At the time during the mistreatment, the family member usually is experiencing personal stresses in addition to having to care for the older adult. These problems can include alcoholism, substance addiction, marital problems, or difficulties on the job. Interestingly, the abuser often was abused as a child by the parent, according to one government study (Roybal, 1985).

An ominous development has emerged concerning elder abuse, and is occurring with increasing regularity, particularly in poor, rural communities and at larger urban hospitals. Elderly and debilitated patients are being brought to hospital emergency rooms and virtually abandoned by families who no longer can afford to cope with the aged person. This previously unrecognized issue has not as yet been addressed by governmental agencies, but it promises to become a matter of intense social concern within the next few years (Hasson, 1991).

This forecast is supported by the steady climb of the number of elderly who are dependent on their children for support. Government figures project that between the years of 1985 and 2030, the proportion of those 65 to 79 years old who rely on younger family members for care and the necessities of life will increase to nearly 26% of the total in that age category (Siegel and Davidson, 1984). This growing dependency by the older citizenry inevitably will lead to greater incidences of elder abuse. That government agencies have not responded as yet to prepare for this threat can be seen in the fact that the average state budget for child protective services in 1984 was 20 times the amount set aside for similar care of the elderly (Roybal, 1985).

The elderly are starting to impact significantly on the American economic scene. One positive way, as described earlier, is the contribution they may be making by remaining in the labor force. But as dependents, they are altering lifestyles of those who must care for them, and thus are creating hardships for younger members of society. Because longevity is becoming the rule, 95% of all 40-year-old people now have at least one living parent, as do 80% of all 50-year-olds. Nearly 25% of the total number of workers in business and industry must provide care, either personal or financial, to an aging parent. Three-quarters of the individual or hands-on care given to the elderly is done by women. This has created such high stress levels, that 25% of all female care-givers have been forced to take time off from a job in order to fulfill their obligations to aging parents, while 12% have had to leave their employment in order to render elder-care services (Highton, 1989).

Too often the women who must deliver eldercare are within the age ranges of 30 to 45, have children of their own at home, have ongoing personal and family concerns, and may be involved in a career of their own, on either a full-time or part-time basis. These females represent a new dilemma in the American social order, that of a grown child with outside adult interests and ambitions being forced to care for homebound aging parents. Caught between their own family needs and the requirements to be a care-giver, this "sandwich generation" is itself at risk (Sheras, 1990). There is evidence that one-third of the adults who are involved in eldercare experience a deterioration of their personal health, including signs of nervous tension, depression, and stress. A quarter of those who have an outside job report they are less efficient at work. Another quarter suffer a serious worsening of their financial situation resulting from the additional expenses involved in providing services to their aging wards and the subsequent loss of income when unable to work outside the home (Cadmus, 1984; Shapiro, 1989).

Nationally, governmental agencies have not grasped the impact being made on individual families or the pending crunch that will be experienced by entitlement programs early in the next century. Industry will be affected as staffing needs will be challenged by the lack of younger workers and the abundance of older persons who may need special inducements to remain on the job after reaching retirement age. Health-care financing and insurance subsidies will need to be restructured, care facilities will need to be provided, and consideration will have to be given to younger working family members who are required to provide care to elderly loved ones.

VISION SERVICES

Debilities of various kinds are the consorts of advancing age. All sensory functions are affected to a greater or lesser extent, with the quality of life being influenced most adversely by losses in areas of vision (Verma, 1989). Fewer than 50% of Americans under the age of 40 years wear ophthalmic prescriptions, but nearly nine out of ten who are in their fifth decade or beyond need some form of lens correction, if for no other reason than to counteract the inevitable onset of presbyopia (Herrin, 1990).

A recent survey (Bertz, 1989) found that at least 50 million Americans, or about one-fifth of the population, did not avail themselves of adequate eye and vision care. Most were either indifferent, taking the visual process somewhat for granted, or simply failed to recognize a problem when it existed. Many also were poorly informed about presbyopia; 49% of those polled believed that high blood pressure placed one at greater risk than did aging. One-third of the respondents did not know the symptoms of presbyopia despite recognizing the term, while a third also failed to understand the function of a bifocal lens. The fact that bifocal contact lenses are available also was unknown to many, while 29% believed that medical or surgical procedures could relieve a presbyopic status.

Why does the living organism age? No one theory seems to explain adequately the human aging process, and other than being intrinsic, ubiquitous, and progressive to all ethnic groups, little else is agreed upon. Hypotheses that address causes of the aging mechanism include the possibility of genetic programming or spontaneous cellular mutations that may occur over a lifetime. Environmental conditions have been targeted, including background radiation effects and trace metals and free radicals in the diet. Enzymatic changes may contribute, along with the accumulation of metabolic waste materials in cells such as lipofuscin. A definite epoch may be inherent to all species in the form of a regulatory influence that allows cells, either individually or when situated within a tissue mass, to replicate by mitosis only a certain number of times before the process is halted. Mitochondrial failure in the process of protein synthesis and other regulatory mechanisms in cell life may contribute to aging. Most authorities agree that the entire aging function has a multiplicity of causes, all of which have not been identified as yet (Weale, 1982; Rumsey, 1988).

Primary care optometrists are responsible for the total health scene of their patients, from infancy through maturity. Brown and Hawkins (1991) list 11 specific areas of primary health-care concern that optometrists should be ready to address. Among these are several issues particularly applicable to adults and the elderly, including the early detection and appropriate referral of ocular and systemic diseases, the amelioration of refractive and binocular dysfunctions, the maintenance of a satisfactory health status through proper diet and exercise regimens, and the analysis of environmental factors that might adversely affect health and sensory mechanisms or job and recreational performances.

While it is tempting to generalize when discussing primary vision care services for the elderly, the fact is that people become more diverse as they grow older. Moreover, profound differences exist when it comes to the availability of professional care for selected groups in American society. In particular, rates of blindness and visual disorders are significantly higher among Black populations than among Caucasians. Such problems as age-related cataracts and open-angle glaucoma are leading causes of visual loss within minority groups, and yet both conditions can be managed successfully by a primary care optometric practice. Other health issues common to Black Americans, such as hypertension and diabetic visual complications likewise can be monitored appropriately by the primary care practitioner (Borska, 1991).

One issue that a large number of seniors face, regardless of ethnic lineage, is that of maintaining safe driving skills. When vision problems begin to curtail mobility, the elderly experience an enforced change in a life-style that most Americans take for granted. The unfettered access to an automobile is held to be a status of freedom and individuality in this country. In truth, many times, the use of a car is essential for reaching work sites and obtaining basic necessities such as food, clothing, and medical care, and for recreation purposes. Denying the elderly driving privileges restricts their independence, and causes them to rely on friends or relatives for transportation. In the process, much of the initiative for the scheduling and control of their personal lives thereby is lost (Wright, 1987).

Stereotypes notwithstanding, older drivers do not account for a high percentage of vehicular accidents. Elderly motorists, in fact, rank second behind younger drivers who are 16 to 24 years old in the number of accidents per mile driven. The younger driver often is at fault because of exercising poor judgment, such as speeding or tailgating. Older drivers are prone to disregard stop signs, may fail to yield right-of-way, and experience awareness problems resulting from reduced vision and hearing abilities. The implications for optometric services are obvious, and certain states such as Florida now are requiring all applicants for automobile driver relicensure to pass both a written and a road performance test (Ketner and Johnson, 1987; Carney, 1989).

While optometry long has been concerned with the presbyopic and elderly patient (Jaques, 1936; Hirsch and Wick, 1960), not all practitioners enjoy working with the older adult (Cole and McConnaha, 1986; Klein and Klein, 1987).

Yet the expanded scope of primary practice has moved the profession so far beyond earlier goals and legal limitations that senior citizens cannot be excluded from the general practice of optometric primary care. Before attempting to evaluate the unusual, however, the optometrist must understand what is expected to occur in the more-or-less normal course of events during the aging process. Mancil and Owsley review the changes that can be anticipated to the eye and adnexa as a person gradually becomes older (Mancil and Owsley, 1988). Other references cover this subject as well (Klopfer et al., 1990; Sekuler et al., 1982). (See Chapter 6.)

Knowing what is considered to be within normal limits regarding age-related changes (Keeney and Keeney, 1985; Williamson and Caird, 1986), the primary care optometrist then can make a differential diagnosis when something unusual is observed (Kornzweiz, 1979). The prevalence of eye pathology increases from a low of about 1% in the general population during preschool ages to a high of about 85% for individuals 65 years old or older (Morse et al., 1987). Various texts discuss diagnostic and therapy options for anterior and posterior ocular segment morbidity (Catania, 1988; Fedukowicz and Stenson, 1985; Bell and Stenstrom, 1983).

An area of care used more often by older patients than younger persons is that of low vision. Approximately 60% of low vision patients are between the ages of 65 and 84 years, and most low vision services are provided by private practitioners rather than at health-care clinics or in other institutional settings. Greater use by low vision specialists of community service resources, such as mobility training, living assistance, and psychological counseling for visually impaired patients has been urged (Lightman and Rosenbloom, 1991). (See Chapters 13 and 15.)

LEGAL ASPECTS

Optometry has struggled to legitimatize itself in the field of health-care delivery since before the start of the present century (Penisten, 1991). Curricula in the professional educational institutions have been strengthened, and state laws have been enacted to permit increasingly the delivery of a higher standard and quality of optometric vision services. A major impetus that has worked to push the profession into the primary care arena, however, has been that of economics. In the 1960s, there began an increasing demand for health-care services of all kinds, as the post-war baby-boomers began to reach adulthood. Costs escalated and consequently began to place access to many health-care systems beyond the financial reach of a number of low- to middle-income American families. Alternative providers were sought, and optometry recognized the need and moved to fill a void. By providing primary health services at less cost and in more geographic areas than more traditional specialties, optometry made a commitment that has broadened the legal base upon which the profession rests (Dupuis, 1987; Hopping, 1987).

As of 1986, the term "primary care" was written into an optometric law only for the state of Florida. The American Optometric Association had published reference materials and guidelines for primary optometric care by the mid-1970s (A.O.A., 1977). In trying to define the concept, this document identified the primary care optometrist as the health-care practitioner who first is contacted by a patient needing some form of attention, who then makes the initial evaluation and assessment of the patient's needs, who coordinates subsequent patient care based on the original visit and work-up, who maintains contact with the patient and monitors the resulting services, and who then assumes ongoing responsibility for continued health care (Classe, 1986).

Baldwin (1987) is more specific. He remarks that the optometrist is obligated by state laws to monitor, consult, and refer patients to others within the health-care system, as the situation might require. Again, where permitted by local jurisdictions, the optometrist must either manage and treat certain anterior segment pathologies when they fall within the scope of the practitioner's expertise, or place that patient in the hands of a competent secondary-level provider. These comments are consistent with Bartlett's definition, which implies that primary care is the practice of managing or treating most of the health problems that most of the patients have most of the time (Bartlett, 1986). Baldwin continues by noting that the didactic and clinical training of today's optometry students equips them to provide preventive health-care services, selected diagnostic and treatment regimens, vision and health screenings, rehabilitative and visual enhancement services, and patient health education information. The obvious conclusion to be drawn is that failure to exercise these professional prerogatives and responsibilities places the practitioner in legal jeopardy.

In 1971, Rhode Island was the first to enact a state law permitting the use of diagnostic pharmaceutical agents in optometric practice. All 50 states and the District of Columbia now likewise allow, or do not prohibit, the employment of diagnostic drugs by qualified optometrists. In 1976, West Virginia became the first jurisdiction to allow optometry to use therapeutic pharmaceuticals, and 15 years later, more than one-half of the various states had followed suit.

These moves to expand the scope of optometric services have sobering implications. First, the optometrist, who by law is responsible for the detection, referral, and in certain locations the treatment of ocular pathologic entities, now has the tools by which these duties may be discharged most efficiently. Second, stature and credibility is added to the optometric profession, as it now has been moved from the "detect and refer" status to that of "diagnosis and manage" (Bartlett, 1986). Third, the optometrist now not only is mandated legally to use every means at his or her disposal to evaluate the patient's ocular health status, but, in many instances, is provided with the means to intervene directly regarding the care and management of certain ailments.

When situations exist that could lead to the impairment of visual functions, it is the examiner's duty to warn the patient of the problem and of any attending health risks that might be present. Liability for failure to advise patients regarding existing health hazards had been extended to optometry from medicine, where physicians have been held responsible for protecting their patients from unreasonable harm. In instances of cataract or macular degeneration, it is obvious that prudent counsel would be necessary because the patient needs to be warned that progressive loss of vision is a possibility. Particularly regarding the elderly, either the patient or a responsible family member or guardian should be briefed on dysfunctions that could impose visual limitations or restrictions. However, even transient impairments or inconveniences may be included in this category, for it is the duty of the optometrist to warn patients to expect such annoyances as photophobia or blurred vision as a result of routine dilation procedures (Classe, 1986a).

As the profession has expanded to incorporate concepts of primary care, a new set of responsibilities has accrued that traditionally have not fallen within the realm of optometric practice. A notable example is the increasing involvement of optometrists in the handling of ocular emergencies and trauma. Classe (1986b) has reviewed several categories of such cases and outlines the standards of care to which optometrists have been held. In addition to the professional's duties, office staff also must shoulder a significant burden, especially when recording telephone assessments and patient contacts of those who present with ocular crises. The importance of documentation is emphasized, particularly the need to obtain a detailed case history, which can be critical in helping to make a differential diagnosis when the patient is first seen (Eagling and Roper-Hall, 1986). Classe (1986) discusses the liabilities involving the management of foreign bodies, retinal detachments, corneal abrasions, and acute glaucomatous attacks. These are episodes to which the elderly in particular are subject, and the primary care optometrist therefore may expect to be confronted with an increasing number of such events as the population ages.

The application of contact lenses (see Chapter 9) to the older patient is of mounting interest to the vision care specialist. Hanks (1984) reports that there are approximately 48 million presbyopes in the United States who are potential contact lens wearers. A variety of fitting techniques may be used (Mandell, 1988), ranging from rigid bifocal designs to soft bifocal contact lenses and monovision procedures. This last approach is discussed in detail by Josephson, et al. (1990).

Before 1980, only 16 states had adult protective service laws. By 1985, a total of 37 states and the District of Columbia had adopted mandatory reporting provisions regarding suspected cases of elder abuse. In spite of this, abuse of the elderly through various physical and psychological embarrassments is an increasing national disgrace. Primary care practitioners must be alert to signs of elder abuse, and be advised that some states may require that suspected cases be reported to a county district attorney's office or to the regional Department of Human Services. Failure to do so is a misdemeanor in some jurisdictions. At the same time, the practitioner most commonly is protected from legal repercussions and has immunity from civil or criminal liability if the practitioner, acting in good faith, can be shown as exercising due care and regard for the patient's welfare when reporting cases of suspected elder abuse (Oklahoma State Statutes, 1977).

EDUCATIONAL ISSUES

As the elderly in America live longer and lead more vigorous lives, they consume more of the health-care expertise and current financial resources than any other population group, testimony that the needs and requirements of older Americans are different from those experienced by the rest of the nation. In this regard, the primary vision care of older patients mandates the practitioner to master a more sophisticated knowledge base than that which is demanded in order to serve a younger clientele. Physical and psychological needs of the elderly call for a more holistic approach from the primary vision care specialist. The most appropriate time for the optometrist to gain insights regarding the primary health-care needs of the elderly is during professional training (Potter, 1985).

The term geriatrics, referring to care of the elderly, was not used until 1909, when it was coined by a Viennese physician, Dr. I. L. Nacher. The first scientific group to devote itself to gerontology, or the study of the aging process, was the British Club for Research in Aging, established in 1939. A similar organization began in America that same year. In 1940 the United States Public Health Service opened its first bureau whose task it was to be concerned about the elderly. The University of Chicago introduced the first gerontology research program into higher education in the mid-1940s. As Decker notes, the study of gerontology largely is a post–World War II development (Decker, 1980).

Health care professionals have not been exposed to rigorous training in the past to prepare for serving the needs of our elderly population. Many medical schools, for instance, have given geriatrics short shrift as a discipline, leaving physicians somewhat unprepared for the influx of older patients that appeared in the last decade (Rosenbloom, 1982). These shortcomings currently are being redressed at all levels in the preparation of health care providers.

Recognizing the importance of geriatric care, organized optometry has made positive efforts to prepare its students to serve the elderly. In 1986, the Association of Schools and Colleges of Optometry established an Optometric Gerontology Curriculum Development Committee. Supported by a grant received in 1987 from the Administration on Aging of the Department of Health and Human Services, the Committee assembled a modular course outline for the teaching of geriatrics and gerontology in optometric institutions. After holding regional workshops during the latter part of 1988 and into 1989, the Committee published a final version of the curriculum in 1989. Copies are available through the Association of Schools and Colleges of Optometry's office in Rockville, Maryland (Aston, et al., 1989).

The educational process is a continuum. While the profession trains its students in the art and science of primary vision care, the optometrist then is in a position to constantly educate his or her patients regarding health maintenance and life-styles. Regarding this last point, there are numerous innovations that can be beneficial to older patients who have suffered sensory or mobility debilities. Such items as communication enhancement devices, cooking aids, recreation materials, and special clothing for the handicapped are available. Many impaired elderly are not aware of the existence of such resources. In addition, there are instruments and equipment available for professional offices that can amplify voice communications between the doctor and a hearing-handicapped patient, as well as enhance television and video sound for in-office instructional and educational purposes. A wealth of inexpensive optical aids are on the market that can be used by the visually limited person to enlarge television screens and computer display terminals, along with other devices for magnifying print and various reading materials (Lunzer, 1989; MAXIAIDS).

Nowhere is the axiom that "optometry treats the whole person" more apparent or applicable then during the care of the geriatric patient. Optometry's educational response to this cresting wave of older health-care claimants is accelerating, and will test the resiliency and innovative thinking of this constantly evolving profession.

COMANAGEMENT CONSIDERATIONS

As a primary care provider, the optometrist has responsibilities both in health education and health promotion (Newcomb, 1990). As one approach, all patients can be provided with a wide variety of health-related printed materials, many of which can be made available in the waiting room or reception areas. Audiovisual presentations also can be used. These range from slide projection and video film displays to cassette tapes, a wide selection of which is available from the American Optometric Association (A.O.A., Order Department).

On a more personal level, the case history is an excellent vehicle by which the practitioner can identify health concerns and communicate with patients about such matters, particularly the elderly (Cole and McConnaha, 1986). Questions concerning specific health conditions such as blood pressure, family and individual histories of diabetes, cardiovascular complications, ocular pathologies, medication regimens, and psycho-social conditions can be explored and serve as educational overtures for the clinician.

The optometrist may be the only primary health-care practitioner seen on a regular basis by a patient. The insidious and deleterious effects of elevated blood pressure, a condition that is correlated positively with increased age, can go undetected by the average person. The optometrist represents a first line of defense in detection of hypertension and other such circulatory dysfunctions (Good and Augsburger, 1989). Concerning a related issue, open-angle glaucoma is an incurable anomaly, yet it can be controlled when diagnosis and management are instituted at the earliest possible time. Optometric practitioners again represent a first line of defense for the elderly against this debilitating ocular dysfunction (Stelmack, 1987).

For persons having a known diabetic condition of four or more years, annual ocular health evaluations are recommended, which would include (among other probes) an updating of the patient's case history, visual acuity assessments, intraocular pressure measurements, and a dilated fundus examination (Special Medical Reports, 1988). Procedures as these can be undertaken easily by the primary care optometrist. Moreover, an increased incidence of elevated intraocular pressure not uncommonly is associated with diabetic conditions, at least in selected minority populations (Krieger, et al., 1988).

While one-quarter of America's population lives in rural communities, only 12% of all practicing medical physicians reside and practice in small towns. There is a disturbing maldistribution of traditional health-care providers throughout the United States, a situation that has placed more than 2,000 small communities in jeopardy regarding conventional access to the health-care delivery system. During the 1980s, for example, 698 community hospitals closed, either because of a lack of professional staffing or for financial reasons, with half of these facilities being located in rural and farming communities. This trend has continued, for in 1989, 44 of the 80 hospitals that ceased operations were in non-urban locations (Rakstis, 1991).

The United States Public Health Service claims that 12.5 million residents of small towns have no community-based, primary, medical health-care practitioner available to them. Specialists are in equally short supply; 52% of all counties in the United States have no office-based obstetrician in residence. Ancillary and support personnel also are lacking because there is a nationwide shortage of 150,000 registered nurses, the scarcity being most critical in our rural areas. As the population ages, the indigent, poor, and elderly increasingly are threatened with having to forego primary health-care services unless other providers can be found (Rakstis, 1991). If one considers their availability and more general distribution throughout the country, their level of training, and the obvious need for services, then the rationale for optometrists to practice primary health care seems self-evident.

While Medicare is in the process of reducing significantly the levels of financial remuneration that medical eye health professionals will be receiving, a congressional panel, The Physician Payment Review Commission, has recommended in its report of December 7, 1990 that starting January 1, 1992, services of equal kind that are rendered by optometrists be compensated at the same level as when performed by doctors of medicine and osteopathy (Soroka and Warner, 1991). Despite a lingering disdain held by many medical personnel for any health-care training outside the purview of a medical jurisdiction, optometry has made positive, albeit slow, progress toward parity in ocular health care.

Of course, not all instances of ocular pathology that are seen in optometric offices require outside consultation or comanagement services. One survey found that of the 500 optometrists who responded, an increasing number were treating pathologic conditions on a primary care level. It has been estimated that the average general practice optometrist who has therapeutic pharmaceutical privileges now sees one treatment-related case for every 13 office visits, which translates into slightly more than 7% of a patient load (News Review, 1991).

It is well to keep in mind a working definition of primary care. Wilson and Hoffman (1989) have described this as largely an ambulatory service activity, being initiated for the most part by patient self-referral. The primary care practitioner usually is the first professional who is contacted within the health-care delivery system by a patient. The primary health-care provider then evaluates the patient's health status, discovering, categorizing, and prioritizing the dysfunctions as they become known. Those situations that can and should be treated immediately are done so by the provider, while conditions that fall beyond the scope of the primary care practitioner are referred for secondary or tertiary level care.

Comanagement begins when such referrals are made. The comanagement of health problems may be as simple and routine as the regular monitoring of a patient's blood pressure (Good and Augsburger, 1989), or as complex as the referral and management of so obscure a condition as Behcet's disease (Peplinski, 1989). As Wilson and Hoffman remark, secondary level care often is conducted on a hospital or medical outpatient basis. The appointment for such care can be made by the primary level practitioner, and represents one means of the practitioner controlling the patient's progression through the health delivery system. Tertiary care consists of more intensive and extensive service, often requiring multidisciplinary, hospital-based expertise, but still incorporates the primary care practitioner's controlling judgment regarding the referral process (Wilson and Hoffman, 1989).

In the past, optometrists tended to work outside the mainstream of health-care delivery. This attitude has undergone a dramatic change over the past 15 years, and with the advent of primary care services, the optometrist now is much more in harmony with the health-care delivery system. Exemplifying this maturity is the growing acceptance of optometrists as hospital staff members. There are numerous advantages both to a community and to the practitioner for an optometrist to be extended hospital privileges (Bartlett, 1988; Myers, 1988; Blackman, 1988). Primary health care cannot be rendered from an arm's-length distance, but rather the practitioner must be an integral member of the delivery team. Obtaining hospital privileges by the optometrist constitutes a significant step toward the realization of this status.

More specifically, most optometrists have participated on an individual and local level with community ophthalmologists in the comanagement of patients who have been referred for secondary surgical or medical care. For the most part, these relationships at least have been workable, if sometimes not totally satisfactory from the optometrist's point of view. During the past few years, however, a new concept has evolved that provides the optometric practitioner more immediate input and subsequent control over the patients referred for higher levels of ocular care. Termed comanagement centers, the general format consists of a central medical complex wherein one or two ophthalmologists provide secondary and tertiary eye care for a surrounding network of participating optometric offices. These medical specialists serve also as consultants, with the patients being returned to the optometrists for monitoring and follow-up care once the secondary or tertiary services have been provided. Typically, such comanagement centers have a board of directors that establishes overall policy, an optometrist who serves as executive director, and one or more staff optometrists who provide professional support to the resident medical staff, conduct continuing education courses, and serve as educational mentors to students and residents who might rotate through the center on externships (Bartlett, 1988).

As with any administrative scheme, there are both advantages and disadvantages to optometric comanagement centers. On the positive side, the optometrist has a coterie of medical experts to whom patients can be referred with confidence, knowing then that those patients will be returned once the required secondary-level care has been supplied. Full and complete reports concerning the diagnostic work-up, therapy regimen, status, and prognosis of the patient will be supplied to the primary care practitioner, with the optometrist remaining in control of the entire referral process. The comanagement center can be identified and presented to the public as being an integral part of the primary care provider's practice, and, hence, the image of the optometrist's ability to provide full-scope eye health care can be enhanced. Continuing education can be obtained on a personalized basis, all being geared toward maintaining and upgrading the primary care practitioner's skills while maintaining good interprofessional relationships with the medical specialists at the center. Telephone consultations are available. In general, the participating optometrist has the opportunity to become an active member on a health-care delivery team in which the optometrist has a proprietary interest, and need no longer feel isolated from other health-care delivery disciplines (Nussenblatt, 1988).

However, a certain degree of independence may be lost by the optometrist who affiliates with a comanagement center. Anyone participating in the referral system of a comanagement organization must submit to the quality assurance guidelines of that center. In certain instances, this may require an updating of skills and the acquisition of new techniques on the part of the practitioner, whose practice and discipline now will come under the scrutiny of the comanagement center administrators as referrals are made. Minimum costs are imposed for the privilege of membership and participation. Finally, it may be necessary to refer to the center those patients who otherwise would have been sent to another practitioner, one with whom the optometrist had established good working relationships over a period of time (Nussenblatt, 1988a).

REFERENCES

1. A.O.A. Order Department. (Catalogue, current edition). 243 N. Lindburgh Blvd., St. Louis, MO, 63141.
2. A.O.A. *Reference Materials on Primary Care Optometry.* St. Louis, MO. American Optometric Association, 1977.
3. A.O.A. "Simple Steps for Targeting Your Primary Eye Care Communications." *American Optometric Association Supplement to Optometric Economics,* St. Louis, MO, December 1990, p. 8.

4. *A.O.A. News* 29 (17) (1991): 1.
5. *Aging America: Trends and Projections.* Special Committee on Aging. United States Senate. United States Government Printing Office, Washington, D.C., November 1989, pp. 78–79.
6. *Aging America: Trends and Projections.* U.S. Senate Special Committee on Aging. U.S. Department of Health and Human Services, Washington, D.C., 1985–1986 edition, p. 1.
7. Altergott, K., and C. E. Vaughn. Themes and Variations: Social Aspects of Aging. In: A. A. Rosenbloom, Jr. and M. W. Morgan, (eds). *Vision and Aging: General and Clinical Perspectives.* New York: Professional Press Books, Fairchild Publications, 1986, p. 19.
8. Aston, S. J., D. A. DeSylvia, and G. L. Mancil. "Optometric Gerontology: State of the Art in Schools and Colleges of Optometry." *J. Optom. Ed.* 14, no. 1 (1988): 8–12.
9. Aston, S. J., D. A. DeSylvia, and G. L. Mancil. *Optometric Gerontology: A Resource Manual for Educators.* Rockville, MD: ASCO, 1989.
10. Baldwin, W. R. "Scope of Optometric Practice: Trends, Portents, and Recommendations." *J. Optom. Ed.* 13, no. 2 (1987): 77–79.
11. Barresi, B. J. "Will Medicare's New Fees Help Your Bottom Line?" *Rev. Optom.* (February 1991): 46–47.
12. Barrow, G. M. *Aging: The Individual and Society,* 3rd. ed. New York: West Publishing Company, 1986.
13. Bartlett, J. D. "Optometry: The Primary Eye and Vision Care Profession." *J. Am. Optom. Assoc.* 57, no. 7 (1986): 495–496.
14. Bartlett, J. D. "Optometry in the Multidisciplinary Setting." *J. Am. Optom. Assoc.* 59, no. 8 (1988): 586–587.
15. Bell, F. C., and W. J. Stenstrom. *Atlas of the Peripheral Retina.* Philadelphia: W. B. Saunders, 1983.
16. Bertz, K. "Harris Poll: Americans Neglect Eye Care." *Optom. Management* (August 1989): 4.
17. Bevan, John (ed.) *Essentials of Pharmacololgy.* New York: Harper and Row, 1969, p. 207.
18. Billig, N., J. H. Fox, and B. Reisberg. "Diagnostic Dilemma: Is It Dementia?" *Patient Care* 23 (1989): 192–220.
19. Bingaman, J. Statement made during hearings before the Special Committee on Aging, United States Senate. In: *Healthy Elderly Americans; A Federal, State, and Personal Partnership.* Washington, D.C.: United States Government Printing Office, 1985, p. 3.
20. Bird, C. "The Jobs You Do." *Modern Maturity* (December 1988–January 1989): 40–46.
21. Blackman, G. L. "Why Should Optometry Become Involved in the Hospital Setting?" *J. Am. Optom. Assoc.,* 59:8 (August 1988), 603–604.
22. Blanchine, J., G. Niholas, and B. Andresen. "Current Concepts on Geriatric Medicine." *SCOPE Publications.* Kalamazoo, MI: The Upjohn Company, 1981, p. 18.
23. Borska, L. "Can Anyone Solve the Black Vision Crisis? *Rev. Optom.* (May 1991): 50–54.
24. Botwinick, J. *Aging and Behavior.* New York: Springer Publishing Company, 1978, pp. 25–29.
25. Bowker, M. "Retires for Hire." *Kiwanis Magazine* (March 1989): 25–27, 53.
26. Brown, B. M., and W. Hawkins. "A Descriptive Study Examining Primary-Level Prevention Activities of Oregon Optometrists." *J. Am. Optom. Assoc.* 62, no. 4 (1991): 296–303.

27. Broyles, G. "Guardianship Puts Elderly at Mercy of Unscrupulous." *Tulsa World* 83, no. 7 (1987), Sec. A-1.
28. Bruce, M. L., and P. J. Leaf. "Psychiatric Disorders and 15-Month Mortality in a Community Sampling of Older Adults." *Am. J. Pub. Health* 79, no. 6 (1989): 727–730.
29. Cadmus, Robert R. *Caring for Your Aging Parents.* New Jersey: Prentice-Hall, Inc., 1984, p. 6.
30. Califano, J. A., Jr. *America's Health Care Revolution.* New York: Random House, 1986, p. 178.
31. Carney, J. "Can a Car Driver Be Too Old?" *Time Magazine* (January 16, 1989): 28.
32. Cason, A., and V. Thompson. "Working with the Old and Dying." *Inst. J. Psychol.* 1 (1980), 58–69.
33. Catania, L. *Primary Care of the Anterior Segment.* Norwalk, CT: Appleton and Lange, 1988.
34. Christensen, B. "Primary Care: Your Income and the Future of Optometry." *Optom. Management* (April 1990): 23–28.
35. Classe, J. G. "The Right to Practice Primary Care." *J. Am. Optom. Assoc.* 57, no. 7 (1986): 549–553.
36. Classe, J. G. "Optometrist's Duty to Warn of Vision Impairment." *South. J. Optom.* 4, no. 1 (Winter Quarter 1986a): 65–69.
37. Classe, J. G. "Liability for Ocular Urgencies and Emergencies." *South. J. Optom.* 4, no. 4 (Winter Quarter 1986b): 65–69.
38. Classe, J. G. "1989 Legal Review: In the Eyes of the Law." *Optom. Management* (February 1990): 51–57.
39. Cole, K., and D. L. McConnaha. "Understanding and Interacting with Older Patients. *J. Am. Optom. Assoc.* 57, no. 12 (1986): 920–925.
40. Comfort, A. *A Good Age.* New York: Crown Publishers, 1976.
41. Cowan, E. Background and History: The Crisis in Public Finance and Social Security. In: Boskin, M. J. (ed.). *The Crisis in Social Security.* San Francisco: Institute for Contemporary Studies, 1977, Chapter 1.
42. Crooks, L. "Older Americans in a Changing Society." *Vital Speeches* 60, no. 18 (1989): 556–558.
43. DeSylvia, D. A. "Low Vision and Aging." *Optom. Vis. Sci.* 67, no. 5 (1990): 319–322.
44. Decker, D. L. *Social Gerontology.* Boston: Little, Brown, and Co., 1980, pp. 5–6.
45. Denzer, S. "Do the Elderly Want to Work?" *U.S. News and World Report* (May 14, 1990): 48–50.
46. Dupuis, S. L. "Projected Changes in the Health Care Delivery System." *J. Optom. Ed.* 13, no. 2 (1987): 82–83.
47. Eagling, E. M., and M. J. Roper-Hall. Eye Injuries: An Illustrated Guide. Philadelphia: J.B. Lippincott Co., 1986.
48. Edmondson, J. M. *Home Safety: It's No Accident.* Kalamazoo, MI: Upjohn Healthcare Services, Inc., 1983.
49. Fedukowicz, H. B., and S. Stenson. *External Infections of the Eye,* 3rd ed. Norwalk, CT: Appleton-Century-Crofts, 1985.
50. Fowles, D. G. *A Profile of Older Americans.* Washington, D.C.: American Association of Retired Persons, Dept. D-996, (Publication PF 3049:1085).
51. Garnett, W. R., and W. H. Barr. *Geriatric Pharmacokenetics.* Kalamazoo, MI: The Upjohn Company, 1984, p. 14.
52. *Geographical Mobility: March 1986 to March 1987.* Population Characteristics, Series P-20, 430. United States Department of Commerce, Bureau of

Census. Washington, D.C.: United States Government Printing Office, 1988, pp. 11–12, 101.
53. Good, G. W., and A. R. Augsburger. "Role of Optometrists in Combatting High Blood Pressure." *J. Am. Optom. Assoc.* 60, no. 5 (1989): 352–355.
54. Grad, S. *Income of the Population 55 and Over: 1984.* United States Department of Health and Human Services. Washington, D.C.: United States Government Printing Office, (December 1985), 2.
55. Gramm, S., and A. Barker. "Sensory Deprivation Training for Your Office Staff." *J. Am. Optom. Assoc.* 53, no. 1 (1982): 53–54.
56. *Graying of Nations, The.* Hearing before the Special Committee of Aging, U.S. Senate, 99th Congress, July 12, 1985. Washington, D.C.: U.S. Government Printing Office, 1986, pp. 4–8.
57. Guralink, J. M., and G. A. Kaplan. "Predictors of Healthy Aging: Prospective Evidence from the Alameda County Study." *Am. J. Pub. Health* 79, no. 6 (1989): 703–708.
58. Hajnosz, J. T., and T. Nishimoto. "Safety of Geriatric Patients in Optometric Clinics." *South. J. Optom.* 6, no. 3 (1988): 12–15.
59. Hamada, K. "Creating the 'Look of the '90's'." *Optom. Econ.* 1, no. 2 (1991): 35–36.
60. Hanks, A. J. "Contact Lenses for Presbyopia." *Eye Contact* 1, no. 1 (1984): 9–14.
61. Hanlen, H. P. Medicare Is Here to Stay. *Opt. Econo.* 1, no. 3 (1991): 11–13.
62. Hanlen, H. P. "'Physician Payment Reform' Translated Means a Fee Schedule." *Opt. Econ.* 2, no. 12 (1992): 41–43.
63. Hasson, J. "Families Abandoning Elderly in Hospital Emergency Rooms." *Muskogee Phoenix* 42, no. 15 (April 15, 1991): Sec. A-6.
64. Heckheimer, E. F. *Health Promotion of the Elderly in the Community.* Philadelphia: W. B. Saunders, 1989, Chapter 17.
65. Henig, R. M. *The Myth of Senility.* Glenwood, IL: Scott Foresman and Company, 1985, pp. 112, 127.
66. Herrin, S. The Surprising '90's. *Rev. Optom.* (January 1990): 32–32.
67. Highton, M. "Business and Eldercare." *Braniff Magazine* (June 1989): 48–53.
68. Hirsch, M. J., and R. E. Wick. *Vision of the Aging Patient.* Philadelphia: Chilton Company, 1960.
69. Hopping, R. L. "The Impact of the Projected Trends and Changes in the Health Care Delivery System on the Optometric Profession. *J. Optom. Ed.* 13, no. 2 (1987): 85–88.
70. Hussar, D. A. *Geriatric Drug Interactions.* East Hanover, NJ: Sandoz Pharmaceuticals Corporation, 1987.
71. Jaques, L. *Fundamental Refraction and Orthoptics.* Los Angeles: Globe Printing Company, 1936, pp. 47–59, 178–184.
72. Jolley, J. L., D. Lewis, and W. Reinertson. Third-Party Payment Programs. In: Robert D. Newcomb and E. C. Marshall, (eds.). *Public Health and Community Optometry.* Boston: Butterworth, 1990, pp. 185–187.
73. Josephson, J. E., et al. "Monovision." *J. Am. Optom. Assoc.* 61, no. 11 (1990): 820–826.
74. Keeney, V. T., and A. H. Keeney. Emotional Aspects of Visual Impairment in the Population Over Sixty Years of Age. In: Marvin L. Kwitko and F. J. Weinstock, eds. *Geriatric Ophthalmology.* Orlando: Grune and Stratton, 1985, Chapter 1.
75. Ketner, J. L., and C. A. Johnson. Visual Function, Driving Safety, and the Elderly. *Ophthalmology* 94, no. 9 (1987): 1180–1188.

76. Klein, S. D., and R. E. Klein. "Delivering Bad News: The Most Challenging Task in Patient Education." *J. Am. Optom. Assoc.* 58, no. 8 (1987): 660–663.
77. Klopfer, J., R. Rosenberg, and S. B. Verma. Geriatric and Rehabilitative Optometry. In: Newcomb, Robert D. and E. C. Marshall. *Public Health and Community Optometry,* 2nd ed. Boston: Butterworth, 1990, pp. 341–346.
78. Kornzweiz, A. L. The Eye in Old Age. In: Isadore Rossman (ed.) *Clinical Geriatrics* 2nd ed. Philadelphia: J. B. Lippincott, 1979, Chapter 20.
79. Krieger, N., G. Ketcher, and G. Fulk. "Physiological Variables Affecting Intraocular Pressure in a Population Study." *Am. J. Optom. Physiol. Opt.* 65, no. 9 (1988): 739–744.
80. Lightman, J. M., and A. A. Rosenbloom. "Geriatric Optometry Questionnaire." *J. Am. Optom. Assoc.* 62, no. 6 (1991): 472–474.
81. Lublen, J. E., P. G. Weiler, and I. Chi. Health Practices of the Elderly Poor. *Am. J. Pub. Health* 79, no. 6 (1989): 731–733.
82. Lunzer, F. Z. "Small Gadgets Than Can Change Lives." *U.S. News and World Report* (March 6, 1989): 58–60.
83. Mancil, G. L., and C. Owsley. "Vision Through My Aging Eyes Revisited." *J. Am. Optom. Assoc.* 59, no. 4 (1988): 288–294.
84. Mandell, R. B. *Contact Lens Practice,* 4th ed. Springfield, IL: Charles C. Thomas, 1988, Chapter 29.
85. *MAXIAIDS: Aids and Appliances.* 86–30 102d Street, Richmond Hill, New York, 11418.
86. McGoldrick, A. E. Stress, Early Retirement, and Health. In: Markroles, K. S., and C. L. Cooper (eds.). *Aging, Stress, and Health.* New York: John Wiley and Sons, 1989, Chapter 5.
87. "Medicare Reforn is Kind to Optometry, Primary Care." *A.O.A. News* 29, no. 24 (1991): 1–2.
88. *Medicare Handbook.* Aetna Medicare, 701 N. W. 63d Street, Oklahoma City, Oklahoma, 73116, 1990, pp. 1–2.
89. "Medicare Reform: Major Changes on Schedule for '92." *A.O.A. News* 29, no. 20 (1991): 1, 13.
90. Michaels, D. D. *Visual Optics and Refraction: A Clinical Approach,* 3rd ed. St. Louis: C. V. Mosby, 1985, p. 417.
91. Morse, A. R., R. Silberman, and E. Trief. Aging and Visual Impairment. *J. Visual Impairment and Blindness* (September 1987): 308–312.
92. Myers, K. J. "Hospitals and Optometry: An Evolving Relationship." *J. Am. Optom. Assoc.,* 59:8 (August 1988), 586–587.
93. Newcomb, R. D. Health Education and Promotion. In: R. D. Newcomb and E. C. Marshall (eds.). *Public Health and Community Optometry,* 2nd ed. Boston: Butterworth, 1990, Chapter 20.
94. News Review. "Drugs Become a Greater Part of Practice." *Rev. Optom.* (March 1991): 7, 9.
95. Nussenblatt, H. "Optometric Utilization and Level of Satisfaction with a Comanagement Center." *J. Am. Optom. Assoc.* 59, no. 10 (1988): 767–772.
96. O'Hara-Devereaux, M., Andrus, L. H., and Scott, C. D. (eds.). *Eldercare.* New York: Grune and Stratton, 1981, p. 51.
97. Oklahoma State Statutes, Title 43A. Mental Health Law: Protective Services for the Elderly and Incapacitated Adults Act (1977). Oklahoma City, OK: Oklahoma Department of Human Services, Publication #88–13.
98. Owens, A. "1995: Who Will Be Your Patients?" *Med. Econ.* (March 31, 1986): 35–53.
99. Packard, R., and S. H. Klinment (eds.). *Architectural Graphic Standards: Student Edition.* Abridged from 7th ed. New York: John Wiley and Sons, 1989.

100. Pastalan, L. A. Environmental Design and Adaptations to the Visual Environment of the Elderly. In: Robert Sekuler, D. Kline, and K. Dismukes, (eds.). *Aging and Human Visual Function. Modern Aging Research,* vol. 2. New York: Alan R. Liss, 1982, pp. 323–333.

101. Penisten, D. "Optometry's 100-Year Wars." *Rev. Optom.* (January 1991): 40–43.

102. Peplinski, L. S. "Ocular Involvement in Behcet's Disease." *J. Am. Optom. Assoc.* 60, no. 11 (1989): 854–857.

103. Potter, J. "Optometry and Gerontology: A Vital Link." *J. Optom. Ed.* 2, no. 2 (1985): 4.

104. Rakstis, T. J. "Wanted: Small-Town Health Care." *Kiwanis Magazine* 76, no. 5 (1991): 30–33.

105. Reisner, R. "Two Professions: Two Perceptions." *Optom. Management* (September 1990): 19–26.

106. "Rising Medicaid Costs Worry Budget-Plagued States." *A.O.A. News,* 29, no. 18 (1991): 2.

107. Rosenbloom, A. A. "A Proposed Curriculum Model for Geriatric Optometry." *J. Optom. Ed.* 11 (1985): 22–24.

108. Rosenbloom, A. A. "Optometry and Gerontology." *Optom. Monthly* (March 1982): 143–145.

109. Roybal, Edward R. (Chairman). *Elder Abuse: A National Disgrace.* A Report by the Chairman of the Subcommittee on Health and Long-Term Care of the Select Committee on Aging, House of Representatives. Washington, D.C.: United States Government Printing Office, May 10, 1985, pp. 1–21.

110. Rumsey, K. E. "Implications of Biological Aging to the Optometric Patient." *J. Am. Optom. Assoc.* 59, no. 4 (1988): 295–300.

111. Schmitt, E. P. "Sensory Deprivation and Remediation Among the Elderly. *Newsnet* 1 (January 1990) Oklahoma Geriatric Education Center, Oklahoma, City, Oklahoma, p. 3.

112. Sekuler, R., D. Kline, and Key Dismukes (eds.). *Aging and Human Visual Function. Modern Aging Research, VII.* New York: Alan Liss, 1982, Chapters 2 and 3.

113. "Senility Reconsidered: Treatment Possibilities For Mental Impairment in the Elderly. Special Communication." *JAMA* 244, no. 3 (1980): 259–263.

114. Shapiro, Joseph P. Economic Outlook. *U. S. News and World Report* (August 28–September 4, 1989), 92.

115. Sheras, Virgina. The 'Sandwich Generation' Cares for Aging Parents. Aging Arkansas, Arkansas Aging Foundation, Inc., Little Rock (September 1990), 2.

116. Siegel, J. A., and M. Davidson. *Demographic and Socioeconomic Aspects of Aging in the United States.* United States Department of Commerce. Washington, D.C.: United States Government Printing Office, 1984, p. 108.

117. Soroka, M. "A Comparison of Charges by Optometrists and Ophthalmologists Under the Medicare Program." *J. Am. Optom. Assoc.* 62, no. 5 (1991): 372–376.

118. Special Medical Reports. "A.O.A. Releases Guidelines for Eye Care in Patients with Diabetes Mellitus. *Am. Fam. Physician* 40, no. 1 (1988): 270–271.

119. Stelmack, T. R. "Management of Open-Angle Glaucoma." *J. Am. Optom. Assoc.* 58, no. 9 (1987): 716–721.

120. Stevens, T. (Chairman). Technology and Aging in America. Office of Technology Assessment. Congress of the United States. U.S. Government Printing Office, Washington, D.C. (June 1985), 249.

121. Swisher, K. (ed.). *The Elderly: Opposing Viewpoints.* San Diego: Greenhaven Press, 1990.

122. Taeuber, C. M. *America in Transition: An Aging Society.* U.S. Department of Commerce, Washington, D.C.: U.S. Government Printing Office, 1983, p. 3.
123. Templeman, J. "Grappling with the Graying of Europe." *Business Week* 3095 (March 13, 1989): 54–56.
124. Verma, S. B. "Vision Care for the Elderly: Problems and Directions." *J. Am. Optom. Assoc.* 60, no. 4 (1989): 296–299.
125. Villaneuva, W. "OD's Play Key Role in Detecting Signs of Drug Abuse." *Optometry Times* 3, no. 12 (December 1985).
126. Weale, R. A. *A Biography of the Eye: Development, Growth, Age.* London: H. K. Lewis and Co., Ltd., 1982, pp. 13–18.
127. Williamson, J., and Caird. Epidemiology of Ocular Disorders in Old Age. In: F. I. Caird and J. Williamson (eds.). *The Eye and Its Disorders in the Elderly.* Bristol, England: John Wright and Sons, 1986, Chapter 1.
128. Wilson, R. J., and D. J. Hoffman. "Optometry in the Multidisciplinary Health Care Setting." *Optom. Vis. Sci.* 66, no. 12 (1989): 859–863.
129. Winslow, C. "Second Annual Expense Survey: OD's Fight to Hold the Line." *Rev. Optom.* (January 1991): 44–47.
130. Wright, I. E. "Keeping an Eye on the Rest of the Body." *Ophthalmology* 94, no. 9 (1987): 1196–1198.
131. Wright, J. "Days Inn Policy Proves Value of Senior Workers." *Tulsa World* (March 17, 1991): Sec. D-3.

2

Ocular Implications of Systemic Disease in the Elderly

David M. Cockburn

Man's allotted span of three score years and ten remains little altered since biblical times, the most significant change being that many more people live out this span to reach four score years, and then confirm the further prophecy that these years shall be lived in sorrow and pain. The age-related changes in bodily function appear to take place in a linear manner, interrupted at times by disease, which then superimposes a steplike deterioration. Disease in the aged is frequently a complex of multiple disease states, perhaps commencing with one organ system but affecting other systems in a cascading sequence of secondary complications. The visual system, of course, is included in these processes. The burden of disease, added to the social and mobility problems of the aged, bring in turn depression, mental deterioration, and rapidly increasing senile changes. Indeed, the first manifestations of systemic disease in the elderly are likely to mimic senility, but they have the potential to be reversed by appropriate medical care.

Problems that occur in the diagnosis of disease in the aged include a tendency for elderly patients to ignore the symptoms because they believe these are inevitable consequences of aging. Decreased cognizance and flattened affect, which are often early signs of systemic disease, also may cause patients to ignore their symptoms and fail to seek attention. The mode of presentation of both systemic and ocular diseases is likely to be different in the aged patient from that which is typical in younger subjects. This is particularly true of diabetes, drug intoxication, and thyroid disease. Another group of diseases is common only in elderly patients and occurs only rarely in the mature or younger age groups; examples of these diseases are basal cell carcinoma, Paget's disease, Parkinson's disease, and temporal arteritis. A well-designed program of screening for disease in the elderly must reflect these special age-related factors.

Samples of patients seeking optometric care are not necessarily similar to those seeking general medical, hospital, or even ophthalmologic care; in consequence, epidemiologic data derived from these sources may not apply to optometric patients. Patients of optometrists tend to be older than the general population; a consecutive series of patients of one optometrist in private practice had a mean age of 55.2 years (Cockburn, 1982), whereas the community from which it was drawn had a mean age of 32 years (Cameron, 1982). It is also reasonable to expect that patients of optometrists are more healthy than those seeking other health care, since they are a self-selecting group who are not yet subject to being monopolized by the medical system. These unique characteristics of optometric patients point to the need to be aware of the very early signs and symptoms of the diseases that are likely to occur in the aged. Of course, special attention should be given to the detection of the ocular signs that suggest systemic disease.

The selection of diseases to be discussed in this chapter was influenced by a number of factors, which include the following:

- The disease should be significantly associated with the processes of aging and be found most commonly in the aged.
- The samples of patients attending optometrists should contain a reasonable yield of the disease state.
- The disease should be capable of being recognized during an optometric examination by techniques that are appropriate to the optometric role in the health-care services of developed countries.
- The disease should have a potential to cause significant morbidity or mortality.
- Some form of effective therapy to cure or relieve the effects of the disease should exist.

Optometrists have an obligation to insure that their patients do not suffer any avoidable visual loss or systemic effects of diseases that can be recognized during the ocular examination and that can be treated successfully. To fulfill this obligation requires a detailed knowledge of the diseases of the elderly and constant clinical vigilance.

CARDIOVASCULAR DISEASE
Stroke

Stroke is the condition in which failure of cerebral vascular supply results in permanent neurologic damage. This may be through embolism of cerebral arteries or as a result of hemorrhage. Stroke has an incidence of approximately one case in every 500 people each year (Howells, 1982; McDowell, 1975; Warlow, 1981), and it is more likely to occur in older age groups. Some 92% of all strokes occur in patients aged 50 years or older (McDowell, 1975). One-third of stroke cases recover to the extent that they can resume a normal life, one-third are seriously and permanently incapacitated, and one-third die (McDowell, 1975; Warlow, 1981). Cerebrovascular disease is the cause of approximately 13% of all deaths, based on the 1979 international classification of diseases. It was second only to ischemic heart disease as a cause of death in Australia during 1980 to 1981, and 85% of these deaths occurred in subjects aged 65 years or older (Howells, 1982).

Many subjects who subsequently develop stroke experience early symptoms over a period of time; these symptoms result from brief episodes of cerebral ischemia of a duration or extent that falls short of causing permanent neurologic damage. The attacks last from a few minutes to several hours: they are characterized by their sudden onset, patterns of neurologic involvement, and complete recovery. Often the attacks are repeated several or many times in an individual. These episodes of cerebral vascular insufficiency are referred to as transient ischemic attacks (TIAs).

There is ample and convincing evidence that TIAs are forewarning of more serious cerebrovascular compromise that leads to permanent stroke-related morbidity (Acheson and Hutchinson, 1964; Duncan et al., 1976; Fein, 1978; Field and Lemak, 1976; Herman et al., 1980; Wishnant et al., 1973). There is a special risk of stroke in the first few weeks following the initial TIA (Warlow, 1981).

The effectiveness of treatment to prevent stroke in patients having TIAs is still subject to controversy (Muuronen and Kaste, 1982). However, there is evidence that anticoagulation therapy — usually aspirin in small quantities — is effective (Harrison et al., 1971; Muuronen and Kaste, 1982; Olsson et al., 1976), especially in males (Canadian Cooperation Study Group, 1978). Surgical repair of atheromatous lesions at the bifurcation of the common carotid artery (carotid endarterectomy) can be effective in eliminating TIAs and in delaying or preventing the completed stroke (McDowell, 1975). However, in the United States, it has been claimed that the procedure has been over used in an estimated 32% of cases on the basis of inappropriate reasons, such as minimal stenosis of the artery. The appropriate indications for endarterectomy are still the subject of debate, but the emerging consensus appears to be that surgery is justified when there is carotid insufficiency with proven artery stenosis beyond about 75% accompanied by TIAs and in an otherwise healthy subject. In the elderly, frail patient, the improvement in terms of stroke-free survival following surgery becomes less certain and antiplatelet therapy may carry a better prognosis. As with all forms of treatment, the risks of surgery must be balanced against the risk of conservative management for the individual patient.

Vascular supply to the brain derives from the right and left internal carotid arteries anteriorly, whereas the posterior portion is supplied by the vertebral arteries, which join to form the basilar artery. Insufficiency of supply in one of these vessel systems results in neurologic deficits, the nature of which is determined by the watershed of the involved artery. However, the signs and symptoms are modified by the availability of an alternative blood supply through anastamosing vessels distal to the site of obstruction. The most important anastamosis, which is at the base of the brain, takes the form of the arterial circle of Willis, by way of the two posterior communicating arteries and the anterior communicating artery. These communicating arteries effectively link the vertebrobasilar and carotid artery systems to continue vital circulation should one or other of these major supply routes be lost. Likened to building practices, it could be said that this arrangement is architecturally brilliant, but the plumber misread the plans, since the communicating arteries are frequently absent or so poorly represented that they are ineffective should one of the major channels be blocked (Sedzimer, 1959). There is also considerable anatomic variation in the vascular arrangement of many of the major cerebral vessels, which restricts their ability to compensate for deficiencies elsewhere (Riggs and Rupp, 1963).

The signs and symptoms of TIA are determined by the cerebral distribution of the affected vessel and the extent to which alternative blood supply is available. It follows that attacks experienced by an individual follow a similar pattern, but that attacks vary between individuals, even when the site of obstruction is similar.

Visual symptoms frequently are experienced during TIAs, a fact that might be expected in view of the extreme sensitivity of the visual system to oxygen deficits and its dependence on both the vertebrobasilar system and the carotid arteries for supply. The classic TIA of carotid origin is ipsilateral amaurosis fugax and contralateral paresthesia, or paresis of the face and upper or lower limbs. When the dominant hemisphere is involved, speech disorders are also common (dysarthria). These symptoms do not necessarily occur at the same time. In verte- brobasilar-induced TIA, the visual disturbance tends to take the form of homony- mous hemianopias or photopsias as a result of cortical ischemia; the non-visual symptoms are chiefly the result of brain stem ischemia and involve the disruption of muscle coordination. Drop attacks commonly occur in basilar territory TIAs; the patient falls without losing consciousness because of loss of postural tone in the leg muscles. Figure 2.1 illustrates the signs and symptoms that might be expected in TIAs associated with insufficiency of the individual cerebral arteries. Table 2.1 shows the prevalence of the various signs and symptoms of

Table 2.1   Prevalence of the symptoms of TIAs and of cervical bruits detected in 82 patients selected from 1,000 consecutive patients aged 50 or older

Symptom	Prevalence	Percentage of Sample
Cervical bruit (carotid, 27; transmitted, 3)	30	3.0
Paresthesia of hands or feet	28	2.8
Drop attacks	23	2.3
Transient visual field disturbance	22	2.2
Dysarthria	20	2.0
Paresis	18	1.8
Amaurosis fugax	17	1.7
Dizziness	6	0.6
Syncope	6	0.6
Numbness of lips or tongue	4	0.4
Ischemic pain	3	0.3
Diplopia	1	0.1
Hearing loss	1	0.1
Memory loss	1	0.1

Source: Adapted with permission from Cockburn, D.M., "Signs and Symptoms of Stroke and Impending Stroke in a Series of Optometric Patients." *Am. J. Optom. Physiol. Opt.* 60, no. 9 (1983): 749–753.

CAROTID ARTERY SYSTEM
T.I.A. INVOLVING UNILATERAL
HEMIPLEGIA ETC. ISCHEMIC PAIN

Middle cerebral artery
Homonymous hemianopia with splitting of fixation
Hemiplegia or hemiparesis, hemi- paresthesia of contralateral face, hand or arm

Anterior cerebral artery
Hemiplegia or hemiparesis, hemi- paresthesia of contralateral leg

Ophthalmic artery
Amaurosis fugax or unilateral blindness
Central retinal artery occlusion
Venous stasis retinopathy
Ischemic optic neuropathy
Unilateral cataract
Rubeosis irides

VERTEBRO-BASILAR SYSTEM
T.I.A. INVOLVING
HOMONYMOUS FIELD LOSS

Posterior cerebral artery
Homonymous hemianopia with sparing of fixation
Disturbance of visual recognition and memory

Basilar artery
Dizziness
Diplopia
Vertigo
Drop attacks
Oscillopsia
Nystagmus

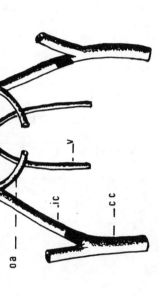

pc —
post c —
mc —
b —
ant c —
ac —
oa —
ic —
v
cc

Figure 2.1. Schematic drawing of the cerebrovascular arterial supply showing common sites for occlusions to develop (solid black) and the signs and symptoms resulting from occlusions of major arterial branches. pc = posterior cerebral artery; post c = posterior communicating artery; mc = middle cerebral artery; b = basilar artery; ant c = anterior communicating artery; ac = anterior cere- bral artery; oa = ophthalmic artery; ic = internal carotid artery; v = vertebral artery; and cc = common carotid artery.

TIAs and of cervical bruits experienced by 82 subjects selected from 1,000 consecutive patients aged 50 years or older who visited an optometrist (Cockburn, 1983).

Details of symptoms of TIA are unlikely to be volunteered by patients during history taking, particularly when the symptoms are other than visual in nature. Even previous attacks of amaurosis fugax, frightening though they may be at the time, are readily forgotten by the patient. Only in one of 17 cases having amaurosis fugax was this symptom volunteered prior to the clinician asking a specific question relating to the symptom (Cockburn, 1983). If patients having TIAs are to be identified, it is important that history taking include questions designed to elicit the symptoms of TIA, including those having a transient visual nature.

Showers of emboli derived from ulcerated atherosclerotic lesions of the heart or great vessels proximal to the cranium may cause stroke or TIAs when they lodge in cerebral vessels. Those that traverse the carotid system may enter the ophthalmic artery to cause temporary, permanent, or incomplete blockage of the short posterior ciliary arteries or the central retinal artery. The emboli that lodge in the ciliary and choroidal vessels cause anterior ischemic optic neuropathy (Hayreh, 1975), since the laminar region of the optic disc depends principally on the choroidal circulation for its nutrition. Emboli that reach the central retinal artery may be seen as white fibrinous deposits in the vessel wall (Fisher plugs) or as bright crystals of cholesterol typically lodged at bifurcations of minor retinal arterioles (Hollenhorst's plaques) (Figure 2.2).

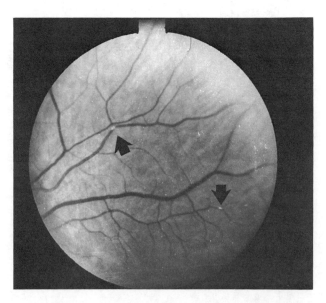

Figure 2.2. Bright refractile cholesterol emboli (Hollenhorst plaques) located at the bifurcation of the retinal arterioles (arrows).

Larger emboli lodging in the central retinal artery cause sudden stoppage of the blood supply and visual loss. The ophthalmoscopic picture is that of a white, infarcted, inner retinal layer with retention of the normal red color at the macula as a cherry red spot and segmented retinal artery blood columns. The emboli that cause these occlusions may be seen at major bifurcations, but they usually lyse rapidly and disappear after several days (Figure 2.3).

Atherosclerotic lesions may affect that intraocular portion of the central retinal artery close to the disc because this portion of the vessel retains a lamina. These lesions occasionally appear as dense yellow sheathing that replaces the normal vessel wall; the lumen of the vessel may remain patent, although no blood column is visible (Figure 2.4). A normal artery wall is not visible by ophthalmoscopy; only the blood column is seen, so these regions of opaque artery wall appear to be wider than the blood column. The finding of atherosclerotic changes in retinal vessels suggests widespread intracranial atherosclerosis.

A gradual reduction of the arterial supply to the retina may lead to retinal ischemia and venous stasis retinopathy (VSR). The most common cause of this restriction of blood flow is atheromatous disease of the carotid artery, which results in ipsilateral ocular ischemia that resembles central retinal vein thrombosis. The retinal veins are dilated and tortuous, and often have hemorrhages lying parallel to their courses. Other retinal hemorrhages (predominantly dot and blot hemorrhages in the deeper retinal layers) together with microaneurysms and cotton wool patches complete the retinal picture of VSR. The optic disc is usually hyperemic (Figure 2.5). Central vision may be quite good in spite of the vascular problem.

The absence of hard exudate and the unilateral presentation should differentiate VSR and diabetic retinopathy. Although VSR can present in bilateral

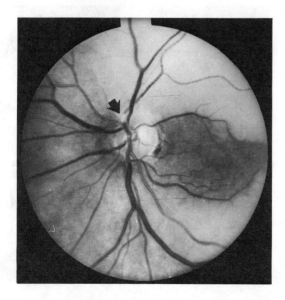

Figure 2.3. Large, yellow embolus lodged at the superior temporal artery bifurcation (arrow). The embolus had moved from the first bifurcation of the central retinal artery where it had caused a central retinal artery occlusion with white infarcted retina.

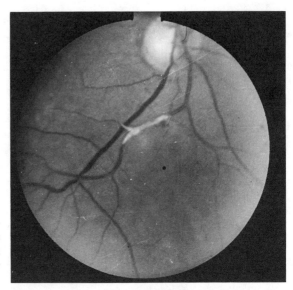

Figure 2.4. Bright, yellow scintillating opacifications of the arteriolar wall. The vessel lumen may be patent or occluded by this process.

form, it usually is unilateral, at least at first presentation. Diabetic retinopathy, on the other hand, would be bilateral in presentation at this florid stage of development (Kearns and Hollenhorst, 1963). The clinician should consider a diagnosis of carotid artery insufficiency when these signs are present. Retinal signs of vascular insufficiency were found in 24 of 1,000 consecutive patients aged 50 or over; the prevalence of individual signs is shown in Table 2.2.

The most consistent clinical finding in atheromatous disease of the carotid artery is the presence of a carotid bruit (Wilson and Ross-Russell, 1977). This is a

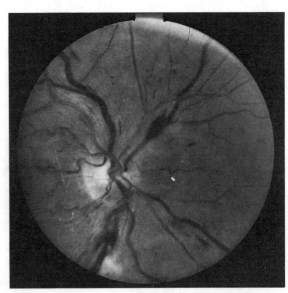

Figure 2.5. Venous stasis retinopathy resulting from restriction of the internal carotid artery. Note the dilated retinal veins, nerve fiber layer hemorrhages, and a cotton wool patch inferior to the disc.

Table 2.2 Prevalence of retinal signs of vascular insufficiency detected in 24 of 1,000 consecutive patients aged 50 years or older

Sign	Prevalence
Hollenhorst's plaques	6
Venous stasis retinopathy	5
Central retinal artery plaques or emboli at, or proximal to, second bifurcation	5
Central retinal vein thrombosis	4
Occlusion of central retinal artery	3
Occlusion of branch retinal artery	3
Tributary retinal vein thrombosis	2
Hemorrhage on the disc	1

sound that is heard on auscultation of the region overlying the carotid artery bifurcation just lateral to the thyroid cartilage. This sign was detected in 61 (6.1%) of the 1,000 patients 50 years or older (Cockburn, 1983). These sounds may be caused by a lesion in the carotid artery or be transmitted from the heart, aorta, or innominate or subclavian arteries. The distinction is usually possible on the grounds that a bruit of carotid origin is loudest over the site of bifurcation in the neck, whereas transmitted bruits are heard with greater intensity lower in the artery and at a maximum in the region of the subclavian fossa at the base of the neck. Of the carotid bruits just mentioned, 44 (4.4%) were carotid; the remaining 17 (1.7%) were judged to be transmitted. In 27 cases of carotid bruit, the patient also experienced TIAs. The high yield of this important sign in an aging population of patients of an optometrist justifies the inclusion of carotid auscultation in the examination of patients, especially those in older age groups and those having additional risk factors for stroke. However, it has been established that in the absence of symptoms, carotid bruits carry a relatively low risk of stroke and that carotid angiography and surgery are not warranted. Optometrists may wish to advise the patient's physician of the presence of a bruit, particularly if there is any evidence of additional risk factors for stroke, or there is evidence of TIA.

There are a number of risk factors for, or causes of, stroke. The more common being atherosclerosis; diabetes; hypertension; heart disease, including dysrhythmias; and the various forms of peripheral arteritis (Kannel, 1971; McDowell, 1975; Veshima et al., 1980; Warlow, 1981). Atherosclerosis, probably a universal and inevitable aging change in the major arteries, is undoubtedly the principal cause of nonhemorrhagic stroke. Atheromatous disease is often present in an advanced form in association with both diabetes and hypertension. In fact, diabetes or hypertension is present in more than two-thirds of all stroke patients (McDowell, 1975). It follows that all patients having these diseases, especially patients of advanced years, should be carefully examined for evidence of impending stroke. This implies a careful evaluation of the history in searching for TIAs, routine cervical auscultation, and evaluation of fundus signs of vascular changes.

The clinician who is aware of the risk factors of stroke and who carefully assesses elderly patients will be rewarded by a relatively high yield of positive findings; as a result of appropriate referral and treatment, the optometrist retains a grateful patient whose declining years are more likely to be accompanied by retained physical and mental faculties.

Hypertension

Because hypertension is a disease defined in terms of a continuous variable (blood pressure), its prevalence in a community will depend largely on the definition adopted for hypertension. The World Health Organization (WHO) (1962) recommends the adoption of a broad standard in which hypertension is defined as systolic pressure of 160 mm Hg or more and/or diastolic pressure of 95 mm Hg or more. The results of surveys of the prevalence of hypertension will be influenced by the selection of subjects; the methods used to measure blood pressure; and environmental, psychological, and geographic considerations. It is also necessary to take into account subjects who are being treated for the condition and whose pressures would be classed as within normal limits as a result of successful therapy. A survey of adults in the small community of Queenscliff, Australia, encompassed 74% of the population of 1,456 adults. Using the WHO criteria and including hypertensive patients already under treatment, it was found that 437 (30%) were hypertensive; of these, 161 (11%) of the sample were previously unaware of their condition (Christie et al., 1976). In the United States, the situation is similar. Stamler (1970) summarizes the evidence of several surveys as follows: "Of the almost 20 million persons with hypertension in the United States, about half are undetected; of the half known, no more than half are receiving long term care from physicians; and of those on therapy, only about half are receiving satisfactory care in terms of the simplest minimum criterion, reduction of blood pressure below hypertensive levels."

The prevalence of hypertension is related to age: in the Queenscliff study, the prevalence was lowest in the group aged 25 to 34 years (4.8%); it rose to 24.4% in the group aged 55 to 64 years, but declined again to 19.6% in subjects aged 65 years or older. Especially in its early years, hypertension is symptomless: the patient is comfortable and appears to be well. This benign presentation, together with the high prevalence of hypertension, insures a continuing diagnostic challenge and reservoir of potential hypertensive people. The significance of this challenge will depend on the morbid effect that untreated hypertension has on its victims and the success of treatment in delaying or preventing these effects. In the special case of the aged, practitioners should examine critically the diagnostic criteria, signs, prognosis, and treatment of hypertension, since these may not be the same as in young and middle-aged subjects.

The levels of both diastolic and systolic blood pressures have long been recognized by life insurance companies as an excellent predictor of life expectancy. Actuarial figures indicate that there is no point at which increased risk of death commences; the risk of cardiovascular-related mortality simply increases as blood pressure rises. The lowest mortality was found in subjects having systolic pressures 5 to 15 mm Hg below average for their age and among those having below-average diastolic pressures (Society of Actuaries, 1959). There is simply no dividing line between normotension and hypertension (Pickering, 1972).

The problems of establishing treatment strategies for hypertension are compounded by the rise of diastolic and, more particularly, systolic pressures with age (Page and Sidd, 1972), as well as the fact that women have a higher threshold for resultant cardiovascular damage than men. The actuarial figures relate to predictions mainly for young to middle-aged men. However, these figures show that for moderate to severe hypertension, the risk for aged subjects, as a percentage of increased mortality, is actually less than for the younger subjects (Society of Actuaries, 1959). It is as though high blood pressure in youth and middle-age imposes a serious threat to middle and long-term survival because of the length of time it has to cause complications, whereas its acquisition in old age is less serious, since other causes of death intervene before hypertensive complications occur. It appears that there is a well-established association between high blood pressure and increased morbidity, but does this association imply a true cause-and-effect relationship? Does the reduction of blood pressure improve the patient's prognosis, and does any improvement extend to the aged hypertensive?

Treatment of moderate to severe hypertension in men has been shown to markedly reduce cardiovascular-related morbidity (Veterans Administration, 1970). However, it should be noted that in this trial the treated subjects had a mean age of 50.5 years, and treatment appeared to benefit those subjects under 50 years of age more than those aged 50 or over. Similar trials conducted in samples drawn from an aged population are not available, and we must rely on clinical experience rather than firm evidence to evaluate the benefit of reducing blood pressure in the aged patient. Chalmers (1977) advises treating diastolic pressures in excess of 110 mm Hg "except perhaps [in] the very old"; Beevers (1982), while pointing out that there is no evidence to suggest that treatment is beneficial in the age group over 70 years, also recommends treating diastolic pressure in excess of 110 mm Hg. Treatment of hypertension in the age group over 70 years old frequently is administered because of symptoms that are not related to the hypertension; in fact, these symptoms can be made worse by potent hypertensive drugs (Peart, 1975). Some physicians believe that in the absence of proof of treatment effectiveness, raised blood pressure in aged patients should not be treated unless it is the result of malignant hypertension. This advice is underscored by the finding that 10% of all admissions to geriatric departments in the United Kingdom were caused by drug side effects, and that it is not uncommon for geriatricians to find that their greatest therapeutic successes are achieved by stopping drugs prescribed by other physicians (Denham, 1981). The opposing view is that hypertension in the elderly should be reduced to around 160/90 mm Hg (Niarchos, 1980), and that this therapy will reduce the incidence of stroke and congestive heart failure (Welzel, 1982).

The controversy surrounding treatment of an elderly patient must be resolved by the attending physician after the patient's overall condition has been considered rather than a set of numbers representing blood pressure. To make correct decisions, the physician needs as much evidence as is available on the state of the organs that are the targets for damage caused by hypertension. The retinal tissues and their supporting vascular system are such a target organ and provide a unique opportunity for direct and noninvasive assessment of complications. The ability to make useful assessments of this kind is built upon continuing experience in examining the fundus, reinforced by knowledge of intercurrent disease, level of blood pressure, and the patient's age. Upon weighing these factors, the optometrist is in a position to assist the physician in the assessment and management of the elderly hypertensive patient.

Ocular Involvements

The retina is limited in its response to the various insults to which it can be subjected by disease; as a consequence, no ophthalmoscopic signs can be said to be pathognomonic of systemic hypertension. Moreover, many of the signs that in the more youthful eye have high specificity for hypertension are commonly found in the eyes of elderly patients having blood pressure at or below mean levels for their age. Similarly, an acute rise in blood pressure may affect younger, more adaptable retinal arterioles in a quite different fashion from that of the sclerosed vasculature of the aged fundus. The indications of damage sustained by the retinal vasculature in the aged are therefore somewhat different from those found in the young and middle-aged hypertensive patient. Table 2.3 lists the retinal signs of systemic hypertension, together with indications of the probable efficiency of each sign in ophthalmoscopic detection of hypertension and its allied conditions. The table shows these estimates for young to middle-aged and elderly patients separately.

In the aged patient, the most significant hypertensive retinal signs are those that demonstrate advanced damage to the vessels. These may be the direct result of hypertension, or be the result of arteriosclerosis and arteriolarsclerosis, metabolic disease, or disorders of blood constituents. Whereas cotton wool patches and papilledema are the hallmarks of severe and malignant hypertension, these developments are exceedingly rare in the elderly (Hodkinson, 1981). The valuable signs of vascular breakdown are those that herald impending thrombosis of the veins or occlusion of arteries. Therefore, the practitioner should search carefully for banking of the retinal veins distal to arteriovenous crossings, arterial/arteriolar plaques, the development of shunt vessels, or microaneurysms. When the blood-retinal barrier already has been compromised, the important and more common signs in the aged retina are hemorrhages of both dot and blot and nerve fiber layer types, although the latter are the more typical of hypertensive damage. Macular edema also may be caused by a breakdown of the normal blood-retinal barrier. This takes the form of leakage of retinal vessels; however, it is also likely that the source of this problem is the result of senile changes in Bruch's membrane, the retinal pigment epithelium or both, leading to a failure of the elimination of metabolic by-products from the retina. Venous thrombosis typically results in sheathing of the vessel, which remains long after compensation

Table 2.3 Ocular fundus signs of hypertension and related systemic disease showing the pathophysiologic correlates of the signs and an estimate of diagnostic efficiency for subjects young to middle-aged and the elderly

Ophthalmic Sign of Hypertension or Associated Condition	Pathophysiologic Correlates	Efficiency as a Sign in Young to Middle-Aged	Efficiency as a Sign in the Aged
Diffuse arteriolar narrowing	Narrowing due to spasm of the vessel wall. Potentially reversible in young subjects.	A difficult sign to evaluate.	Attenuation of vessels occurs commonly with age. Not a reliable indicator.
Focal constriction of arterioles	Localized regions of passive arteriolar dilation alternating with local spasm.	A very specific and sensitive sign of hypertension in this age group.	Aged but otherwise healthy vessels often have this sign. Not a reliable indicator.
Straightening of arterioles	Occurrence in conjunction with diffuse narrowing from constriction of vessel; also secondary vascular occlusion and following compensation. May also occur in toxic states.	Only reliable if comparison is possible with previous appearance.	Not a reliable indicator.
Venular tortuosity	Stasis of flow through arterial insufficiency or venous occlusion. May signify macular edema when at posterior pole.	Difficult to evaluate, but very significant when present. Occurs in diabetes and many blood dyscrasias.	A reliable sign, especially in association with other signs (banking and hemorrhages).
Silver wire reflexes	Reflection of light from arteriolar wall accentuated in sclerosis of the vessel, which often is associated with hypertension.	Very poor specificity and difficult to assess. Of use only when noted in younger subjects.	Occurs in age as a senile change.

(continued)

Table 2.3 continued

Ophthalmic Sign of Hypertension or Associated Condition	Pathophysiologic Correlates	Efficiency as a Sign in Young to Middle-Aged	Efficiency as a Sign in the Aged
Arterial/arteriolar plaques	Atheromatous change in the artery on the disc or adjacent to the disc. Thrombi from heart carotid or great vessels. Arteriolar sclerosis due to hyalinization of vessel wall.	Very important indication of vascular damage, often associated with hypertension.	An important and reliable sign. Treatment of associated hypertension is justified.
Sheathing of veins	Fatty degeneration of vein following an occlusion or inflammation. The channel may recanalize and be associated with the development of shunt vessels.	Venous occlusions occur commonly in association with hypertension. An important sign of local and/or systemic disease.	An important indicator of hypertensive or associated disease.
Microaneurysms	Localized ballooning of the capillaries, venules, or arterioles. Occurs in diabetic retinopathy and following venous occlusions.	Uncommon in hypertension alone, but very common in diabetes. A useful sign of possible accompanying hypertension in diabetes and other vascular disorders. A highly significant sign.	An important sign that requires investigation.

Arteriovenous nicking (Gunn's sign)	Vein compressed at the point of arteriovenous crossing by a sclerosed arteriole or venule. The vein may be depressed into the retinal layers, which obscure it at the point of opacification of the arteriolar wall. Due to hyaline changes that obscure the vein.	Has poor specificity for hypertension unless accompanied by banking (see the next category).	Occurs in almost all senile fundi. Of little use as an indicator of disease unless associated with banking.
Banking	Restriction of the venous return distal to the site of arteriovenous crossing. Causes distension of the vessel. Commonly precedes thrombotic occlusion.	Confirms Gunn's sign (see the previous category) and is a very reliable sign of impending retinal vascular damage, which is often due to hypertension or related disease.	An important sign, as it is in younger eyes.
Shunt vessels	Dilation of capillary channels to form shunts to compensate for partial or total venous occlusions. Often seen in association with banking or sheathing.	Indicates serious previous or current vascular insufficiency. Often associated with hypertension.	Indicates need for treatment of any associated hypertension.
Dot and blot hemorrhages	Leakage of blood into the outer plexiform layer or nuclear layers of the retina. Indicates breakdown of blood retinal barrier in the deep capillary plexus.	Common in diabetes and in venous thrombosis. These diseases commonly are associated with hypertension. An important sign that requires evaluation.	An important sign, as it is in younger subjects.

(continued)

Table 2.3 continued

Ophthalmic Sign of Hypertension or Associated Condition	Pathophysiologic Correlates	Efficiency as a Sign in Young to Middle-Aged	Efficiency as a Sign in the Aged
Flame hemorrhages	Bleeding from superficial capillary layer.	Hypertension is the most common cause, but it also occurs in diabetes, venous thrombosis, anemia, papilledema, papillitis, sickle cell disease, and the blood dyscrasias.	An important sign of hypertension or another, often related disease.
Subretinal hemorrhages	Leakage of blood through Bruch's membrane from a choroidal source or from new vessels that have penetrated under the retinal pigment epithelium.	A serious sign often indicating the onset of disciform degeneration. May be associated with hypertension.	An indication of serious underlying vascular disturbance. May be associated with hypertension.
Preretinal hemorrhages	Hemorrhages that are usually the result of rupture of newly formed vessels arising from the retina or the disc, and occasionally caused by breakthrough by a large choroidal hemorrhage.	Part of the spectrum of diabetic retinopathy. Diabetes and hypertension often coexist, making this an important sign. May occur subsequent to venous thrombosis.	Proliferative diabetic retinopathy is rare in the elderly. Usually denotes old venous thrombosis or fragility of retinal vessels from arteriosclerosis; both may be associated with hypertension.
Papilledema	Noninflammatory swelling of the nerve head because of stasis of circulation, interruption of axoplasmic transport, or both. Commonly associated with increased intracranial pressure.	Rarely seen in clinical practice as a sign of hypertension, but is a serious sign in advanced cases. Other causes should be assumed in mild to moderate hypertensives.	In the elderly, it probably never occurs as a result of hypertension. Seek other causes.

Cotton wool patches (soft exudates)	Edema of the nerve fiber layer resulting from microinfarcts of this region. Potentially reversible.	Most common cause is accelerated hypertension and diabetes. Not likely to be found in mild to moderate hypertension. Also occurs in venous stasis retinopathy, papilledema, and systemic lupus erythematosus.	Not found in the moderately elevated blood pressures usual in the aged. However, it is a sign that requires investigation.
Hard exudates	Serum lipid deposits in the outer plexiform layer or partly phagocytosed remains of this layer. May remain permanently or resolve over a long period.	Most common in diabetes, but they appear also in hypertension, when they appear more white than the yellow deposits found in diabetes. A significant sign, since the damage is irreversible. In the absence of diabetes, they may be due to vascular occlusions associated commonly with hypertension.	Relatively common in the elderly patient having multiple-system disease, which may include hypertension.
Retinal edema	Leakage of serum from retinal vessels or from the choroid through Bruch's membrane.	An occasional complication of untreated hypertension, more common in diabetes.	An occasional complication of untreated hypertension, more common in diabetes.

has taken place (Figure 2.6). Should these signs be discovered in an elderly patient, the attending physician should be informed of the findings in order to review the patient's overall condition in light of this reliable evidence of vascular involvement.

Whether or not to treat the elderly hypertensive and to what therapeutic goals remain a matter of controversy. However, in view of the general clinical impression that lowering of the blood pressure reduces vascular and renal complications, it appears reasonable to lower pressures gradually in the elderly patient (Tucker, 1980). A general guide might be to treat patients having diastolic pressures of 105 mm Hg or greater and those having diastolic pressures between 90 and 104 mm Hg if there is established target organ damage; a family history of hypertensive complications, diabetes, raised cholesterol levels, elevated systolic pressures; or if the patient smokes (Lucas and Omar, 1980). The therapeutic aims of the internist should be a symptom-free patient having blood pressure around 160/90 (Niarchos, 1980).

Infective Endocarditis
Bacterial Endocarditis

Infective endocarditis is a disease in which there is inflammatory involvement of the heart endocardium, the heart valves, or the aorta. There is usually a focus of infection lodged at the site of previous damage to these structures. The most common infective organisms are streptococci or staphylococci, although other bacteria and fungi are becoming increasingly implicated (Gribbin, 1983).

Until fairly recent times, infective endocarditis was chiefly a disease seen in adolescents or young adults as a sequel to previous attacks of rheumatic fever or congenital heart defects. Better control of these predisposing causes has dramatically reduced the number of young people at risk of infective endocarditis, espe-

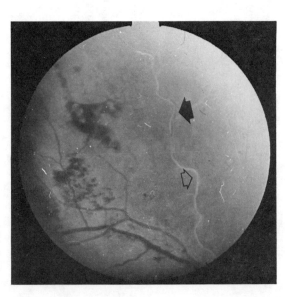

Figure 2.6. Sheathing of a branch retinal vein following occlusion of the vessel, showing both pipestem sheathing (open arrow) and parallel sheathing (solid arrow).

cially in developed countries. However, the increasing number of older people having open heart surgery, including the insertion of prosthetic heart valves, has created a new high-risk population in which the disease occurs much later in life (Geddes, 1982). This vascular surgery creates scar tissue and distortion of vessels, which create pockets in which infective organisms can lodge and multiply. The clinical features of infective endocarditis in the elderly differ from the classical descriptions of the disease in the younger age groups. In young patients, the organisms that affect the heart and great vessels are most commonly introduced during dental surgery and lodge at sites of previous damage to the heart. For this reason, both young and elderly patients having a history of rheumatic fever or congenital heart defects should have prophylactic antibiotic cover prior to undergoing even simple dental procedures. In aged patients, especially males, the introduction of the infection commonly follows urinary tract instrumentation (Gribbin, 1983).

The probable overall incidence of infective endocarditis in the United Kingdom is 6 per 10,000 per annum. However, these figures vary in different socioeconomic settings, with the areas having less, well-developed medical services tending toward a greater incidence and a lower age of onset for the disease. The course of infective endocarditis usually is categorized as acute or subacute, although no clear-cut difference exists over a spectrum of clinical presentation. The chief non-ophthalmic signs and symptoms are fever, headache, malaise, muscle and joint pains, nausea, and heart murmurs. Osler's nodes (small, raised, and tender nodes approximately 5 mm in diameter) may develop on the pads of the fingers or toes in approximately 5% of cases, and small hemorrhagic lesions (Janeway's lesions) appear on the palms of the hands and the soles of the feet in a similar proportion of patients (Gribbin 1983). There may be splinter hemorrhages in the fingernails, and in chronic disease, the fingers are clubbed. Neurologic involvement may occur in as many as one-third of patients, and this is particularly likely in elderly patients (Geddes, 1982), mainly as a result of embolic occlusions of ocular or cerebral vessels.

In the eye and its adnexa, petechial hemorrhages are common in the conjunctiva, and similar lesions may appear in the mouth. Hemorrhages are found in the retinal nerve fiber layer and are commonly associated with a white exudative center (Roth's spot; see Figure 2.7). In addition to these ocular signs, Duke-Elder (1976) lists spastic mydriasis, optic neuritis, venous thrombosis, and choroiditis as occasional complications of infective endocarditis.

Infective endocarditis is not rare in the elderly, although its presentation is frequently atypical and difficult to recognize. The elderly patient may be lethargic, confused, and disoriented, with loss of short-term memory, a combination that may lead to an incorrect diagnosis of senile dementia or Alzheimer's disease. Any fever may be slight or intermittent in aged subjects, so it is easily overlooked. A heart murmur is very common and usually can be heard during routine cervical auscultation as a transmitted bruit, particularly over the common carotid bifurcation on the patient's left side. The erythrocyte sedimentation rate (ESR) may be raised, appetite is diminished, and weight loss occurs in chronic dis-

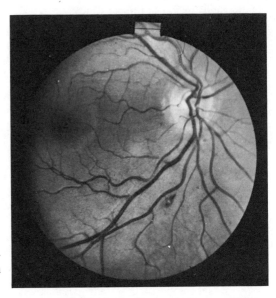

Figure 2.7. Small splinter hemorrhage in the nerve fiber layer with Roth's spot.

ease in the elderly. These findings in elderly patients should suggest the possibility of infective endocarditis, especially when there is history of previous heart damage or open heart surgery; a careful search for conjunctival and retinal hemorrhages could provide valuable corroborative diagnostic evidence. Prompt referral to a physician will enable effective treatment to be given and avoid the very high mortality associated with untreated infective endocarditis.

Treatment of infective endocarditis consists of antibiotic administration, preferably using drugs specifically chosen for their effectiveness against the invading pathogen that is identified by pathology specimens. Surgical repair of underlying physical heart abnormalities may be appropriate in some cases.

Carotid Artery/Cavernous Sinus Fistula

A fistula of the internal carotid artery may develop within the cavernous sinus as a result of the rupture of a small, previously asymptomatic intracranial aneurysm. Middle-aged and elderly women are particularly susceptible, although the more common cause in younger patients is trauma. Because the cavernous sinus serves the ophthalmic venous drainage system and also contains both the ocular motor nerves and the ophthalmic and maxillary divisions of the trigeminal nerve, there is potential for diverse ocular signs and symptoms following rupture of the internal carotid artery within the sinus.

A fistula between the artery and the sinus allows arterial blood to enter the sinus at higher pressure than is normal in the sinus and thus raise the venous pressure to near-arterial values. The increased venous pressure is transmitted as back pressure to the ophthalmic venous system, causing conjunctival congestion, chemosis, dilation of the conjunctival veins, and raised episcleral venous pressure, which, in turn, causes raised intraocular pressure.

A dramatic feature of the disease is a pulsating exophthalmos, which is usually unilateral at first but eventually becomes bilateral, because the sinuses are joined by the connecting circular sinus, and the effect of raised venous pressure is thereby transmitted to both sinuses. In the retina, the veins become dilated and tortuous as a result of back pressure, microaneurysms develop, leading to intra-retinal hemorrhages and the typical picture of venous stasis retinopathy.

The marked changes in hemodynamics that result from carotid cavernous sinus fistula give rise to a bruit with a swishing or blowing character that can be heard by auscultation over the orbit or brow. A pediatric stethoscope attachment, because of its small size, allows a neat fit over the globe and is ideal for auscultation of the orbit. The patient also may be aware of this sound, particularly when lying in bed. The bruit is synchronous with the heart beat and disappears when the ipsilateral carotid artery in the neck is compressed.

When the intra-sinus course of the oculomotor nerves is affected by the increased intra-sinus pressure, diplopia may result from paresis of the muscles, most commonly affected is the lateral rectus. Facial and ocular pain also occurs because of the effect on the sensory nerves as they traverse the sinus.

The differential diagnosis of carotid artery cavernous sinus aneurysm should include cavernous sinus thrombosis; however, this disease occurs most commonly as a complication of well-established and serious sepsis, which spreads through the cerebral and intracerebral veins or from adjacent structures.

A carotid cavernous sinus fistula may heal spontaneously; however, the prognosis usually is poor in untreated cases, and treatment is not without hazard. Treatment consists of carefully graded, partial ligation of the cervical portion of the internal carotid artery on the same side as the fistula. This reduces the arterial pressure within the sinus and, provided there is sufficient collateral vascular supply available to the ocular and cerebral structures, the signs and symptoms are relieved and sufficient circulation is maintained to preserve normal function.

VASCULAR OCCLUSIVE DISEASE

Cranial Arteritis (Temporal arteritis, giant cell arteritis, or Rumbold's disease) is a self-limiting form of generalized granulomatous arteritis that has a special predilection for the carotid arteries and their cranial branches. It is rare in patients under 50 years of age, and most affected patients are between 60 and 80 years of age (Cogan, 1974). Both sexes are affected equally. When the symptoms of cranial arteritis occur in their classic form, it is more likely that the patient will seek medical rather than optometric treatment, and the relatively low incidence of the disease insures that optometrists do not see many cases. However, on occasion, the ocular symptoms may be the first to appear and cause the patient to seek optometric advice. These early symptoms may occur singly or in various combinations, concurrently or at different times. This symptom diversity and the very high risk of blindness from untreated cranial arteritis demands vigilance on the part of the optometrist.

The pathologic features of cranial arteritis consist initially of degeneration of the smooth muscle cells of arteries, followed by damage to the elastic lamina and generalized inflammation of the wall of the vessels (Reinecke and Kuwabara, 1969). Macrophages respond to these changes by conversion to giant cells within the artery wall; fibroblasts proliferate, and consequently there is restriction or total occlusion of the lumen of the affected artery (Greer, 1972). These changes may be present in patches only, or over the entire course of the major arteries, including the aorta and hepatic and renal vessels (Beeson, 1975).

In the classic presentation of the disease, the watershed of the facial artery and, particularly, the superficial temporal artery becomes extremely tender to the touch. The superficial temporal artery becomes prominent as a tortuous, beaded, and swollen vessel under locally reddened skin. These signs and symptoms are not necessarily found in all cases and, indeed, probably occur in only about half the cases of cranial arteritis. Early signs and symptoms of cranial arteritis are a general malaise, low-grade fever, weight and appetite loss, and a headache that may be very severe and unresponsive to analgesic treatment (Beeson, 1975). Headaches are a relatively uncommon symptom in the elderly, so it follows that all elderly patients who complain of recent onset headache should be further investigated with cranial arteritis in mind.

Insufficiency of arterial supply caused by the vascular changes of cranial arteritis may give rise to ischemic ocular pain or pain in the face, jaw, tongue, temple, or neck. Many patients report pain in the jaw on chewing as an early sign; this condition is brought about by the failure of an adequate vascular supply to the muscles used in mastication. The tongue may become sore or even necrotic, and gangrene of fingers and toes has been reported (Andrews, 1966).

The extraocular muscles are affected by the disease in approximately 15% of patients (Gombos, 1977), causing paresis or paralysis of any or all of these muscles. A diagnosis of cranial arteritis should be considered in all elderly patients having diplopia of recent onset.

Retinal complications of cranial arteritis are common and occasionally may be the presenting signs. These most commonly occur in the first one to four weeks of the disease and are caused by vascular insufficiency brought about by occlusion or significant restriction of the ophthalmic, central retinal, or short posterior ciliary arteries. The classic fundus picture of central retinal artery occlusion consists of a pale, infarcted, inner retinal layer; grossly attenuated arterioles; and a red macula. The resulting gross visual loss is a common tragic feature of this disease. Central retinal artery occlusion sometimes occurs despite treatment (Beeson, 1975), and, on occasion, as an initial sign. When the short posterior ciliary arteries are occluded, there may be pale overall or sectorial swelling of the optic disc, with a few retinal hemorrhages and choroidal infarction at the posterior pole. The disc becomes pale and atrophic following regression of the inflammatory process. On the rare occasions when the iris is affected by the ischemic process, rubeosis irides and secondary glaucoma may follow (Gartner and Henkind, 1978). A pseudo Foster-Kennedy syndrome may arise in the situation where one eye has been affected by anterior ischemic optic neuropathy early in the disease process and optic atrophy has supervened. Should the second eye then become involved, its pale swelling simulates papilledema and completes the illusion of a Foster-Kennedy syndrome.

Occult cranial arteritis may occur in elderly patients when the presenting symptom is a sudden loss of vision and there is either an absence of other signs and symptoms or only vague indications of the underlying arteritis. Cullen (1967) considers the occult form to be a common cause of blindness in the elderly and considers that the occult form of cranial arteritis occurs more frequently than the well-recognized classic presentation. It follows that recent central retinal artery occlusion in the elderly should be a considered to be a signal of the possibility that the underlying disease could be cranial arteritis even when there are no other symptoms of this disease.

The diagnosis of cranial arteritis is confirmed by the finding of a raised ESR and a biopsy of the temporal artery that demonstrates the presence of giant cells, histocytes, lymphocytes, and other evidence of vascular inflammation. A raised ESR may occur in many conditions other than arteritis, and an artery biopsy may be negative because of the patchy nature of the arterial inflammation in some cases (Eshaghian, 1979). Treatment relies on the use of 60 to 90 mg of prednisone daily, and a tapering of this dose after several weeks (Field and Lemak, 1976). Treatment should be continued for several months. Unfortunately, blindness from arterial occlusion may occur in spite of this treatment and may be in the contralateral eye rather than in the eye that apparently is involved clinically (Merck Manual, 1982). Bilateral blindness is not uncommon in patients having cranial arteritis.

ENDOCRINE DISEASE
Diabetes Mellitus

Rather than a specific disease, diabetes mellitus is a complex syndrome of biochemical anomalies caused by a deficient production of biologically active insulin or a resistance of its action at the receptor sites on cell membranes. Whereas the signs and symptoms of this disease are protean and encompass a great many aspect of medicine, the predominant clinical feature is hyperglycemia. In addition to its role in the metabolism of glucose, insulin also is essential for amino acid and lipid uptake, storage, and later release for use. Insulin is also a messenger involved in the function of other endocrine systems. The spectrum of the diabetes syndrome as determined by these metabolic dysfunctions ranges from clearly normal to levels incompatible with life. Between these two extremes lies an area in which a precise diagnosis is not possible. Blood glucose levels either during fasting, after meals, or following challenge by large doses of sugar are used by the clinician in diagnosing diabetes. The presence of other abnormal signs or symptoms makes this judgment more reliable in the event that blood assays are within

Table 2.4 Diagnostic levels of capillary blood glucose (millimoles per liter)

Diagnosis	Fasting Level	Random Blood Glucose Test Level (Postabsorptive)	2-hour Blood Glucose Level Following 75 g Oral Glucose
Normal	—	<6	<6
Equivocal	—	6–10*	—
Impaired glucose tolerance	—	—	6–12+
Diabetic	≥ 8	>11	>12

*Requires 2-hour blood glucose screening test.

+ Requires standard glucose tolerance test.

the equivocal range. Table 2.4 shows the generally accepted values of blood glucose for the clinical diagnosis of diabetes (Keen, 1981).

Diabetes is now classified as insulin-dependent diabetes mellitus (IDDM) or non-insulin dependent diabetes mellitus (NIDDM); this replaces the previous classification of juvenile or mature age onset diabetes (National Diabetes Data Group, 1979). Table 2.5 shows the further subclassification of diabetes. There are shortcomings to this classification because the underlying cause has not yet been elucidated, and individual cases may change in status between and within the two major classifications during the natural course of the disease.

Diabetes is clearly an inheritable disease (Urrets-Zavalia, 1977); concordance for diabetes in identical twins approaches 100% for NIDDM acquired in later life; however, for IDDM acquired in early life, the concordance is somewhat less. Subjects at special risk are those having two parents with diabetes, those with

Table 2.5 Classification of diabetes mellitus

1. Insulin-Dependent Diabetes Mellitus (IDDM)

2. Noninsulin-dependent Diabetes Mellitus (NIDDM)
   Nonobese
   Obese
   Secondary NIDDM
     Pancreatic disease
     Hormonal disorders
     Drug induced
     Insulin receptor abnormalities
     Genetic syndromes
     Miscellaneous

3. Impaired glucose tolerance
   Nonobese
   Obese
   Drug or disease induced

Source: Adapted with permission from H. Keen, "The Nature of the Diabetic Syndrome." *Int. Med.* 8 (1981): 328.

a diabetic family history, or those who are the identical twin of a diabetic. Whereas the propensity for diabetes appears to be inherited, it frequently is precipitated through over-nutrition; 90% of NIDDM patients are overweight at the time of diagnosis (Merck Manual, 1982).

The true prevalence of diabetes mellitus is difficult to establish because of the lack of universally accepted diagnostic criteria, the differing susceptibility of racial groups, and the variations in the age of the samples surveyed for the disease. Reports of the prevalence of the disease among Caucasian samples vary from 1.5% through 6% (Cahill, 1975; Fisher and Vavra, 1969; Foster, 1980) although they are much higher in Pima Indian (McDonald, 1970), Nauraun (Guthrie et al., 1977), and Australian Aborigine (Bastian, 1979) populations. A survey conducted in two Australian provincial cities provided figures of the prevalence of diabetes of 2.2% and 1.08%, respectively. The patients of optometrists are probably a relatively fair sample of the overall population and a series of 3,798 consecutive patients yielded a prevalence of 2.6% diabetics (Cockburn, 1987). Increasing age brings a greater risk of diabetes, which rises from 2.4% for people aged 21 years and over, to 7% to 8% in those over 70 years of age (Welborne, 1991).

Because diabetes has a peak age of onset that coincides with the onset of presbyopia, optometrists have the opportunity to recognize this condition in its early stages. Indeed, in the study cited previously (Cockburn, 1987), seven of the 100 diabetics were previously undiagnosed. These seven patients ranged in age from 49 to 81 and had a mean age of 63 years.

The eye, brain, kidney, and lower limbs appear to be major targets for the pathologic changes of diabetes. Diabetes is the most important systemic disease leading to blindness, and the majority of diabetic blind patients are middle aged or elderly (Caird et al., 1969). Ocular involvement may occur in the early stages of diabetes; indeed, between 20% and 40% of diabetic patients had ocular involvement at the time of diagnosis of their disease (Caird et al., 1969). The high prevalence of diabetes in an aging population, together with frequent and early ocular involvement, justifies the inclusion in the eye examination of a specific search for the signs and symptoms of diabetes.

History Taking
History taking provides a useful guide to the presence of diabetes. All patients should be questioned routinely for a family history of diabetes; when the answer is positive, they should be questioned further to find evidence of other relevant symptoms. The early diabetic may have an increased fluid intake (polydipsia) and consequent increased micturition (polyuria). Younger patients especially have an increased appetite (polyphagia). In spite of the increased food intake, untreated diabetics may lose weight although they generally remain obese. Fluctuating vision and changes in refractive errors are fairly common in uncontrolled diabetics. The change in refraction is cyclical and but not necessarily in phase with blood glucose levels; as a general rule the change is toward increasing hyperopia in untreated diabetics, although myopic shift also is observed. The induced

hyperopia may remain for some weeks after normal blood glucose levels have been obtained (Pascoe and Vaughan, 1982).

The optometric history taking should include an investigation of the patient's current medication, since glucose tolerance may be reduced significantly by the action of a large number of therapeutic substances. These drugs include many of the commonly prescribed diuretics; mood-altering drugs; hormones (particularly the glucocorticoids); indomethacin (which is used for the treatment of osteoarthritis); and neurologically active drugs, including levodopa, which is used to treat Parkinson's disease (Treleaven, 1982). Even niacin, a vitamin complex frequently prescribed for psychopathologic conditions, is implicated in the impairment of glucose tolerance (Duke-Elder, 1971). Elderly patients are particularly at risk for iatrogenic precipitation of diabetes because of their lowered tolerance to toxicity and the common use of these classes of drugs in the aged population.

Although it is not a common manifestation of diabetes, a form of neuropathy may involve the nerves serving the extraocular muscles and the iris. Complaints by elderly patients of difficulties related to binocular vision, especially frank diplopia, should initiate a search for diabetes. The neuropathy involving the extraocular muscles usually resolves spontaneously after about 12 weeks.

Cataracts

Cataracts occur in a high proportion of elderly, non-diabetic patients, making this a poorly sensitive sign of diabetes. However, diabetes appears to accelerate the progression of cataracts so that they appear at an earlier age than usual or are more advanced for the patient's age than would be expected. The acute onset of snowflake opacities that characterize the true form of diabetic cataract occurs only in diabetics under 30 or 40 years of age and is usually reversible when the blood glucose level is brought under control. An increase in the density of the lens nucleus is the cause of the refractive shift mentioned earlier. Although these myopic changes occur in many elderly, non-diabetic patients, a special search for diabetics is warranted when the change is noted.

Duke-Elder (1969b) cites a number of studies that demonstrate that asteroid bodies frequently are associated with abnormal glucose tolerance or frank diabetes. In spite of the continuing controversy regarding this association (Topilow et al., 1982), asteroid bodies are sufficiently unusual to make reasonable special efforts to seek other signs of diabetes in patients having this sign.

The retinal vasculature is commonly, if not invariably, involved in diabetic angiopathy. These changes occur predominantly in the small vessels of the retina and involve loss of the nuclei of the intramural pericytes, which interferes with the normal structural properties of the capillaries (Cogan and Kuwabara, 1963). At the same time, the basement membrane of capillaries becomes thickened, the lumen narrows, and occlusions of these small vessels becomes common (Scheie and Albert, 1977). These processes lead to a relative breakdown of the blood-retinal barrier and retinal ischemia culminating in the characteristic fundus lesions of diabetic retinopathy. Similar vascular changes have been noted in the choroid of diabetics (Saracco et al., 1982).

Diabetic Retinopathy

Diabetic retinopathy generally is classified as pre-retinopathy, simple or background retinopathy, and proliferative retinopathy. However, it might prove useful for clinical purposes to include a transitional stage between simple and proliferative retinopathy, which would include retinas that possess the hallmark of the transition from the simple to the proliferative stage since the treatment of proliferative retinopathy is most successful if applied at an early stage of this complication (Hercules et al., 1977). It could be argued that the transitional phase of retinopathy represents the most important clinical diagnosis and warrants separate and special emphasis. Table 2.6 summarizes the clinical signs associated with the various forms of diabetic retinopathy and includes notes regarding their treatment.

The onset of diabetic retinopathy is closely related to the duration of the diabetes (West et al., 1980) and tends to occur after a shorter duration in the elderly than in younger patients. It is common after 10 years and almost universally present after 20 years' duration. Its incidence does not appear to be related to the severity of the diabetes (Newell, 1982) or the method of blood glucose control. In many cases, retinopathy occurs and continues to progress in spite of good blood glucose control. However, there is a strong clinical impression that good early control of blood glucose levels delays or reduces the extent of retinal dam-

Table 2.6 Classification of diabetic retinopathy based on clinical data and showing appropriate treatment

Diabetic Complication	Description (In Most Common Sequential Order)	Treatment
Pre-retinopathy	Dilated tortuous veins, venous loop formation	None
Simple (background) retinopathy	Retinal microaneurysms, dot and blot hemorrhages	None
	Yellow, hard exudates near avascular zone, macular edema and retinal thickening	Grid pattern laser photocoagulation
Transition stage	Exacerbation of above signs plus venous beading and cotton wool patches	Pan retinal photocoagulation
Proliferative retinopathy	New vessels on the disc and elsewhere, pre-retinal hemorrhages	Pan retinal photocoagulation
	New vessels on iris or in anterior chamber angle, neovascular glaucoma	Pan retinal photocoagulation, glaucoma medication
	New vessels in vitreous, fibrinous vitreous strands, retinal detachment	Vitrectomy, detachment surgery

age (Kohner et al., 1969). The Steno Study Group (1982) reported that continuous infusion of insulin had considerable value in the control and prevention of diabetic retinopathy. However, this question of the effect of control cannot be considered to be settled, since Lawson et al. (1982), in a similar study, found that in spite of good blood glucose control, the treatment did not provide protection against, or reduce the effect of, diabetic retinopathy. Unfortunately, for approximately one-third of diabetics, ocular involvement occurs, with the aged diabetic being affected after a shorter duration of the disease than are younger patients. However, this statement should be put into perspective for diabetics as a whole, since, in spite of this involvement, the majority of diabetics do not have significant loss of vision when compared with age-matched controls (Cockburn, 1987).

Pre-retinopathy

Pre-retinopathy is difficult to identify, because the definitive signs of dilated veins and tortuosity are common in normal subjects and in eyes of patients having other vascular diseases. It is probably safe to make this diagnosis only for a confirmed diabetic or for a patient for whom there is a fundus photographic record that establishes a change in the form of retinal vessels.

Simple Retinopathy

Simple retinopathy occurs in approximately 26% of diabetic seen in optometric practice (Cockburn, 1987) and is heralded by the appearance of microaneurysms (Chuna-Vaz, 1978), preferentially in the area outside the capillary-free macular zone and extending for about 10 degrees from the posterior pole. The microaneurysms may appear in clusters or as isolated, dense, dark-red spots, which are easily overlooked unless specifically sought. Later, dot and blot hemor-

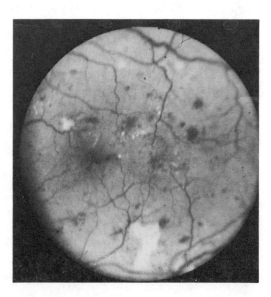

Figure 2.8. Advanced simple diabetic retinopathy featuring microaneurysms, multiple dot and blot hemorrhages, exudates, and cotton wool patches.

rhages and hard, yellow, diabetic exudates appear (Figure 2.8). Retinal hemorrhages are confined by the orientation of the tissues into which the blood seeps; in the outer plexiform layer, this pools the blood into vertical columns, which then appear as dark-red, discrete dots (dot hemorrhages). The loosely packed and predominantly horizontally coursing fibers in the nuclear layers allow the blood to spread irregularly and form thin sheets (blot hemorrhages), which are lighter in color. Leakage of lipid-rich serum may occur in some eyes as a result of damage to the retinal vessels. The intra-retinal escape of serous fluid causes micro-cystic macular edema with retinal thickening, which is a common cause of visual loss in diabetics. Hard, yellow, diabetic exudates form in the macula, particularly near the fovea from which they tend to migrate outward to lie as a rough annulus typically about 10 degrees from the fovea. Hard exudates near the foveal avascular zone pose a serious threat to vision and should be treated by grid photocoagulation of the surrounding macula.

Although diabetes appears to affect the deep capillary layers preferentially, signs of retinal nerve fiber layer involvement in the form of flame hemorrhages and cotton wool patches are not unusual. These, along with exacerbation of the size and number of deep retinal hemorrhages and microaneurysms, may herald the onset of the proliferative stage of retinopathy.

Proliferative Retinopathy

The prevalence of proliferative diabetic retinopathy in a diabetic sample varies according to the nature of the sample; it rarely occurs in less than 15 years' duration of the diabetic condition when the disease is acquired in childhood or adolescence. Thereafter, it becomes more common, and in older diabetics, the interval between the diagnosis of diabetes and the onset of retinopathy is shorter, with proliferative retinopathy developing in a smaller proportion of patients but after a shorter duration than in younger diabetics. Type 1 diabetes is more likely to lead to proliferative retinopathy than type 2 diabetes (Bodansky et al., 1982) but is by no means restricted to this form of the disease. Reports of the prevalence of proliferative retinopathy in studies carried out in specialist retinal clinics or dedicated diabetic centers can be distorted by the tendency of diabetics with serious visual problems to be overrepresented through self-selection and referral of difficult cases to these institutions. A more reliable figure for the prevalence of proliferative retinopathy can be obtained from studies that seek this complication in an overall population. In a rural population in Canada, Collaritis et al. (1984) found that 1.8% of 624 diabetics had proliferative retinopathy and Mitchell (1980) found 36 (2.8%) in 1,309 diabetics in the Hunter River region of Australia. Patients attending an optometrist are likely to under-represent serious or late diabetic eye disease but more closely mirror the overall diabetic population than those attending ophthalmologic centers. An Australian optometrical sample of 100 diabetics contained two patients having proliferative retinopathy (Cockburn, 1987).

The development of new blood vessels marks the transformation to proliferative diabetic retinopathy and may commence as new vessels on the disc and within a disc diameter of the disc (NVD), or in any portion of the retina, including the periphery when it is termed new vessels elsewhere (NVE) (Figure 2.9). It is believed that a vasogenic factor, which so far has not been identified, is produced in response to retinal ischemia; this originally is brought about by closure of large areas of the retinal capillary bed. These areas of retinal capillary non-perfusion can be seen in fluorescein angiograms as dark patches (hypofluorescence) that replace the usual mottled fluorescence of the normally perfused retina (Figure 2.10).

Newly formed vessels in proliferative diabetic retinopathy are immature and readily break down to cause serum extravascation, pre-retinal hemorrhages (Figure 2.11) and vitreal hemorrhages if the blood has penetrated the vitreous. Any growth of new vessels into the vitreous is accompanied by a fibrous matrix, which after resolution of the vessels, may remain dense strands (Figure 2.12). Contraction of these strands causes retinal detachment and further extensive retinal and vitreal hemorrhages in the later stage of proliferative retinopathy.

The stimulus for neovascularization may affect the iris, beginning with the pupillary margin and spreading radially to invade the anterior chamber angle. Unlike normal iris vessels that have a fibrous coat that makes them difficult to see, these new channels lie on the surface of the iris and are bright red. The vessels in the angle develop on a fibrovascular membrane similar to that which appears in association with vitreal neovascularization. This membrane may occlude the trabecular spaces, denying access of aqueous humour to the canal of Schlemm and causing a steep rise in intraocular pressure. The form of secondary glaucoma is particularly difficult to treat, but it may respond to panretinal photocoagulation, which reduces the vasoproliferative stimulus produced by the anoxic retina. As a

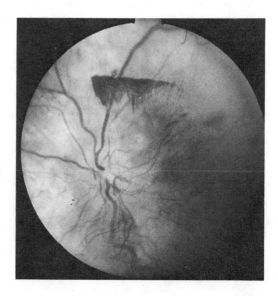

Figure 2.9. Early proliferative diabetic retinopathy in a 32-year-old woman. Numerous new vessels arise from the optic disc, and a preretinal hemorrhage lies superior to the disc.

A

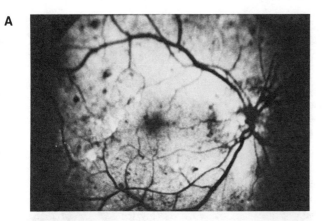

B

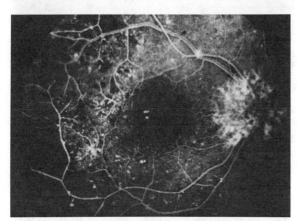

Figure 2.10 A and B. Red free photograph of an eye having proliferative diabetic retinopathy and showing proliferation of blood vessels at the optic disc (A). (B) is a fluorescein angiogram of the same eye showing hyperfluoresence surrounding the new vessels and dark areas representing capillary nonperfusion particularly in the temporal fundus.

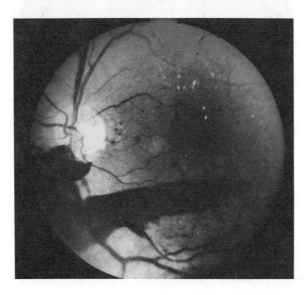

Figure 2.11. Large preretinal hemorrhage in the same patient as illustrated in Figure 2.9 as seen 12 months later. Note that the hemorrhages overlie all retinal features.

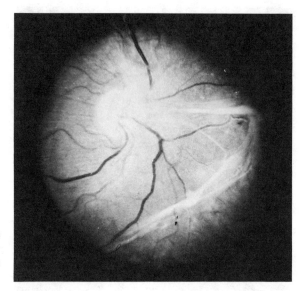

Figure 2.12. Fibrous vitreous strands in an eye with partly resolved proliferative diabetic retinopathy.

temporary relief, direct goniophotocoagulation of the vessels as they cross the scleral spur may be effective or pancryotherapy applied (Wand, 1982).

It is fortunate that the proliferative form of diabetic retinopathy occurs only in a relatively small proportion of the overall diabetic population. It is chiefly confined to IDDM patients in whom the disease becomes manifest before age 40 and then after many years of its duration. The majority of older diabetic patients (approximately two-thirds of all diabetics) have the NIDDM form of the disease, and it is not common for elderly subjects to develop this added complication; their visual loss, if any, is more commonly due to macular edema.

Treatment

Elderly NIDDM patients are treated with oral hypoglycemic drugs, which include sulfonylurea, biguanides, and sulfapyrimidine derivatives. Apart from occasional gastrointestinal side effects, these drugs are well tolerated and do not appear to cause ocular side effects.

Optometric Management of the Diabetic Suspect

Although there is at present no effective treatment for simple retinopathy, the physician in charge of overall management of the patient should be informed of the ocular status and be assured of cooperation should retinopathy progress to the proliferative stage or the onset of retinal edema or exudates threatening the fovea. During the course of background diabetic retinopathy, the patient should be reviewed at not less than 12 monthly intervals. Patients should be referred to a retinal specialist if they develop retinal thickening, microcystic edema, or hard exudates on or close to the foveal avascular zone. These complications are treated by application of a pattern grid laser photocoagulation, which appears to stimulate the retinal pigment epithelium to reduce edema and remove the exudates. At the first indication of the transition stage, or the appearance of frank proliferation, the patient should be referred to an ophthalmologist for consideration of treatment by panretinal photocoagulation designed to reduce retinal oxygen demand.

Arguably, the most important role for the optometrist is the early detection of previously undiagnosed diabetes at a stage before it causes brain, kidney, or eye damage or an acceleration of atherosclerosis with its consequences for stroke and coronary disease. Vigilance in the history taking and ophthalmoscopy may be complemented by the use of blood glucose estimates. Instruments for this purpose are readily available, simple to use, and provide valid and reliable estimates. However, whenever any doubt remains, the patient should be referred for a standard glucose tolerance test. Figure 2.13 is an algorithm intended as a guide to the extended investigation of the person suspected of having diabetes and using blood glucose analysis as a diagnostic criterion.

Hyperthyroidism (Thyrotoxicosis, Toxic Goiter, Basedow's Disease)

Thyroid hormones control the metabolism of oxygen and the synthesis of proteins; as a consequence, they regulate the metabolic activity in most of the body's tissues. This system is influenced and controlled by the pituitary gland through the production of thyroid-stimulating hormone (TSH), which, in turn, is subject to modulation according to the level of circulating hormones. Other organ systems, notably the liver, are involved in this regulatory system, the nature of which is not yet fully understood. Considering the complexity of the system, it is hardly surprising that the cause of many of the thyroid abnormalities is not yet clear. In clinical terms, thyroid disease is classified as hyperthyroidism or hypothyroidism (myxedema) and a number of less common varieties such as Hashimoto's thyroiditis, virus-induced granulomatous thyroiditis, tumors of the thyroid, and euthyroid goiter in which there is painless and symptomless enlargement of the thyroid gland despite normal concentrations of thyroid hormones. The ocular signs of interest to the optometric clinician may occur in either hyperthyroidism or, less commonly, in hypothyroidism and in the euthyroid state. The term Graves' disease is appropriate when ophthalmic symptoms occur in any form of thyroid disease (Duke-Elder, 1976). Table 2.7 lists both the ocular and general signs and symptoms of Graves' disease.

The peak age of onset of thyroid disease is 30 years to 50 years. The disease has an incidence of 3 per 10,000 adults per year, and a female-to-male ratio of 5 to 1 (De Groot, 1975). However, some 15% of patients having hyperthyroidism are aged 65 or older (Merck Manual, 1982); in this age group, the classic signs may be confined to a single organ system to produce a confusing clinical picture referred to as occult or masked thyrotoxicosis. The diagnosis is easily missed,

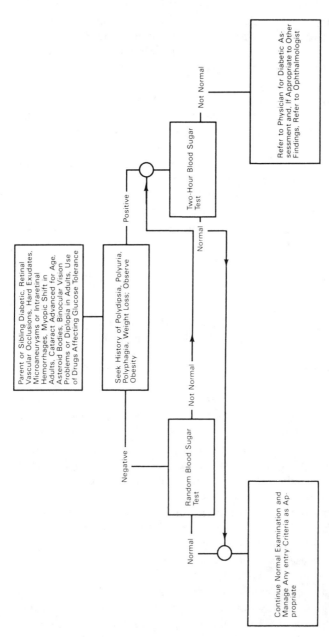

Figure 2.13. Algorithm showing suggested management of ophthalmic patients having risk factors for diabetes.

Table 2.7 Ocular and general signs and symptoms of hyperthyroidism (Graves' disease), with the special diagnostic indicators of the occult form found in aged patients

Ocular Signs	General Signs	Occult Form Signs
Lid retraction and staring gaze	Weakness, fatigue, weight loss, breathlessness on exertion	Muscle weakness
Lid lag on downward gaze		Depression
Proptosis	Insomnia	Inactivity
Reduced blink rate	Hyperactivity	Apathy
Lid edema	Tremor	Mental confusion, senile-dementia-like state
Bulbar and conjunctival swelling or hyperemia	Excessive perspiration, moist fine skin	
Tearing or burning sensation	Thinning hair, brittle nails	Low-grade fever
	Heat intolerance, cold tolerance	Wizened, wrinkled appearance
Exposure keratitis, corneal ulceration	Swelling of thyroid gland	Weight loss
Weakness of convergence	Heart palpitations, systolic murmur	Congestive heart failure
Diplopia, phoria, or ophthalmoplegia	Tachycardia, arterial fibrillation	Arrhythmias, atrial fibrillation
Retrobulbar pain	Abdominal pain, loose bowel motions, pruritus	Constipation
Reduced visual acuity		Liver enlargement
Retrobulbar neuritis (central and arcuate)	Absence or irregularity of menstrual periods	Bone pain
Visual field defects	Anxiety, restlessness	
Papilledema	Absence of forehead wrinkling on upward gaze	
Secondary glaucoma		

especially when there are no signs of thyroid enlargement; therefore, the presence of any ocular signs in Table 2.7 should raise the issue of thyroid disease in the differential diagnosis. Other signs that may support a diagnosis of occult thyrotoxicosis are tachycardia (which should be detected during carotid auscultation) and a aged patient who is wrinkled, apathetic, lethargic, and apparently prematurely senile. These and other signs and symptoms more common in the aged thyrotoxic patient are shown separately in Table 2.7. Note that in the aged subject, inactivity rather than hyperactivity is common.

In the more common form of presentation of hyperthyroidism, the variety and combinations of symptoms and signs bear no relationship to the metabolic state (Sachdev et al., 1979) and may precede, occur in conjunction with, or only become manifest, after remission of the hormonal disturbance. Furthermore, the ocular signs may recede or progress in spite of treatment that normalizes the thyroid hormonal balance (Bouzas, 1980). The rare, but important, complication of optic neuropathy should be considered when visual field losses are discovered. These defects may be central scotomas or nerve fiber bundle defects (Henderson, 1958). The increased bulk of retrobulbar tissue that gives rise to the proptosis so common in thyrotoxicosis also may restrict the episcleral vessels, which, in turn, compromises aqueous outflow. The resulting increase in intraocular pressure may be sufficient to lead to secondary glaucoma (Stone, 1982). Temporary and less serious increases in intraocular pressure tend to occur when the patient attempts eye movements against the restrictions imposed by extraocular muscle hypertrophy and orbital adhesions. The optometric review of these patients should include a search for signs of optic nerve compression. When the disease presents in a classic form, diagnosis may be simple. However, it should be confirmed by the physician after laboratory testing; this is particularly important in the aged patient having atypical signs or the occult form of hyperthyroidism.

Propranolol is effective in controlling tachycardia, tremor, and psychiatric symptoms. However, it must be used with caution in patients having a tendency to congestive heart failure. Otherwise, treatment involves the use of radioactive iodine and other thyroid suppressants (Merck Manual, 1982). Support treatment by the optometrist may be directed toward correcting any ocular muscle defects, using prisms where appropriate, and providing methylcellulose drops for any dry eye problem that is caused by exposure during proptosis. Drying of the cornea may occur during sleep from a failure of lid closure. The patient may benefit from the use of a shield similar to a Buller's shield, which fits closely over the eye to maintain high humidity and prevent corneal dehydration. Less severe cases can be treated by application of methylcellulose ointment at night and drops by day.

NEUROLOGIC DISEASE
Parkinson's Disease (Paralysis Agitans)

Parkinson's disease is a term that embraces a group of neurologic disorders involving degeneration of the region of the brain stem, particularly the substantia nigra (Escourolle and Poirer, 1978). It is said to have a prevalence of 1,000,0000 cases in the United States, with an additional 50,000 new cases each year. The disease has an insidious onset in later years, usually becoming manifest between the ages of 50 and 65 (Yahr, 1975). The mean age of onset of Parkinson's disease is between 58 and 62 years but with an increasing incidence in the aged population, particularly in those aged over 70 years, when it is present in approximately 1.5% (Selby, 1991).

Disease that occurs at the extrapyramidal level involves the complex of nerve fibers and nuclear masses that runs from the motor cortex to the brain stem from which motor fibers then descend the spinal cord to control muscle activity. Lesions at the extrapyramidal level cause a delay in the initiation of, and poverty of, movement, together with a large-amplitude tremor and repetitive involuntary movements (MacLeod, 1979). It generally is held that lesions of the extrapyramidal pathways interfere with involuntary and stereotyped movements without being directly involved with voluntary movements (Barr, 1979).

The clinical picture of Parkinsonism is unmistakable. An early and obvious sign involves a coarse, repetitive movement of the thumb across the tips of the fingers in a "pill rolling" movement that ceases when the patient attempts a voluntary movement involving the hands. The resting tremor of Parkinson's disease, which resolves on attempted movement, helps differentiate this condition from that of essential tremor (senile, familial, or juvenile tremor) in which there is typically little or no tremor at rest, but the tremor commences or worsens on initiation of movement (Morris, 1991). The patient's face tends to be expressionless, with the facial muscles smoothed out and almost immobile. Speech is slow and monotonous, yet occasionally interspersed with a very rapid series of words, the whole delivered at such a low level that it may be impossible to hear. The blink rate is much reduced, yet the glabellar tapping blink reflex is exaggerated. In the normal patient, repetitive tapping over the bridge of the nose results in the patient blinking synchronously for the first five or six taps and then reverting to the normal blink pattern. The Parkinsonian patient will continue to blink synchronously for as long as the tapping is continued.

The gait of patients who have Parkinson's disease is characteristic: they tend to lean forward and almost fall from one short, shuffling step to the next while their hands are held flexed and at their sides. There is a pronounced slowness of all voluntary movements and, frequently a muscular rigidity in passive movements that results in a series of jerks as a limb is moved (cogwheel rigidity). The patients also tend to be unable to continue or initiate a movement; this may be quite striking when they attempt to walk but then find that they are unable to move their feet for some time.

The tremor characteristic of Parkinson's disease has a rate of between four and eight cycles per second; it is most severe at rest and when the patient is fatigued but will diminish with voluntary movement and disappear when the patient is sleeping (Merck Manual, 1982). It may affect the mouth or tongue with resulting rhythmic sucking, whistling, or lip movements. The patient's handwriting may deteriorate, causing previously flowing writing to become spidery, diminished in size, and wandering from straight lines.

In addition to alteration of the blink reflex, other ocular signs are common in Parkinson's disease. A form of facial spasm affects some patients. The lids are clamped tightly together, and other facial muscles develop irregular jerks without order or rhythm; this performance is repeated at regular intervals interspersed with periods of repose. The optometric examination of these patients can be most frustrating; however, a show of impatience by the clinician will only worsen the problem.

Frequently, a paresis of the upper lids causes them to remain fixed when the patient looks downward. When the lower lids are affected also, the eyes adopt the staring appearance of the typical Parkinsonian faces. By way of contrast, in some patients, ptosis may result from rigidity of the levator muscle (Treleaven, 1982).

Ocular movements may become involved in the disease so that eye movements become slow and irregular, with a slowing of saccades and deficiency of convergence. Patients having Parkinson's disease frequently have difficulty turning their eyes upward; this may be noted when the optometrist attempts to instill eye drops. Eventually, myostatic paralysis may cause the eyes to assume a locked position in which any attempt at voluntary movement gives rise to ineffective cogwheel movements (Duke-Elder, 1973).

Medical Treatment and Prognosis

Levodopa, the metabolic precursor of dopamine, relieves the symptoms of Parkinson's disease, presumably through replenishment of dopamine, which is deficient in the corpus striatum of patients having the disease. Carbidopa inhibits the breakdown of levodopa in extracerebral tissues, thus making more levodopa available to the brain. Treatment consists of using levodopa alone or in combination with carbidopa titrated to achieve satisfactory control of symptoms. The dosage may be reduced in geriatric patients with liver or kidney disease, since these organs are responsible for the breakdown and excretion of dopamine. Because dopamine, in turn, is the precursor of epinephrine and norepinephrine, this drug tends to dilate the pupils and may precipitate angle closure glaucoma in susceptible patients, especially when used in combination with monoamine oxidase inhibitors (Mandelkorn and Zimmerman, 1982). Management of patients with Parkinson's disease is very complex and should be under the direction of a competent physician who may elect to withhold treatment in the early stages because the effect of the drugs appears to diminish with long-term use and side effects can be serious.

The Parkinson Study Group (1989) has reported the results of a placebo-controlled, 12-month trial of deprenyl (Selegine; FDA Investigational New Drug 28,477; Hoffmann-LaRoche USA) in the early treatment of Parkinson's disease. There was a marked symptomatic improvement in these mildly affected patients using the drug, with less risk of having to cease employment than in the control group. The effect appeared to continue for at least one month after discontinuing treatment, but it is still unclear whether the drug counters the long-term effect of the disease process.

Optometric management is largely supportive but requires initiative in meeting the special needs of these patients. Bifocal segments may be placed much higher than is usual to allow effective use of the reading segment, since a forward head tilt usually is adopted by the patient. A stand on which reading material can be rested will relieve the problem of shaking from tremor of the upper limbs. Fixed-focus stand magnifiers also should be considered for people with low vision. Binocular vision problems may be alleviated initially by the use of prisms, but monocular occlusion is probably a better solution in advanced cases. Ocular lubricants will provide relief from the discomfort of dry eyes resulting from the paucity of blinking.

Levodopa may produce side effects including sleep disturbance, increased libido, nausea, and reduced appetite. Anticholinergic drugs on the other hand cause dryness of the mouth, reduction in accommodation, memory impairment, hallucinations, difficulty in commencing micturition, and constipation. The examination should include gonioscopy to identify anterior chamber angles at risk of occlusion because of drug treatment. Patients having very narrow angles should be referred for laser iridotomy to prevent this occurrence.

PSYCHIATRIC ILLNESS

Psychopathology is the study of the abnormal function of personality (abnormal in that the expression is an exaggeration of characteristics present in the normal personality). It follows that the clinical appearance of psychiatric illness is a continuum from that which would be regarded as a clearly normal personality to frank psychotic behavior in which all contact with reality has been lost. Optometrists occasionally are consulted by patients having psychiatric illness in early or moderately advanced form; however, the visual problems of these people generally differ little from those of other patients. Patients having psychiatric disorders may have functional visual defects in the form of lowered visual acuity or visual field defects. These symptoms are unresponsive to spectacle or placebo treatment and persist for lengthy periods (Kathol et al., 1983). Because the possibility of an unrecognized underlying organic disorder always exists, it is important that these patients receive a complete ophthalmic assessment.

Patients of optometrists tend to include a high proportion of elderly people because some degree of failing sight is almost universal in the aged. Advanced age brings not only failing sight, but also increasing forgetfulness, lethargy, and an inability to adjust to change. These characteristics are largely accepted as a natural and inevitable part of aging; however, at some point that is almost impossible to define, these and other behavioral characteristics decline to the point where the patient is said to suffer dementia. Although there are no ocular changes specific to the condition, and indeed there are simply no physical clinical markers whatsoever, the optometrist needs to recognize dementia to successfully manage these patients' visual problems.

Senile Dementia and Alzheimer's Disease

Dementia is a state in which there is a reduction of intellectual ability from a previous stable level. In the early stages, it manifests itself as defective self-criticism or capacity to make fine discriminations involving moral and social issues and as a lessening of the ability to use abstract concepts or to learn new procedures. Short-term memory loss is an early and obvious feature of dementia. In the aged, these initial changes may be quite subtle and the progress of the condition so gradual that the individual and the family adapt to the changes without difficulty. The majority of patients finally die from an unrelated cause without serious behavioral problems having arisen. However, approximately 6% of people aged 65 years or older suffer from advanced dementia and require constant supervision or institutional care.

The clinical course of Alzheimer's disease and senile dementia differ only in that the disease process occurs at an earlier age in Alzheimer's disease and usually progresses more rapidly. Differentiation is only possible at autopsy, when Alzheimer's disease is characterized by extensive plaque development within cortical tissue and intracellular neurofibrillar tangles. Areas 18 and 20 of the cortex are concerned with higher-order visual processing and are grossly affected by these plaques and tangles, while the primary visual cortex (area 17) is only mildly affected. In some patients, this allows retention of the ability to recognize single letters but may inhibit the process of making sense of what is being read. In Alzheimer's disease, the patient may still be able to write but be unable to read (alexia without agraphia), probably as a result of selective damage to higher-order processes. These cortical changes also cause visual agnosia and homonymous visual field neglect (Cogan, 1985).

Because of the similarity in the clinical presentation and course of senile dementia and Alzheimer's disease, the two conditions will be considered together. The course of dementia may be interrupted by a sudden exacerbation following an increase in emotional or physical stress. Usually, this additional life stress is caused by bereavement, the onset of physical disease, trauma, ingestion of medication having CNS effects, or drastic changes in living patterns.

With worsening of the dementia, there may be serious lack of initiative, apathy, depression, a deterioration of personal hygiene, and a worsening memory problem. Abstract concepts become more difficult to grasp; verbal communication tends to be introspective and repetitive, and often fails to reach the intended conclusion because the subject loses the thread of the original thought. Emotional instability may be manifest as fits of anger or euphoria, sometimes inappropriate or paradoxical, although apathy and depression are most common. The patient may fail to answer questions or answer only after several repetitions of the question, after which the reply may be inappropriate as the result of the patient's diminished capacity for judgment and expression.

As dementia progresses, the patient's previous character traits tend to become exaggerated. For example, an exacerbation of previous obsessive states of hyperchondriasis could lead the patient into a miserable existence, which, in turn, could accelerate the dementia through added emotional stress and the use of drugs intended to manage the obsessive symptoms. Advanced dementia imposes nearly intolerable burdens upon family, friends, and health-care practitioners. However, the reactions of people close to the patient are crucial to the containment of dementia; kindness, understanding, and gentle persuasion reduce the rate of deterioration, whereas the opposite occurs when the subject is abandoned by family and friends.

Obviously, the patient with dementia will cause special problems for the optometrist. During the ocular examination, the patient is in an unfamiliar place surrounded by complex equipment and is subjected to a history taking that taxes the patient's defective memory for details that cannot be recalled. The patient is required to maintain a fixed posture and attention while unfamiliar procedures are performed. During the subjective refraction, the patient is expected to remember and follow complex sequential instructions and to make many fine discriminatory judgments in rapid succession. These requirements are all severely limited by the disease process so it is hardly surprising that patients having even a minor degree of dementia retreat into an apathetic state and either fail to provide answers or provide quite unreliable responses to the questions directed to them during subjective refraction.

When examining an elderly patient having dementia, the optometrist should adapt the investigation to the intellectual capacity of the subject. History taking can be made to appear a relatively casual series of questions asked intermittently during the course of the examination rather than a rapid-fire preliminary to the physical examination. The information being sought should be relevant to the patient's special circumstances; it need not necessarily explore for conditions usually found in younger subjects nor search for hereditary ocular disease that would have become manifest many years earlier.

During the physical examination, the patient may have difficulty maintaining concentration or keeping the eyes in a fixed position. Elderly patients tend to slump during subjective refraction, and if they are placed behind a phoropter, they frequently begin to look through the extreme lower edge of the lens or even slip into a position where they cannot see through the lens aperture at all. The use of a trial frame during both retinoscopy and the subjective refraction reduces this problem and also allows large changes of lens power to be introduced in a single step and with greater speed.

The patient having dementia may be dissatisfied in spite of appearing to have reasonable vision with glasses. Reading requires a high level of intellectual capacity and concentration, which the patient may lack because of the changes that occur with dementia. To the patient and the immediate family, it seems most likely that a reading difficulty is caused by poor vision; they can be disappointed when new spectacles do not allow easy reading. The optometrist should be sure there is an appreciable benefit from changes made to spectacles and that the use of any special devices is within the capacity of the patient.

Although at present there is no effective drug treatment for dementia, the optometrist should insure that these patients are under medical care, since almost identical changes can be caused by subdural hemorrhage, alcohol abuse, lead and carbon monoxide poisoning, and inappropriate drug therapy. A clinical picture similar to that seen in dementia is also found in Pick's disease, Creutzfeldt-Jacob disease, Parkinson's disease, and, occasionally, as a result of viral encephalitis. A step-like deterioration of intellect may accompany multiple infarcts of the brain caused by intermittent showers of small emboli. Early recognition and treatment of the underlying cause may prevent serious brain damage and death. Because dementia may be secondary to a treatable disease, patients not already under medical care should be referred for examination by a physician. Even in cases where no causative disease can be found, antidepressant drugs may be valuable and intercurrent medical problems managed to the overall benefit of the patient's life-style; hence, an improved prognosis may be possible for the dementia itself.

Although there are no physical markers for dementia, a test for this condition is detailed in Table 2.8. The entire test need not be administered to optometric patients, and useful information can be obtained by using the three-object, short-term registration and recall test; the sequential instruction test; and the

Table 2.8 Mini-mental state examination

ORIENTATION
What is:
  The year?
  Season?
  Date?
  Month?
  Score 1 for each correct answer.
Can you tell me what state of Australia we are in?
What city are we in?
What are two main streets nearby?
What is the address or name of this place?

REGISTRATION
Score 1 for each correct answer.
I am going to name three objects. After I have said them, I want you to repeat them. Remember what they are because I am going to ask you to name then again in a few minutes.
Please repeat these three objects to me.
  "Apple. . . Table. . . Coin"
  Score first attempt and repeat objects until all are learned.
  Score 1 for each correctly repeated word.

ATTENTION AND CALCULATION
Will you subtract 7 from 100 and then subtract 7 from the answer you get and keep on subtracting 7 until I tell you to stop?
  Record (93) . . . . (86) . . . . (79) . . . . (72) . . . . (65) . . . .
  Score 1 for each correct answer.

LANGUAGE
Now I am going to spell a word forward and then I want you to spell it backwards. The word is WORLD, W-O-R-L-D.
  Print letters _____
  Repeat if necessary, but not after spelling attempt starts.
  Score 1 for correct spelling.

RECALL
Now what were the three objects I asked you to remember?
  Apple
  Table
  Coin
  Score 1 for each item recalled.

LANGUAGE
Show wristwatch. What is this called?
  Score 1 for correct answer.
Show pencil. What is this called?
  Score 1 for correct answer.
I would like you to repeat a phrase after me. "No ifs, ands, or buts." Allow one attempt.
  Score 1 if all words repeated correctly.

Table 2.8 continued
ABILITY TO FOLLOW SEQUENTIAL INSTRUCTIONS
Read the words on this page and then do as it says. (Hand sheet reading "Close your eyes.")
   Score 1 if respondent closes eyes.
Read the following statement and then hand over a piece of paper. "I am going to give you a piece of paper. When I do, take the paper in your right hand, fold it in half using both hands, and put the paper on your lap."
   Takes in right hand.
   Folds paper.
   Puts paper in lap.
   Score 1 for each action correctly taken.

LANGUAGE AND WRITING
Now I would like you to write any complete sentence on this piece of paper. (Hand paper and pen to patient.) The sentence should have a subject and a verb and make sense. Ignore spelling and grammar errors.
   Score 1 if sentence is acceptable.

CONSTRUCTIONAL ABILITY
Here is a drawing. Please copy the drawing onto the paper. (Give subject the drawing below.) Score 1 if the two 5-sided figures intersect to form a 4-sided figure and if all angles in the 5-sided figure are preserved.

NOTE: This test procedure is not diagnostic of mental disorder. However, a score of 20 or less is likely to occur in dementia, delirium, schizophrenia, or affective disorders. Normally, elderly subjects or those having neuroses or personality disorders should achieve higher scores.

Modified from: Folstein, M., J.C. Anthony, I. Parhad, B. Duffy, E.M. Grunberg. "The Meaning of Cognitive Impairment in the Elderly." *J. Am. Geriatrics Soc.* 33 (1985): 228–235; and M.F. Folstein, S.E. Folstein, P.R. McHugh. "Mini Mental State." A Practical Method of Grading the Cognitive State of Patients for the Clinician. *J. Psychiat. Res.* 12 (1975): 189–198.

These tasks test a variety of mental functions under the headings shown. You will require four sheets of paper, an additional sheet of paper on which to record the results, and a pen or pencil. Read the instructions from the form, commencing with: "Now I would like to ask you some questions to check your memory. Most of them will be easy."

construction ability test. The results of these tests usually will provide sufficient insight to assess the patient's ability to respond adequately to a normal, subjective refraction.

Depression

Depression may occur as a result of some real and potent change in the subject's environment, the onset of serious illness, or the death of a friend or family member. Where the depression is within the range of accepted grieving or depressed mood, the term reactive depression is appropriate. On the other hand, some subjects become profoundly depressed although they are unable to give a reason for this mood (primary depression). The underlying cause of primary depression is unknown.

Approximately 20% of people suffer depression during their lifetime, and 10% of the population have depressive symptoms of sufficient severity and duration to make a diagnosis of depressive illness. The lifetime risk of being treated for depression is approximately 12% for men and 25% for women (Burrows, 1991), and there is a lifetime risk of developing a major manic depressive disorder of 3% to 4% for men and 5% to 9% for women (Goodwin and Jamison, 1984). The elderly are particularly at risk of primary depression, which is said to occur chronically in from 5% to 20% of people over the age of 60 years (Gurland, 1976). Depressed people are well recognized to be more likely to attempt suicide, but a less well-known fact is that depressed people are at almost twice the risk of death from all causes than are age-matched controls (Garfinkel and Persad, 1980).

Patients occasionally enter bouts of profound depression when there appears to be no reason for this emotion. They report fatigue, difficulty with concentration, headache, loss of appetite, energy, and sex drive. They are preoccupied with trivial problems of health and obsessive foci of complaints associated with those around them; they especially tend to become hypochondriacal, and this problem is likely to take the form of headaches and symptoms associated with the eyes and vision. These bouts of primary depression are difficult to separate clinically from the depressive phase of manic depression and probably differ only in degree of severity.

Depression is common following stroke in aged patients. It is also a relatively common side effect of drug therapy as liver and kidney function declines to the degree that formerly therapeutic doses become toxic.

Optometrists may find it useful to ask questions of their elderly patients based on a system developed for the identification of depressed subjects. Table 2.9 shows a series of questions developed as a valid and reliable test for depression. In order to detect depression, it is usually only necessary to ask three or four of these questions in a very informal or conversational manner during the examination.

Elderly patients of optometrists who are severely depressed may report difficulty in reading which they believe to be caused by their eyesight but which, in reality, is caused by boredom, a lack of concentration, and loss of interest in the subject matter being read. The resulting failure to continue reading is then blamed on "tired eyes" rather than these signs of depression. Lack of concentration of depressed subjects often leads to difficulty with subjective refraction because inappropriate answers frequently are given, and the patient seems unable to make reliable judgments.

Medical treatment of depression remains a controversial issue. Of course, depression forms a prominent part of the more serious age-related states of senile dementia and Alzheimer's disease, and it is common for depression to be mistakenly diagnosed as either of these dementias. Monoamine oxidaoxidase inhibitors and tricyclic and tetracyclic antidepressants combined with psychotherapy are

Table 2.9 Geriatric depression scale. Score positively when a "no" answer is made to questions 1, 5, 7, 9, 15, 19, 21, 27, 29, and 30, and when any remaining questions are answered "yes." A score of 20 or more suggests depression.

1. Are you basically satisfied with life?	Yes/No
2. Have you dropped many of your activities and interests?	Yes/No
3. Do you feel that your life is empty?	Yes/No
4. Do you often get bored?	Yes/No
5. Are you hopeful about the future?	Yes/No
6. Are you bothered about thoughts you can't get out of your head?	Yes/No
7. Are you in good spirits most of the time?	Yes/No
8. Are you afraid that something bad is going to happen to you?	Yes/No
9. Do you feel happy most of the time?	Yes/No
10. Do you often feel helpless?	Yes/No
11. Do you often get restless and fidgety?	Yes/No
12. Do you prefer to stay at home rather than going out and doing things?	Yes/No
13. Do you frequently worry about the future?	Yes/No
14. Do you feel you have more problems with memory than most?	Yes/No
15. Do you think it is wonderful to be alive now?	Yes/No
16. Do you often feel downhearted and blue?	Yes/No
17. Do you feel pretty worthless the way you are now?	Yes/No
18. Do you worry a lot about the past?	Yes/No
19. Do you find life very exciting?	Yes/No
20. Is it hard for you to get started on new projects?	Yes/No
21. Do you feel full of energy?	Yes/No
22. Do you feel that your situation is hopeless?	Yes/No
23. Do you think that most people are better off than you are?	Yes/No
24. Do you frequently get upset over little things?	Yes/No
25. Do you frequently feel like crying?	Yes/No
26. Do you have trouble concentrating?	Yes/No
27. Do you enjoy getting up in the morning?	Yes/No
28. Do you prefer to avoid social gatherings?	Yes/No
29. Is it easy for you to make decisions?	Yes/No
30. Is your mind as clear as it used to be?	Yes/No

Yesavage, J.A., T.L. Brink, T.L. Rose, et al. "Geriatric Depression Scale Reliability/Validity." *Psychiat. Res.* 17, no. 1 (1983): 37–49.

currently the most beneficial form of treatment of depression. There is a better response to psychotherapy treatment combined with these drugs than to psychotherapy and placebo in the first week, but placebo appears to be almost as effective as the active drugs over longer periods (Shapiro et al., 1983). Occasionally, it may be appropriate for optometrists to help depressed patients by applying a measure of tender loving care in addition to the primary responsibility of helping them back to an interest in life through better vision and a renewed interest in reading.

Tricylic antidepressants are highly toxic in overdose, and the depressed patient with suicidal tendencies is particularly liable to attempt self destruction using this form of medication. There are approximately 10,000 hospital admissions and 400 deaths in the UK yearly from intentional, self-administered overdose of these drugs.

Optometrists will see many patients exhibiting the full range of depression symptoms because of the frequent association of depression with hypochondriasis. Optometric treatment should only be for significant ocular problems and delivered with a frank explanation of what can and what cannot be expected from the treatment. It is disadvantageous to both patient and practitioner to prescribe glasses as placebo treatment for depressed patients, and the patients should be referred for medical management if the depression is judged to be outside the normal response to the precipitating event. A careful history, sympathetic ear, non-judgmental attitude and a willingness to let the patient talk will greatly benefit the patient and establish a lifelong loyalty.

Anxiety

Anxiety is a disorder in which the survival instincts give rise to an inappropriate degree of fearfulness in circumstances where little or no threat exists. During anxiety attacks, the patient becomes breathless, develops a rapid heart rate, perspires, is irritable and easily fatigued. The patient may complain of a tension-type headache.

While anxiety forms part of the symptom complex of almost all psychiatric diseases, including depression, it also may occur alone or in a disproportional degree in minor psychiatric disorders. It is often especially difficult to separate anxiety from phobic neuroses or depression. Some anxious patients commit suicide as a paradoxical means of escaping the misery of their anxiety. The differential diagnosis in anxiety states includes thyrotoxicosis, hypoglycemia in diabetes, overdose of corticosteroids, and epilepsy.

Anxiety may appear during any stage of life and in previously stable and well-balanced personalities. Acute attacks can last for a few minutes to hours without the patient being aware of any cause, and recurrence is a common feature.

Treatment

Mild cases are commonly seen in optometric practice where the patient expresses a fear of blindness or serious eye disease when no grounds for such fear exist. Patients under care frequently are left bewildered and frightened by the lack of explanation given and understanding shown by a specialist who is constrained from providing counselling by an overflowing waiting room. Careful reassurance of the clinical situation, with emphasis on the positive aspects of the prognosis, is valuable therapy. Optometrists should avoid giving the impression that they believe that the patient is imagining the symptoms. On the contrary, the patient should be encouraged to talk about the symptoms and be met with tolerance, understanding, and a plausible explanation of the symptoms when this is possible. As in other psychiatric conditions, optometric management should otherwise be confined to treating existing significant ocular conditions, and the patient should understand the nature, limitations, and likely outcome of such treatment. The length of time between follow-up visits should be determined by the patients who should be invited to return should they feel anxiety concerning their vision.

In anxious states, the physician may use low doses of anti-anxiety agents such as *sodium amytal, diazapam,* or *chlordiazepoxide.* However, it is doubtful if these drugs are much more effective than placebos in uncomplicated anxiety states, and in view of its common association with depression, it is ironic that propranolol is used as a treatment for anxiety when it also is known to be a cause of depressive states in some individuals.

CONNECTIVE TISSUE DISEASE

The connective tissue diseases are a complex and heterogeneous group of diseases in which the common factor is pathologic changes in the main supporting tissues of the body (in particular, skin, tendons, cartilage, bone, and the vascular system). Although the diseases are classified as inflammatory or degenerative, the distinction is seldom clear because prior inflammation renders the supporting tissue vulnerable to the stresses it must bear in its functional role. However, inflammation is a common, if not universal, response to the degenerations resulting from these stresses.

Arthritis

The collagen diseases that have ocular manifestations are chiefly those of the rheumatoid arthritis group and those affecting blood vessels (scleroderma, systemic lupus erythematosus, and polyarteritis). Osteoarthritis is the most common connective tissue disease; it is universally present to some degree in the aged population. Osteoarthritis has no recognized ocular complications. Many of the rheumatoid arthritis group are diseases having an onset in the early or middle years of life; however, the victims of these diseases may carry their disease with its complications into old age, and it is important that the clinician has a knowledge of these signs and symptoms. Table 2.10 lists the ocular complications of a number of the connective tissue diseases.

Rheumatoid Arthritis

Rheumatoid arthritis is an inflammatory disease of unknown cause that principally affects the joints but may result in multi-system complications in which the eyes may be involved. Although any of the synovial joints may be affected, those of the hands, wrists, and feet are involved most consistently. The changes are primarily the result of synovial swelling and the accumulation of granulomatous tissue within the joints. Bone changes consist of periarticular osteoporosis and areas of bone erosion leading to distortion through weakening of their texture and subluxation of smaller joints.

Table 2.10 Ocular complications of selected connective tissue diseases

Ocular Complication	Marfan Syndrome	Pseudoxanthoma Elasticum	Sjögren Syndrome	Systemic Lupus Erythematosus	Dermatomyositis	Myotonic Dystrophy	Myasthenia Gravis	Erythema Multiform	Ankylosing Spondylitis	Rheumatoid Syndrome Juvenile	Rheumatoid Syndrome Adult	Reiter Syndrome	Sarcoidosis	Progressive Systemic Scleroderma
Ectopia lentis	+													
Lens dislocation	+													
Glaucoma	+									+			+	
Retinal detachment	+													
Angioid streaks		+												
Retinal hemorrhages		+		+	+								+	+
Keratoconjunctivitis			+	+	+							+		+
Scleritis or episcleritis			+	+	+			+			+	+	+	+
Cotton wool patches				+	+									+
Optic atrophy				+					+					
Retinal vascular occlusions				+										
Ophthalmoplegia or ocular paresis						+	+				+			
Cataracts	+				+	+		+		+	+		+	
Color vision defects						+								
Peripheral retinal pigmentation						+								
Impaired dark adaptation						+	+							
Ptosis						+								
Uveitis					+			+	+	+	+	+	+	
Symblepharon								+			+		+	
Band-shaped keratopathy								+		+	+		+	
Dry eye			+	+				+			+		+	+
Keratoconus	+												+	
Papilledema														
Keratitis or corneal furrowing				+				+						+
Conjunctival telangiectasis														+

The onset of rheumatoid arthritis is mostly between the ages of 20 and 50 years. However, the disease may appear at any age (Merck Manual, 1982). Although there are no internationally accepted criteria for the diagnosis of rheumatoid arthritis, the four-tier classification of the American Arthritis Association (Rodman, 1973) provides a practical basis for clinical diagnosis. These classifications are classical, definite, probably, and possible rheumatoid arthritis. The non-laboratory criteria for the system are as follows (Arnett et al., 1987):

1. Morning stiffness
2. Pain on motion or tenderness in at least one joint
3. Swelling of one joint, representing soft tissue or fluid
4. Swelling of at least one other joint (soft tissue or fluid) with an interval free of symptoms no longer than three months
5. Symmetrical joint swelling (simultaneous involvement of the same joint right and left)
6. Subcutaneous nodules over bony prominences, extensor surfaces, or near joints

Because of the looseness of the criteria and the lack of an International Standard definition of the disease, the reported prevalence of rheumatoid arthritis varies considerably but appears to be approximately 1% to 2% in men and 2% to 4% in women.

The mode of onset of rheumatoid arthritis varies widely; it may be slow and insidious, or it may occur painfully and precipitously in the course of a single day (Christian, 1975). Up to 75% of sufferers will improve with conservative treatment within a year, 10% to 20% will have virtually complete remissions, and 5% to 10% eventually are disabled by the disease (Merck Manual, 1982).

Clinical Presentation

The small bones of the hands and feet are most commonly first affected in the classical form of rheumatoid arthritis. The finger joints particularly become swollen and distorted (Figure 2.14), the skin becomes fragile, and the hands bruise easily. Firm nodules approximately 1 cm in diameter develop beneath the skin; these may break down, ulcerate, and heal only with difficulty. Systemic complications affect the heart, lungs, and dura mater (Hayson and Grennan, 1983). Entrapment of nerves within the distorted bony tissue may produce neurologic signs, including paresis of muscles; the combination of these changes and loss of mobility of the joints eventually leads to muscle wasting.

Patients suffering from rheumatoid arthritis have more severe pain and stiffness in the morning on rising and after periods of inactivity; these symptoms are worse in cold weather. The patient is fatigued easily; suffers loss of appetite; is more sensitive to cold; and may experience numbness, particularly in the hands and feet.

Ocular Signs

The most common eye complication of rheumatoid arthritis is keratoconjunctivitis sicca, either alone or in combination with paucity of saliva (Sjögren syndrome). The lacrimal secretion reserve may be estimated from the height of the tear meniscus at the lower lid. In the normal eye, this meniscus has a height of approximately 0.1 to 0.3 mm (Lamberts et al., 1979). The Schirmer test usually is considered to be positive if less than 10 mm of the absorbant strip wets within 5 minutes in an eye that is not anesthetized. In dry eyes, Bengal Rose frequently stains the conjunctiva and filamentous threads of mucous secretion; in addition, there may be punctate staining of the inferior portion of the corneal epithelium. Some 10% to 15% of rheumatoid arthritis sufferers develop keratoconjunctivitis sicca, making this disease the most common cause of dry eyes (Pavan-Langston, 1980).

The less common, albeit more serious, ocular complications tend to occur when the disease has been present in severe form for a long time. Table 2.11 summarizes these signs, together with their special features and sequelae. Elderly patients who have rheumatoid arthritis are especially prone to develop scleral nodules. In the early stages, it is difficult to differentiate between relatively benign, although possibly quite painful, rheumatic nodules and early necrotizing nodular scleritis. Both forms are raised yellowish nodules in the sclera surrounded by hyperemic conjunctiva. Rheumatic nodules go through remissions and exacerbations more or less in synchrony with the underlying systemic disease, whereas necrotizing nodules develop into extremely painful areas that become thinned to the degree that the uvea becomes ectatic. Uveitis is common in eyes having necrotizing scleral nodules. The aged patient who has rheumatoid arthritis is at risk of developing scleromalacia perforans. This is an insidious, usually painless condition that develops from a scleral nodule; the sclera melts away, leading to perforation and the complications of cataract, uveitis, panophthalmitis, and glaucoma (Duke-Elder, 1965).

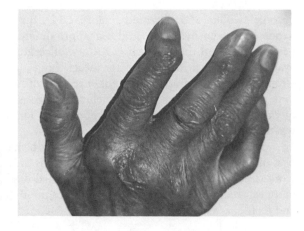

Figure 2.14. Typical changes in the hand of a patient having rheumatoid arthritis. Note the distortion of the joint in the index finger.

Table 2.11 Ocular complication of rheumatoid arthritis, their features, and possible sequelae

Complicaton	Features and Possible Sequelae
Keratoconjunctivitis	Occurrence in 10 to 15 percent of rheumatoid arthritis, lacrimal insufficiency; foamy tears; corneal and conjunctival erosion (part of Sjögren syndrome)
Scleritis and episcleritis	Painful red eye
Rheumatic nodules of sclera	Raised nodules surrounded by hyperemic sclera; pigmented areas on resolution
Necrotizing nodules	Uveitis; gross hyperemia; pain; scleral ectasia
Scleromalacia perforans	Perforation of the globe; panophthalmitis; cataract; glaucoma; often symptomless in early stage
Corneal marginal degeneration	Corneal ulceration; new vessel growth
Band keratopathy	Occurrence in long-standing corneal involvement
Anterior uveitis	Very mild, often symptomless; occurrence in 4 to 5 percent of subjects; usually resolution without serious damage; may be recurrent
Cataract	Complicated cataract; rarely polychromatic
Paresis of extraocular muscles	Usually transient, causing diplopia

Sorsby and Goma in 1946 drew attention to the prevalence of a mild anterior uveitis in patients having rheumatoid arthritis. In their series of 332 subjects, 15 (4.5%) had uveitis. However, it is now believed that uveitis is not more common in arthritic patients than in controls, except when the complication of scleromalacia perforans is present.

Medical Treatment

Because of its largely unpredictable course, the treatment of rheumatoid arthritis is difficult to evaluate. Spontaneous remissions frequently are ascribed to whatever fad diet or conventional or unconventional treatment was in use at the time the improvement commenced. The mainstay of treatment is aspirin (Leak, 1983) because of its combined anti-inflammatory and analgesic properties. Other drugs commonly used include ketoprofen, piroxicam, diflunisal, sulindac, indomethacin, phenylbutazone, chloroquine, hydroxychloroquin sulfate, gold compounds, adrenocorticosteroids, and penicillamine. These drugs may prove useful when salicylates prove ineffective; however, the complications associated with both nonsteroidal anti-inflammatory drugs and the corticosteroids can cause greater morbidity than the disease itself (Christian, 1975). The eyes and vision frequently are involved in these side effects. Corticosteroids may cause sharply increased intraocular pressure (Armaly, 1963; Becker and Mills, 1963) and posterior capsular cataract (Oglesby et al., 1961), as well as precipitate diabetes mellitus in susceptible subjects (Irvine et al., 1974). Indomethacin and chloroquine have been implicated in corneal and retinal damage, particularly in the macular and para macular regions (Burns, 1968). Patients undergoing treatment with these drugs merit careful and regular optometric examination, particularly as the patient ages, and the cumulative effects of these drugs reach a threshold level for morbidity.

Paget's Disease (Osteitis Deformans)

Paget's disease is a noninflammatory, slowly progressive bone disease of insidious onset. It is characterized by an absorption of bone alternating with its replacement by a chemically, structurally, and architecturally abnormal material that produces skeletal deformities. The condition, except for a rare juvenile form, is unknown in patients of less than 30 years of age; it has an increasing prevalence in older age groups, and about 10% are affected by age 90. Both sexes are affected, and it appears to have a peculiar geographic distribution, being unusually common in Australia and New Zealand (Saville, 1975). Patients of optometrists are drawn largely from older population groups and, consequently, provide a sample in which Paget's disease is not uncommon. This trend is exaggerated by the fact that in most patients the disease does not cause mobility problems or intellectual impairment, leaving the patient capable of seeking private eye care rather than that provided in institutions.

Paget's disease has an unknown cause. In spite of a rapid turnover and reabsorption of calcium, serum levels of calcium remain normal, although the serum alkaline phosphatase level becomes elevated (Holvey, 1972). Decalcification of bone results in softening, which in turn causes deformities, especially of the long bones and other weight-bearing structures. This becomes most obvious in a marked bowing of the legs. In advanced cases, there may be spontaneous fractures of these bones. X-ray studies show enlarged and irregular contours, abnormal strands in the bone structure, and dense zones chiefly extending from the ends of the affected bones. Severe impairment of hearing is common.

From the optometrist's viewpoint, the importance of Paget's disease is its frequent involvement of the bones of the skull. These changes may produce headaches, which vary greatly for different patients. They usually are severe and accompanied by back pain and tenderness of other bony structures. The compression of nerves entering the orbit may lead to extraocular muscle palsies and diplopia, the lateral recti being the muscles most commonly affected. In extreme and long-standing cases, the development of bony material along the facial midline causes lateral displacement of the orbits, with a consequential increase in pupillary distances (Duke-Elder, 1974b).

Angioid streaks are a more dramatic ocular manifestation of Paget's disease and occur in about 10% of cases (Cogan, 1974). As the name implies, these streaks have a superficial resemblance to blood vessels in the retina. However, on inspection with the slit lamp and fundus contact lens or pre-corneal lens, they are readily identified as being deep to the retina in Bruch's membrane. The streaks consist of breaks along lines of stress in the fibroelastic layer of this membrane and have a characteristic radiating pattern that tends to originate from an incomplete annulus surrounding and close to the optic disc (Figure 2.15). There may be hemorrhages into the streaks or into the retina at locations away from the streaks

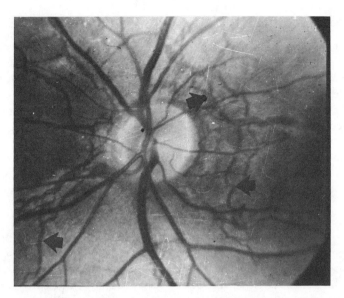

Figure 2.15. Angioid streaks (arrows). These breaks in Bruch's membrane have a superficial resemblance to blood vessels. They occur in some patients having Paget's disease.

indicating that there is probably widespread damage to ocular connective tissue in this disease. There also may be exudation of serum, which leads to sensory retinal detachment or a central disciform macular lesion (Greer, 1972). Angioid streaks are commonly associated with retinal pigment epithelial abnormalities and the formation of drusen.

The diagnosis of asymptomatic Paget's disease is not urgent, since a treatment has yet to emerge; the most effective help to the patient is supportive measures if and when the symptoms develop, as well as treatment of intercurrent disease. Frequently, widespread cardiovascular disease is associated with Paget's disease of long standing, consisting of systemic hypertension, intermittent claudication, and gastrointestinal bleeding (Cogan, 1974). The disease is associated with extensive development of new vascular channels in the bone structure, which leads to high-output cardiac stress and ultimately to death from heart failure (Holvey, 1972).

Treatment consists of the administration of calcitonin, mithramycin, and drugs of the diphosphate group (Greenburg, 1976). Calcitonin is the least toxic of these drugs, and has fewer and usually transient side effects; nevertheless, treatment should be reserved for patients having pain that proves refractory to analgesics and those with neurologic involvement (Peabody, 1980). Patients having angioid streaks require ophthalmologic attention because neovascular tufts within the choroidal break can be destroyed by photocoagulation, thus preventing bleeding and retinal edema.

TUMORS OF THE LIDS, CONJUNCTIVA, AND SKIN

Patients living in, and exposed to, sunny environments are particularly at risk of epibulbar and adnexal tumors (Irvine, 1972), especially aged patients who have been exposed to actinic radiation for many years (MacRae, 1980). Elderly, fair complexioned people, especially men who have worked outdoors in sunny climates for most of their lives, are rarely spared some form of skin lesion. The following discussion will emphasize the commonly seen benign lesions, pre-malignant tumors, and malignant tumors that most commonly occur in the elderly patient.

Tumors of the eyelids, conjunctiva, and the skin surrounding the eyes present a formidable diagnostic challenge, since a clinical differentiation between benign and malignant forms is frequently impossible, and only a biopsy and cytologic study of the tissues will allow identification. In the early stages of tumor growth, the difficulty of diagnosis is even more marked, yet it is at this stage that treatment of malignancies is most effective. Naturally, an advanced fulminating and disfiguring tumor will cause the patient to consult a medical rather than an optometric clinician. The optometrist will be more likely to observe early tumors of which the patient is either unaware or that are not sufficiently advanced to cause concern. For these reasons, optometrists should be alert to the possibility of tumors on and about the eye and accept a relatively high over-referral rate of these lesions in return for the confidence that early treatable cancers are not neglected until they have caused serious damage.

It is customary to classify tumors into the broad categories of malignant and benign. Malignant tumors tend to invade adjacent tissues, they may metastasize, and the cells may become undifferentiated or may revert to more primitive forms than those cells from which they are derived. In contrast, benign tumors do not invade other tissues or metastasize; they more closely retain the characteristics of the cells of origin, and they usually are enclosed in a connective tissue capsule. This classification is not absolute, and some tumors exhibit mixed characteristics.

Tumor types are named according to the cells from which they develop, to which the suffix -oma is added. The term carcinoma denotes that the tumor is epithelial in nature; this term may be interchanged with epithelioma. Thus, basal cell carcinoma is a tumor that arises from the basal cell layer of the dermis. A sarcoma derives from connective tissue. Where the tumor cells can be identified as being of a primitive form, blast is inserted into the description (for example, retinoblastoma), whereas a more mature cell form has the addition of cyto (for example, astrocytoma). If two or more cell types are involved, the less prominent cell type is named first and the more prominent is second (for example, neurofibrosarcoma).

Common Benign Tumors
Papillomas
Papillomas are the most common benign eyelid tumors. They tend to occur on the lid margin as rasberry-like growths or pedunculated (being attached by a stalk) lesions (MacRae, 1980) that have a smooth, flat surface continuous with

the palpebral conjunctiva. They usually cause no symptoms and grow very slowly. Less commonly, fleshy papillomas develop on the conjunctiva, where they appear in villiform (protruding), sessile (being attached by a base), or pedunculated (having a stem-like attachment) configuration. They may have a viral origin (Irvine, 1972). The possibility of misdiagnosis of conjunctival papillomas is greater than for those on the eyelids, and these cases should be referred for further examination. Treatment is by simple excision.

Skin Tags

Skin tags are common in the aged. They are harmless, soft, pedunculated protrusions usually constricted at their base. They usually are found on the upper lid and on the skin of the neck. Treatment is not necessary except for cosmetic reasons.

Seborrheic Keratoses

Seborrheic keratoses are symptomless and harmless, slow growing, flat, fissured, and slightly raised plaques that have a characteristic greasy texture. They are most commonly brownish, appear to be merely stuck to the surrounding skin and, indeed, it is possible to insert the finger nails well under the extremities of the lesion. These keratoses typically reach a size of 1 cm or 2 cm. These are very common in elderly patients and usually occur on the face and arms. They may be removed for cosmetic reasons but frequently re-form after removal.

Keratoacanthoma

Keratoacanthomas usually occur as single lesions on the hands, arms, face, or eyelids of elderly patients. These are rapidly growing, benign tumors growing in an elevated fashion but have a characteristic crusted central crater with a keratinized plug. They resolve spontaneously in approximately 6 to 8 weeks but may leave unsightly scars. They are best removed by simple excision if the scarring is likely to be unacceptable. Keratoacanthoma and squamous cell carcinoma may have a similar appearance (Greer, 1972). Indeed, it is possible that the keratoacanthoma is a self-healing squamous cell carcinoma.

Pingueculae

Pingueculae are yellowish, raised, limbal lesions that are very common in the aged and probably represent a degeneration of subepithelial collagen that results from long exposure to the sun and other irritating factors. Occasionally, the epithelium covering a pinguecula will undergo carcinogenic change (Greer, 1972). A prominent pinguecula may cause the eyelid to rise above a portion of the cornea during blinking. This results in dehydration and thinning of the corneal stroma to form dellen. Dellen are treated readily by eyedrops containing polyvinyl alcohol or methylcellulose. Uncomplicated pingueculae do not require treatment.

Pterygiums

Pterygiums are wedge-shaped degenerative lesions arising from the proliferation of fibrovascular tissue at the limbus, usually from the site of pingueculae (Figure 2.16). A wing of tissue invades the cornea, causing degeneration of Bowman's level and edema of the underlying stromal tissue. To a large extent, the virulence of a pterygium can be judged by the degree of vascularization; rapidly developing lesions have an abundant network of vessels. Infiltration of the stroma is visible as a dark shadow seen with the retinoscope against the retinal reflex. When this shadow extends more than about 1 mm beyond the superficial growth, the pterygium probably is developing rapidly. On the other hand, the presence of a reddish-brown line (Stocker's line) in the corneal epithelium ahead of the leading edge of the pterygium suggests that the pterygium is slow growing or stationary.

Treatment of pterygiums can be delayed in the very old, provided the growth is not rapid and the pterygium is not encroaching on the optic zone of the cornea. Removal should be considered when the lesion is on the only good eye and the growth is rapid. A large change in the cylindrical component of the refractive error is also a good indication that the growth should be removed. The decision regarding removal of pterygiums should take into account the finding that recurrence is common and the re-growth is often more aggressive than the original pterygium (Jaros and De Luise, 1988).

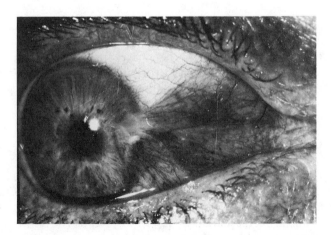

Figure 2.16. Active pterygium accompanied by a prominent tuft of conjunctival vessels.

Common Premalignant Tumors
Solar Keratoses
Solar keratoses take the form of slow developing, multiple, dry, scaly plaques on exposed skin. They are very common in elderly white patients who have been exposed to years of sunlight. The clinician often will feel rather than see the scaly lesions on the forehead while steadying the ophthalmoscope during the ocular examination. Their importance lies in reports that between 12% (MacRae, 1980) and 20% (Greer, 1972) develop into squamous cell carcinomas. Less frequently, basal cell carcinomas may arise from solar keratoses (Boink, 1964). However, this should be balanced by a more recent report of a large-scale prospective study of Australian, white-skinned patients, which suggests that the risk of conversion of solar keratosis to squamous cell carcinoma is only in the region of 1/1,000 per year (Marks and Rennie, 1988). It would seem prudent for all patients having solar keratoses to use ultraviolet-filtering creams on exposed surfaces, and to wear protective clothing and head wear to prevent continued skin damage from actinic radiation.

Carcinoma *in situ* (Intra-epithelial Carcinoma, Bowen's Disease)
A carcinoma *in situ* is a squamous cell carcinoma that is confined to the epithelial layer of the conjunctiva and the cornea. It has a gelatinous, elevated and vascularized appearance with finger-like processes. When on the bulbar conjunctiva, it may resemble a conjunctival papilloma. However, carcinoma *in situ* is found predominantly in elderly men and rarely, if ever, in children, whereas papillomas are relatively common in children (Duke-Elder, 1969a). Although these tumors only occasionally become malignant, they should be removed when they invade the cornea or become particularly exuberant. The differential diagnosis includes papilloma, pterygium, and corneal pannus.

Common Malignant Tumors
Basal Cell Carcinoma
A basal cell carcinoma is the most common malignancy affecting the eyelids and is reported to occur in 0.8% of ophthalmic patients (Morax, cited in Duke-Elder, 1974a). It has a peak incidence in patients between 60 years and 69 years old, and the lower eyelid or medial canthus was the site in 75% of cases (Collin, 1976). Men are said to be more likely to have a basal cell carcinoma than women (Scheie and Albert, 1977), although one large series demonstrated almost equal sex distribution (Payne et al., 1969). The early appearance of a basal cell carcinoma is a raised, pearly nodule or a flat, hard, scar-like plaque; the lesion is symptomless and grows slowly. Eventually, the tumor develops a roughly circular, raised border leaving a central crater that may contain a small scab or frank hemorrhage from the breakdown of a blood vessel within the tumor (Figure 2.17). The edges of the raised tumor are shiny, and small telangiectasias can be seen on slit-lamp examination. If the lesion is pinched between the thumb and

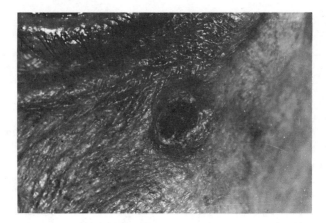

Figure 2.17. A typical basal cell carcinoma located below the lid margin showing raised, crenated, crusty, and pearly edges with a central depression in which there is a blood clot.

index finger, the subcutaneous portion will be found to be harder than normal surrounding tissue.

Errors of diagnosis of basal cell carcinoma are common. In a series of 273 cases of histologically proved basal cell carcinomas, the clinical diagnosis was correct in 60% of the cases. The most common mis-diagnosis was papilloma (Payne et al., 1969). Basal cell carcinomas may contain pigment cells and be confused with malignant melanoma as a result of their dark color. Patients typically seek professional examination when the lesion has been present for approximately 5 years and has reached a diameter of 4 mm or 5 mm. Squamous cell carcinomas, in contrast, grow more rapidly and reach this size in approximately one year. It appears that the size of the tumor is the critical factor in bringing the patient for examination, and careful history taking to assess the duration of the lesion will help the clinician make the correct diagnosis. Discovery of a basal cell carcinoma should alert the optometrist to the likelihood of multifocal tumors; in one series of 30 consecutive, ocular, basal cell carcinoma patients, 18 (60%) had one or more additional lesions (Wesley and Collins, 1982).

Although basal cell carcinomas rarely, if ever, metastasize, they can become locally invasive and cause extensive tissue destruction (Figure 2.18). Lesions that develop in the medial canthus carry the worst prognosis, and the absence of metastasis should not be a cause for complacency, since basal cell carcinoma can still be a fatal disease through tissue destruction and subsequent infection (Collin, 1976).

Treatment of basal cell carcinomas is by excision, preferably under frozen section control by means of which the margins of the excised tissue are examined for abnormal cells during the surgery, and the incision is enlarged until all margins contain normal cells (Doxanas et al., 1981). However, good results also are claimed for cryotherapy (Allen et al., 1979) and radiation treatment (Lederman, 1976).

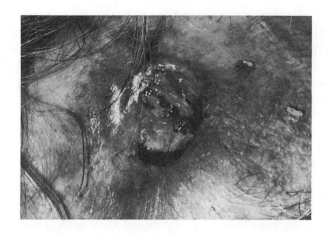

Figure 2.18. Neglected basal cell carcinoma that has extended to cause necrosis and infection of deeper tissues leading to exposure of the frontal bone.

Squamous Cell Carcinoma

The squamous cell carcinoma is another skin tumor that is more common in aged patients (MacRae, 1980), although it is much less prevalent than basal cell carcinomas. It has a predilection for developing on the bulbar conjunctiva, particularly at the transition zone between the conjunctival and corneal epithelium; when it occurs on the eyelids, the upper lid is more likely to be the site of the lesion. As has been noted in the discussion of basal cell carcinoma, this form of tumor grows more rapidly than a basal cell carcinoma, and patients tend to seek examination when the tumor reaches approximately 5 mm and has been present for approximately 12 months.

In its early stages, a squamous cell tumor on the eyelid is similar in appearance to a basal cell carcinoma; it has papular or plaque-like form with an indurated base. However, it is generally whitish and is more likely to be keratinized before the ulcerative stage has been reached. These tumors frequently evoke an inflammatory response, which can lead to the mis-diagnosis of hordeola. Squamous cell carcinomas that develop on the conjunctiva form gelatinous-looking masses, usually at the caruncle or the limbal margin, and they are easily confused with papillomas. Squamous cell carcinomas eventually metastasize by extension through the lymphatic system, where they become rapidly invasive, often causing an inflammatory response and considerable pain (Peabody, 1980). Early treatment of squamous cell carcinoma is desirable and may be by excision, radiation, or chemotherapy (MacRae, 1980).

Merkel Cell Carcinoma

Merkel cells are found in the epidermis, concentrated particularly around touch receptors in the extremities and also are found around the follicles of hair, eyelids, and eyelashes. They are located in close association with touch receptors. The function of these cells is unknown, although they were thought earlier to be part of the touch receptor system or possibly hierarchical cells from which this system is developed. More recently, it has been postulated that they have a role in the nutrition of the touch receptor system, or perhaps that they act as targets for the development of the axons of this system during its development. Merkel cells develop from epidermal stem cells.

Merkel cell tumors are rather rare primary malignant tumors seen more common in women than men and are particularly likely to occur in aged patients, although they have been reported in young adults. About half of these tumors appear in the head and neck, and of these, 10% (or 20% of all Merkel cell tumors) affect the eyelids or periocular region, with the upper lid being the most common site. Typically, the tumor presents as a smooth-surfaced, shiny, painless, bulging, and occasionally lobulated mass on the margin of the upper lid. Its deep red color is the result of proliferation of many dilated blood vessels within the tumor mass. By simple inspection, it may be difficult to differentiate a Merkel cell carcinoma from a Kaposi sarcoma, except that in the latter case, the tumor is associated with HIV infection and usually in younger patients. These tumors also are similar to malignant melanomata, can mimic chalazion, and are frequently mis-diagnosed as undifferentiated carcinoma (Kivella and Tarkkanen, 1990).

Treatment should be prompt in view of the natural history of rapid growth and common occurrence of metastases. These tumors may be removed surgically by wide excision followed by reconstruction surgery when the eyelids are involved. They also respond well to radiation therapy.

Kaposi's Sarcoma

Kaposi's sarcoma is a multifocal malignant neoplasm consisting of fine, anastamosing capillary vessels associated with endothelial and pericyte proliferation. The tumor takes the form of red, brown, blue, or purple plaques or nodules that can remain unchanged, ulcerate, or disappear. The usual course taken by the tumor is indolent and slowly progressive with increasing numbers of lesions occurring. Prior to its appearance in association with autoimmune deficiency syndrome (AIDS), the tumor tended to occur as a rare disease predominantly in elderly male Jews and Italians and in the Bantus of the African Congo, where it is reported to occur approximately equally in the two sexes (Piot et al., 1984). The external presentation of the classical tumor is most commonly on the lower extremities and on the hands, arms, nose, neck, and body at a later stage; ocular or adnexal involvement is rare. Gastrointestinal and lung involvement occurs in many patients, and hemorrhages from tumors at these sites may be severe.

Subjects having AIDS are particularly vulnerable to an aggressive form of Kaposi's sarcoma, and approximately one-third of AIDS victims in the United States have this tumor (Freeman et al., 1984). The high prevalence of the tumor in this younger age group is thought to be due to the virus-causing uncoupling of the cellular contact inhibition process, which normally prevents the proliferation of small blood vessels (Macher et al., 1983). When occurring as part of the AIDS complex, the lesions develop on the face early in the course of the disease and also are found commonly on the conjunctiva, eyelids, and periocular skin. Occasionally, there is spontaneous regression of the lesion (Janier et al., 1985).

It is probable that there will be few cases of AIDS-related Kaposi's sarcomas in the aged because HIV-positive subjects are not thought to have a long life expectancy. Nevertheless, as HIV infection spreads laterally in the heterosexual community, it is possible that the disease also will spread vertically into older age groups, so that Kaposi's sarcoma should be kept in mind when examining skin lesions in older patients. There are a number of conditions having a similar appearance that are relatively common in the aged and which might be mistaken for Kaposi's sarcoma. These include hemorrhagic conjunctivitis, subconjunctival ecchymosis, squamous or basal cell carcinoma, malignant melanoma, bruising, congenital facial hemangioma (Sturge-Weber syndrome), nevus of Ota, and choroidal staphyloma.

MANAGEMENT DECISIONS

When elderly patients have clinical evidence of conjunctival, lid, or skin tumors, the optometrist should temper management decisions with a knowledge of, and experience with, these lesions. When in doubt, it is wise to assume the diagnosis having the worst prognosis, and refer the patient for a second opinion. A very frail, elderly patient having a terminal illness and short life expectancy may elect to remain untreated. Foregoing treatment is reasonable for precancerous lesions and perhaps for early basal cell carcinomas; however, squamous cell carcinoma may cause painful and destructive lesions within 12 months and should not be neglected.

CONCLUSION

No single professional group has the capacity to provide a comprehensive support service for elderly persons. Trained, dedicated, and caring professionals from many disciplines who are prepared to work as a team offer the greatest prospect of meeting the needs of these people. Although high-level technology has a place in some areas of medical care, the instruments of good geriatric medicine are simple and universally available: they are the ears, the heart, and the time of the clinician. In many cases, the ability to listen, empathize, and show concern for the elderly patient is all that is required to produce therapeutic dividends. If the clinician can dispel false apprehensions, add a little genuine reassurance, and accentuate the more positive aspects of the prognosis, the vast majority of aged patients will be helped to live out their last years in tranquility.

Optometrists have the potential to become an important part of the caring team for the aged; they are uniquely equipped to optimize the vision of elderly patients, yet not so remotely professional and exalted that they cannot relate to their patients. Both the value of their contribution and the acceptance of their role depend on the extent of their clinical skills, their humanitarian approach, and particularly their depth of knowledge of the common systemic diseases encountered in age.

The optometrist also must understand and respect the scope of service available through other professionals and be prepared to refer patients when appropriate. Frequently, a decision must be made about whether to advise further medical investigation or treatment of systemic disease noted during the ocular examination, or simply to provide support and comfort without further intervention. The burden of this decision should be shared with patients to the limits of their ability to understand the alternatives, but optometrists must never abrogate their responsibility to fully and accurately inform patients so that the decisions can be soundly based. However, it does no service to the elderly patient to draw attention to, or initiate, uncomfortable procedures merely to confirm the presence of a disease for which treatment is ineffective. The vast majority of the ambulatory elderly who make up patient samples are capable of, and have the inalienable right to, making informed choices involving their own life-styles and health care.

It should be remembered that in age, illness becomes more easily tolerated through the blunting of the senses. Physical incapacity is accepted as the desire for activity diminishes, and even death becomes less frightening when the challenges of life are behind and there is assurance of understanding and caring support in the final years.

REFERENCES

1. Acheson, J., and E.C. Hutchinson. "Observations on the Natural History of Transient Ischemic Attacks." *Lancet* 11 (1964): 871–874.
2. Allen, E.D., et al. "Cryotherapy of Basal Cell Lesions." *Trans. Ophthalmol. Soc. UK* 99 (1979): 264–268.
3. Andrews, J.M. "Giant Cell (Temporal) Arteritis." *Neurology* 16 (1966): 963–971.
4. Armaly, M.F. "Effect of Corticosteroids on Intraocular Pressure and Fluid Deficiencies." *Arch. Ophthalmol.* 70 (1963): 482–499.
5. Arnett, F.C., S.M. Edworthy, D.A. Bloch, et al. "American Rheumatism Association 1987 Revised Criteria for the Classification of Rheumatoid Arthritis." *Arthritis Rheum.* 31 (1988): 315–324.
6. Barr, M.L. *The Human Nervous System,* 3d. ed. Hagerstown, Harper & Row, 1979.
7. Bastian, P. "Coronary Heart Disease in Tribal Aborigines." The West Kimberley Survey." *Aust. N.Z. J. Med.* 9 (1979): 284–292.
8. Becker, B., and D.W. Mills. "Corticosteroids and Intraocular Pressure." *Arch. Ophthalmol.* 70 (1963): 500–507.
9. Beeson, P.B. "Polymyalgia Rheumatica and Cranial Arteritis." In: Beeson, P.B., and W. McDermott, eds. *Textbook of Medicine,* 14th ed. Philadelphia: W.B. Saunders, 1975.
10. Beevers, D.G. "Hypertension." *Intern. Med (Aust. ed)* 19, part 3 (1982): 892–902.
11. Bodansky, H.J., A.G. Cudworth, R.A.F. Whitelocke, J.H. Dobree. "Diabetic Retinopathy and Its Relation to Type of Diabetes. A Review of Retinal Clinic Population." *Br. J. Ophthalmol.* 66 (1982): 496–499.

12. Boink, M. *Ocular and Adnexal Tumors.* St. Louis: C.V. Mosby, 1964.
13. Bouzas, A.G. "Endocrine Ophthalmology." *Trans. Ophthalmol. Soc. UK* 100 (1980): 511–520.
14. Burns, A. "Indomethacin Reduced Retinal Sensitivity and Corneal Deposits." *Am. J. Ophthalmol.* 66, no. 5 (1968): 825–835.
15. Norman, T.R. and Burrows, G.D. "Psychotropic Drugs – Potential Interactions." In: F.K. Judd, G.D. Burrows, and D.R. Lipsitt (eds.). Handbook of Studies in General Hospital Psychiatry. Amsterdam: Elsevier Science Publishers, 1991:153–178.
16. Cahill, G.F. Diabetes Mellitus. In: P.B. Beeson, W. McDermott (eds.) *Textbook of Medicine,* 14th ed. Philadelphia: W.B. Saunders, 1975, pp. 1599–1619.
17. Caird, R.I., M.A. Pirie, and T.G. Ramsell. *Diabetes and the Eye.* Oxford: Blackwell, 1969.
18. Cameron, R.J. *Year Book Australia* No. 66. Canberra: Australian Government Publication, 1982.
19. Canadian Cooperation Study Group. "A Randomized Trial of Aspirin and Sulfinpyrazone in Threatened Stroke." *N. Engl. J. Med.* 299 (1978): 53–59.
20. Chalmers, F.P. "Treatment of Uncomplicated Essential Hypertension." *Aust. Prescriber* 2, no. 1 (1977): 6–8.
21. Christie, D., L. McPherson, and V. Vivian. "The Queenscliff Study: A Community Screening Programme for Hypertension." *Aust. Med. J.* 2 (1976): 678–680.
22. Christian, C.L. In: P. B. Beeson and W. McDermott. *Textbook of Medicine,* 14th ed. Philadelphia: W.B. Saunders, 1975.
23. Chuna-Vaz, J.G. "Pathophysiology of Diabetic Retinopathy." *Br. J. Ophthalmol.* 62 (1978): 351–355.
24. Cockburn, D.M. "The Prevalence of Ocular Hypertension in Patients of an Optometrist and the Incidence of Glaucoma Occurring during Long-Term Follow-Up of Ocular Hypertensives." *Am. J. Optom. Physiol. Opt.* 59, no. 4 (1982): 330–337.
25. Cockburn, D.M. "Signs and Symptoms of Stroke and Impending Stroke in a Series of Optometric Patients." *Am. J. Optom. Physiol. Opt.* 60, no. 9 (1983): 749–753.
26. Cockburn, D.M. "The Prevalence and Expression of Diabetes in a Sample of Optometric Patients." *Clin. Exp. Optom.* 70 (1987): 156–165.
27. Cogan, D.G. "Visual Disturbance with Focal Progressive Dementing Disease." *Am. J. Ophthalmol.* 100 (1985): 68–72.
28. Cogan, D.G. *Ophthalmic Manifestations of Systemic Disease.* Philadelphia: W.B. Saunders, 1974.
29. Cogan, D.G., and T. Kuwabara. "Capillary Shunts in the Pathogenesis of Diabetic Retinopathy." *Diabetes* 12 (1963): 293–300.
30. Collaritis, C.R., R.D. Kiess, A. Das, A.M. Hall, E.I. Jordan, J.E. Donavan. "Diabetic Retinopathy in a Rural Diabetic Population." *Am. J. Ophthalmol.* 97 (1984): 709–714.
31. Collin, J.R.O. "Basal Cell Carcinoma in the Eyelid Region." *Br. J. Ophthalmol.* 60 (1976): 806–809.
32. Cullen, J.F. "Occult Temporal Arteritis." *Br. J. Ophthalmol.* 51 (1967): 513–525.
33. De Groot, L.J. "The Thyroid." In: P.B. Beeson and W. McDermott (eds.) *Textbook of Medicine,* 14th ed., Philadelphia: W.B. Saunders, 1975.
34. Denham, M. "Diagnostic Differences in Old Age." *Med. Austr.* series 1, no. 35/36 (1981): 2578–2580.

35. Doxanas, M.T., W.R. Green, and C.E. Iliff. "Factors in the Surgical Management of Basal Cell Carcinoma of the Eyelids." *Am. J. Ophthalmol.* 91 (1981): 726–736.

36. Duke-Elder, S. *System of Ophthalmology.* Vol. 8, part 2. London: Henry Kimpton, 1965.

37. Duke-Elder, S. *System of Ophthalmology.* Vol. 8. London: Henry Kimpton, 1969a.

38. Duke-Elder, S. *System of Ophthalmology.* Vol. 11. London: Henry Kimpton, 1969b.

39. Duke-Elder, S. *System of Ophthalmology.* Vol. 12. London: Henry Kimpton, 1971.

40. Duke-Elder, S. *System of Ophthalmology.* Vol. 6. London: Henry Kimpton, 1973.

41. Duke-Elder, S. *System of Ophthalmology.* Vol. 13, part 1. London: Henry Kimpton, 1974a.

42. Duke-Elder, S. *System of Ophthalmology.* Vol. 13, part 2. London: Henry Kimpton, 1974b.

43. Duke-Elder, S. *System of Ophthalmology.* Vol. 15. London: Henry Kimpton, 1976.

44. Duncan, G.W., M. S. Pessin, J.P. Mohr, and R.D. Adams. "Transient Cerebral Ischemic Attacks." *Adv. Intern. Med.* 21 (1976): 1–20.

45. Escourolle, R., and J. Poirer. *Basic Neuropathology.* Philadelphia: W.B. Saunders, 1978.

46. Eshaghian, J. "Controversies Regarding Giant Cell (Temporal, Cranial) Arteritis." *Doc. Ophthalmol.* 47 (1979): 43–67.

47. Fein, J.M. "Microvascular Surgery for Stroke." *Sci. Am.* 238, no. 4 (1978): 59–67.

48. Field, W.S., and L.A. Lemak. "Joint Study of Intracranial Arterial Occlusion: Part 9. Transient Ischemic Attacks in the Carotid Territory." *J.A.M.A.* 235, no. 24 (1976): 2608–2610.

49. Fisher, G.T., and H.M. Vavra. *Diabetes Source Book.* Washington, D.C.: US Department of Health Education and Welfare, 1969.

50. Foster, D.W. Diabetes Mellitus. In: Isselbacher K.J., Adams R.D., Braunwald, E., Pertersdorf, R.G., Wilson, J.D., (eds.) *Principles of Internal Medicine,* 9th ed. New York: McGraw-Hill, 1980, pp. 1741–1764.

51. Freeman, W.R., C.W. Lerner, J.A. Mines, et al. "Prospective Study of the Ophthalmologic Findings in the Acquired Immune Deficiency Syndrome." *Am. J. Ophthalmol.* 97 (1984): 133–142.

52. Garfinkel, P.E., E. Persad. In: S.E. Greben (ed.) *A Method of Psychiatry.* Philadelphia: Lea & Febiger, 1980, p. 178.

53. Gartner, S., and P. Henkind. "Neovascularization of the Iris (Rubeosis Iridis)." *Surv. Ophthalmol.* 22 (1978): 291.

54. Geddes, M. "Infective Endocarditis." *Intern. Med* 19, no. 3 (1982): 878–884.

55. Gombos, G.M. *Handbook of Ophthalmological Emergencies,* 2nd ed. Flushing, N.Y.: Medical Examination Publishing, 1977.

56. Goodwin, F.K., K.R. Jamison. "The Natural Course of Manic Depressive Illness. In: R.M. Post, J.C. Ballenger (eds.) *Neurobiology of Mood Disorders.* Baltimore: Williams & Wilkins 1984, pp. 20–37.

57. Greenberg, P.P. "Calcitonin in Paget's Disease." *Aust. Prescriber,* 2, no. 1 (1976): 26–27.

58. Greer, C.H. *Ocular Pathology,* 2nd ed. Oxford England: Blackwell, 1972.

59. Gribben, B. "Infective Endocarditis." In: D.J. Weatherall, J.G.G. Ledingham, and D.A. Warrell (eds.) *Oxford Textbook of Medicine,* Vol. 2. Oxford: Oxford University Press, 1983.

60. Gurland, B.J. "The Comparative Frequency of Depression in Various Age Groups." *J. Gerontol.* 31 (1976): 283–292.
61. Guthrie, W., P. Taft, K. Thomas. "The High Prevalence of Diabetes Mellitus on a Central Pacific Island." *Diabetologia* 13 (1977): 111–115.
62. Harrison, M.J.G., J. Marshall, J.C. Meadows, and K.W. Russ-Russell. "Effect of Aspirin in Amaurosis Fugax." *Lancet* 2 (1971): 743–744.
63. Hayreh, S.S. *Anterior Ischemic Optic Neuropathy.* Berlin: Springer-Verlag, 1975.
64. Hayson, M.I.V., and D.M. Grennan. "Clinical Features of Rheumatoid Arthritis." In: D.J. Weatherall, J.G.G. Ledingham, and D.A. Warrell (eds.) *Oxford Textbook of Medicine.* Oxford: Oxford University Press, 1983.
65. Henderson, J.W. "Optic Neuropathy in Exophthalmic Goiter (Graves' Disease)." *Arch. Ophthalmol.* 59 (1958): 471–480.
66. Hercules, B.L., I.I. Gayed, S.B. Lucas, and J. Jeacock. "Peripheral Retinal Ablation in the Treatment of Proliferative Diabetic Retinopathy: A Three Year Interim Report of a Randomized Study Using Argon Laser." *Br. J. Ophthalmol.* 61 (1977): 555–563.
67. Herman, B., B.P.M. Schulte, J.H. van Luijk, A.C.M. Leyton, and C.W.G.M. Frenken. "Epidemiology of Stroke in Tilbrug, The Netherlands. *Stroke* 2, no. 2 (1980): 162–165.
68. Hinton, D.R., A.A. Saduin, S.J.C. Blank, C.A. Miller. "Optic Nerve Degeneration in Alzheimer's Disease." *N. Engl. J. Med.* 315 (1986): 485–487.
69. Hodkinson, M. "Diagnostic Differences in Old Age." *Med. Aust.* series 1, no. 35/36 (1981): 2578–2580.
70. Holvey, D.N. (ed.). *The Merck Manual of Diagnosis and Therapy,* 12th ed. Rahway, N.J.: Merck, Sharp, and Dohme, 1972.
71. Howells, G., *Annual Report of the Director-General of Health, 1981–82.* Canberra: Australian Government Printer, 1982.
72. Irvine, R. A. "Epibulblar Squamous Cell Carcinoma and Related Lesions." *Int. Ophthalmol. Clin.* 71 (1972): 83.
73. Irvine, W.J., D.R. Cullen, R.B.L. Eward, J.D. Baird, and J.N. Harcourt-Webster. "Diseases of the Endocrine Glands." In: R. Passmore, and J.S. Rotron (eds.) *A Companion to Medical Studies,* Vol. 3. Oxford, England: Blackwell, 1974, pp. 23–76.
74. Janier, M., M.D. Vignon, F. Cottenot. "Spontaneously Healing of Kaposi's Sarcoma." *N. Engl. J. Med.* 312 (1985): 1638–1639.
75. Jaros, P.A., and V.P. De Luise. "Pingueculae and Pterygia." *Surv. Ophthalmol.* 2 (1988): 41–49.
76. Kannel, W.B. "Current Status of the Epidemiology of Brain Infarction Associated with Occlusive Arterial Disease." *Stroke* 2, no. 4 (1971): 295–318.
77. Kathol, R.G., T.A. Cox, J.J. Corbett, and H.S. Thompson. "Functional Visual Loss: Follow-Up of 42 Cases." *Arch. Ophthalmol.* 101 (1983): 735–739.
78. Kearns, T.P., and R.W. Hollenhorst. "Venous-Stasis Retinopathy of Occlusive Disease of the Carotid Artery." *Proc. Mayo Clin.* 38 (1963): 304–312.
79. Keen, H. "The Nature of the Diabetes Syndrome." *Int. Med.* 8 (1981):327–333.
80. Kivella, T., A. Tarkkanen. "The Merkel Cell and Associated Neoplasms in the Eyelids and Periocular Region." *Surv. Ophthalmol.* (1990) 35:171–187.
81. Kohner, E.M., T.R. Fraser, G.F. Joplin, and N.W. Oakley. "The Effect of Diabetic Control on Diabetic Retinopathy." In: M.F. Goldberg and S.L. Fine (eds.) *The Treatment of Diabetic Retinopathy.* U.S. Public Health Service Publication no. 1890. Washington, D.C.: U. S. Government Printing Office. 1969, pp. 119–128.

82. Lamberts, D.W., C.S. Foster, and H. D. Perry. "Schirmer Test after Topical Anaesthesia and the Minimum Height in Normal Eyes." *Arch. Ophthalmol.* 97 (1979): 1082–1085.

83. Lawson, P.M., M.C. Champion, C. Canny, et al. "Continuous Subcutaneous Insulin Infusion Does Not Prevent Progression of Proliferative and Preproliferative Retinopathy." *British J. Ophthalmol.* 66 (1982): 762–766.

84. Leak, A.M. "Advances in the Treatment of Rheumatic Disease." *Practitioner* 227 (1983): 1139–1145.

85. Lederman, M. "Radiation Treatment of Cancer of the Eyelids." *Br. J. Ophthalmol.* 60 (1976): 794–805.

86. Lucas, C.P., and M. Omar. "Pretreatment Assessment." *Geriatrics* 35 (1980): 51–55, 59.

87. McDonald, G.W. "The Epidemiology of Diabetes." In: M. Ellenberg, H. Rifkin (eds.) *Diabetes Mellitus: Theory and Practice.* New York: McGraw-Hill, 1970, p. 462.

88. McDowell, F.H. "Cerebrovascular Diseases." In: P.B. Beeson and W. McDermott (eds.). *Textbook of Medicine,* 14th ed. Philadelphia: W.B. Saunders, 1975.

89. McLeod, J. (ed.). *Clinical Examination,* 5th ed. Edinburgh: Churchill Livingstone, 1979.

90. Macher, A.M., A. Palestine, H. Masur, G. Briant, et al. "Multicentric Kaposi's Sarcoma of the Conjunctiva in a Male Homosexual with the Acquired Immunodeficiency Syndrome." *Ophthalmology* 90 (1983): 879–884.

91. MacRae, D.W. "Tumors and Related Lesions of the Eyelids and Conjunctiva." In: A.P. Gholam, D.R. Sanders, and M.F. Goldberg (eds.). *Principles and Practice of Ophthalmology,* Vol 3. Philadelphia: W.B. Saunders, 1980.

92. Mandelkorn, R.M., and T.J. Zimmerman. "Effects of Nonsteroidal Drugs on Glaucoma." In: R. Ritch and M.B. Shields (eds.). *The Secondary Glaucomas.* St. Louis: C.V. Mosby, 1982.

93. Marks, R., G. Rennie, T.S. Sellwood. "Malignant Transformation of Solar Keratosis to Squamous Cell Carcinoma." *Lancet,* April, 1988: 795–796.

94. *The Merck Manual.* Rahway, N.J.: Merck & Co., 1982.

95. Mitchell, P. "The Prevalence of Diabetic Retinopathy. A Study of 1300 Diabetics from Newcastle and the Hunter Valley." *Aust. J. Ophthalmol.* 8 (1980): 241–246.

96. Morris, J.G.L. Essential tremor. In: T.M. Speight (ed.). *Mims Disease Index.* Crows Nest: IMS Publishing, 1991, p. 183.

97. Muuronen, A., and M. Kaste. "Outcome of 314 Patients with Transient Ischemic Attacks." *Stroke* 13, no. 1 (1982): 24–31.

98. National Diabetes Data Group. "Classification and Diagnosis of Diabetes Mellitus and Other Categories of Glucose Intolerance." *Diabetes* 28 (1979): 1039–1057.

99. Newell, F.W. *Ophthalmological Principles and Concepts.* 5th ed. St. Louis: C.V. Mosby, 1982.

100. Niarchos, A.O. "Hypertension in the Elderly." *Mod. Concepts of Cardiovasc. Dis.* 49 (1980): 49–54.

101. Oglesby, R.B., R.L. Black, L. Allmann, and J.J. Bunim. "Cataracts in Patients with Rheumatic Disease Treated with Corticosteroids." *Arch. Ophthalmol.* 66 (1961): 625–630.

102. Olsson, J.E., R. Muller, and S. Berneli. "Long-term Anticoagulant Therapy for TIAs and Minor Strokes with Minimum Residium." *Stroke* 7, no. 5 (1976): 444–451.

103. Page, L.B.V., and J.J. Sidd. "Medical Progress: Medical Management of Primary Hypertension." *N. Engl. J. Med.* 287, no. 19 (1972): 960–966.
104. The Parkinson Study Group. "Effect of Deprenyl on the Progression of Disability in Early Parkinson's Disease." *N. Engl. J. Med.* 321 (1989): 1364–1371.
105. Pascoe, P.T., and D.G. Vaughan. "Refractive Changes in Hyperglycaemia: Hyperopia not Myopia." *British Journal of Ophthalmology* 66 (1982): 500–505.
106. Pavin-Langston, D. (ed.). *Manual of Ocular Diagnosis and Therapy.* Boston: Little, Brown, 1980.
107. Payne, J.W., J.R. Duke, R. Butner, and D.E. Eifrig. "Basal Cell Carcinoma of the Eyelids: A Long-term Follow-up Study." *Arch. Ophthalmol.* 81 (1969): 553–558.
108. Peabody, R.R. "Angioid Streaks." In: F. Fraunfelder and F.T. Roy (eds.). *Current Ocular Therapy.* Philadelphia: W.B. Saunders, 1980.
109. Peart, W.S. "Arterial Hypertension." In: P.B. Beeson and W. McDermott (eds.). *Textbook of Medicine,* 14th ed. Philadelphia: W.B. Saunders, 1975.
110. Pickering, G. "Hypertension, Definitions, Natural Histories and Consequences." *Am. J. Med.* 52 (1972): 570–583.
111. Piot, P., T.C. Quinn, H. Taelman. "Acquired Immunodeficiency Syndrome in a Heterosexual Population in Zaire." *Lancet* (1984): 65–69.
112. Reinecke, R.D., and T. Kuwabara. "Temporal Arteritis." *Arch. Ophthalmol.* 82 (1969): 446–453.
113. Riggs, H.E., and C. Rupp. "Variation in the Form of Circle of Willis." *Arch. Neurol.* 8, no., 1 (1963): 8–31.
114. Rodman, G.P. (ed.). "Primer on the Rheumatic Diseases: Criteria for the Diagnosis and Classification of Rheumatic Diseases." *J.A.M.A.* 224, no. 5 (1973): 799–800.
115. Sachdev, Y., J.C. Chatterji, and R.C. Sharma. "Heterogenicity of Failure of Visual Acuity in Graves' Disease." *Postgrad. Med. J.* 55 (1979): 241–247.
116. Saracco, J.B., P. Castaud, B. Ridings, and C.A. Ubaud. "Diabetic Choroidopathy." *J. Fra. Ophtalmol.* 5 (1982): 231–236.
117. Saville, P.S. "Paget's Disease of Bone: Osteitis Deformans." In: P.B. Beeson and W. McDermott (eds.). *Textbook of Medicine,* 14th ed. Philadelphia: W.B. Saunders, 1975.
118. Scheie, H.G., and D.M. Albert. *Textbook of Ophthalmology,* 9th ed. Philadelphia: W.B. Saunders, 1977.
119. Sedzimer, C.B. "An Angiographic Test of Collateral Circulation through the Anterior Segment of the Circle of Willis." *J. Neurol. Neurosurg. Psychiatry* 22, no. 1 (1959): 64–68.
120. Selby, G. Parkinson's Disease. In: T.M. Speight (ed.). *Mims Disease Index.* Crows Nest: IMS Publishing, 1991, p. 406.
121. Shapiro, A.K., E.L. Stroening, E. Shapiro, B.I. Milcarek. "Diazapam: How Much Better than Placebo? *J. Psychiatr. Res.* 17 (1983): 51–73.
122. Society of Actuaries. *Build and Blood Pressure Study,* Vols. 1 and 2. Chicago: Society of Actuaries, 1959.
123. Sorsby, A., and A. Goma. "Iritis in Rheumatoid Disease." *Br. J. Med.* (1946): 597–600.
124. Stamler J. *Comprehensive Treatment of Essential Hypertensive Disease: Why, When, and How.* Monographs on Hypertension. Rahway, N.J.: Merck, 1970.

125. Steno Study Group. "Effect of 6 Months of Strict Metabolic Control of Eye and Kidney Function in Insulin Dependent Diabetics with Background Retinopathy." *Lancet* 1 (1982): 121–124.
126. Stone, R.A. "Glaucoma Associated with Systemic Disease." In: R. Ritch, and M.B. Shields (eds.). *The Secondary Glaucomas.* St. Louis: C.V. Mosby, 1982.
127. Topilow, H.W., K.R. Kenyon, M. Takahashi, H.M. Freeman, F.I. Tolentino, and L.A. Hanninen. "Asteroid Hyalaosis: Biomicroscopy Ultrastructure and Composition." *Arch. Ophthalmol.* 100 (1982): 964–968.
128. Treleaven, G.K. (ed.). *Prescription Proprietaries Guide.* Melbourne: Australian Pharmaceutical, 1982.
129. Tucker, R.M. "Is Hypertension Different in the Elderly?" *Geriatrics* (May 1980): 28–32.
130. Urrets-Zavalia, A. *Diabetic Retinopathy.* New York: Masson, 1977.
131. Veshima, H., M. Lida, T. Shimamoto, et al. "Multivariate Analysis of Risk Factors in Stroke." *Prev. Med.* 9 (1980): 722–740.
132. Wesley, R.E., Collins, J.W. "Basal Cell Carcinoma of the Eyelid as an Indicator of Multifocal Malignancy." *Am. J. Ophthalmol.* 94 (1982): 591–593.
133. Veterans Administration Co-operative Study Group on Antihypertensive Agents. "Effects of Treatment on Morbidity in Hypertension: 2. Results in Patients with Diastolic Blood Pressure Averaging 90 through 114 mm Hg." *J.A.M.A.* 213, no. 7 (1970): 1143–1152.
134. Wand, M. "Neovascular Glaucoma." In: R. Ritch and M.B. Shields (eds.). *The Secondary Glaucomas.* St. Louis: C.V. Mosby, 1982.
135. Warlow, C. "Management of Cerebrovascular Disease." *Med. Aust.* 32, no. 3 (1981): 2300–2308.
136. Glatthaar, C., Welborn T.A., Stenhouse, N.S., Garcia-Webb P. "Diabetes and Impaired Glucose Tolerance: A Prevalence Estimate Based on the Busselton 1981 Survey." *Med. J. Aust.* 143 (1985): 436–440.
137. Welzel, G. "Antihypertensive Treatment in the Elderly." *Gerontology* 28, supp. 1 (1982): 83–92.
138. Wesley, R.E., and J.W. Collins. "Basal Cell Carcinoma of the Eyelid as an Indicator of Multifocal Malignancy." *Am. J. Ophthalmol.* 94 (1982) 591–593.
139. West, K.M., L.J. Erdreich, and J.A. Stober. "A Detailed Study of the Risk Factors for Retinopathy and Nephropathy in Diabetes." *Diabetes* 29 (1980): 501–508.
140. Wilson, L.A., and R.W. Ross-Russell. "Amaurosis Fugax and Carotid Artery Disease: Indications for Angiography." *Br. Med. J.* 2 (1977): 435–437.
141. Winslow, C.M., D.H. Solomon, M.R. Chassin, J. Kosecaff, N.J. Merrick, R.H. Brook. "The Appropriateness of Carotid Endarterectomy." *N. Engl. J. Med.* 318 (1988): 721–727.
142. Wishnant, J.P., N. Matsumoto, and L.R. Elueback. "Transient Cerebral Ischemic Attacks in a Community; Rochester, Minnesota, 1955 through 1969." *Proc. Mayo Clin.* 48 (1973): 194–198.
143. World Health Organization. *Arterial Hypertension and Ischemic Heart Disease.* World Health Organization Technical Report no. 231. Geneva. WHO, 1962.
144. Yahr, M.D. "The Parkinsonian Syndrome." In: P.B. Beeson and W. McDermott (eds.). *Textbook of Medicine,* 14th ed. Philadelphia: W.B. Saunders, 1975.

3

Oculomotor Signs of Pathology in the Elderly

David Pickwell

Anomalies of the oculomotor system that affect binocular vision in the elderly patient can require optometric care. In some cases, an anomaly also can be a sign that the patient would benefit from medical attention. It is in the interests of patients that practitioners be able to determine promptly when oculomotor problems are a sign of pathology and the cooperation of a medical practitioner is indicated. In some cases, the primary cause of the disturbance is such that referral to another practitioner is essential before any optometric care proceeds. This chapter is concerned with the differential diagnosis of optometric problems from medical problems in patients in whom an oculomotor anomaly is apparent.

PATHOLOGIC DEVIATIONS

For the purposes of this chapter, the deviations that indicate the onset of an underlying cause requiring medical attention are referred to as *pathologic deviations.* In very general terms, they have two main characteristics. First, the onset is comparatively sudden; second, the deviation and diplopia are usually noncomitant. That is not to say that all deviations with a sudden onset are necessarily pathologic, nor is it true that all noncomitant deviations are a sign of active pathology. However, these two signs are usually present in pathologic deviations, and when they occur, the possibility of pathology should be explored carefully.

A noncomitant deviation varies in angle in different parts of the motor field. The squint may be present when the eyes turn to look in one direction of gaze and absent in all other directions. In other cases, it is present in all directions of gaze but increases in angle when the eyes turn in one direction. Pathologic deviations usually are accompanied by diplopia of sudden, recent onset, and are also noncomitant. In long-standing squint, the sensory adaptations of suppression and anomalous retinal correspondence will have intervened, so the patient is not disturbed by diplopia; the motor anomaly will be observable, but sensory adaptations will have alleviated the symptoms.

INVESTIGATION

Normally, a full, routine, optometric examination will proceed in each case, but particular attention will be given to these aspects outlined in the following sections.

History and Symptoms

From what has been said about the nature of pathologic deviations, it can be seen that history and symptoms become an important aspect of the differential diagnosis. Patients with a dramatic onset of diplopia accompanied by other signs and symptoms of ill health present an obvious picture of suspected pathology. Indeed, it may be so obvious that the patient will consult a medical practitioner rather than an optometrist. It is the more insidious cases that require more care in evaluation. A recent onset of intermittent diplopia associated with headaches during reading could be due to a functional anomaly such as exophoria becoming decompensated with age. It also might be caused by a fourth nerve palsy (Duke-Elder 1973). Although the symptoms need careful evaluation, they must be considered together with the rest of the clinical investigation. The following symptoms are particularly important:

1. *Diplopia.* When diplopia is given as a symptom, the question of comitancy must be explored. The patient may be able to recognize the variation in different parts of the motor field. In pathologic deviations, there is very frequently a vertical element, and sometimes a tilting of one image is reported. It will be appreciated that diplopia in pathologic deviations usually is not associated with any particular use of the eyes, such as reading, but rather with a direction of gaze.
2. *Abnormal head posture.* The patient may be aware that a compensation for the diplopia can be made by holding the head in an abnormal position.
3. *Headache.* The underlying cause of the deviation may cause headaches; for example, it can be present in vascular disturbances, neoplasms, and so on. Other conditions are considered later in this chapter.
4. *General health.* A deterioration in general health may occur when the cause is a metabolic anomaly. The patient may report loss of weight, increased or decreased appetite, general fatigue, loss of muscular ability, tremor of limbs, breathlessness, and so on.
5. *Injury.* In the elderly, an accident such as a fall can be responsible for an intracranial injury that can lead to an oculomotor disturbance, even when the patient has thought it not serious enough to seek medical advice but considered that rest was all that was needed.
6. *History.* The history of the patient's ocular and vision health also will help. When there has been a long-standing squint, an elderly patient usually will know. However, it must not be assumed that when the patient has had a squint throughout life, pathology also cannot occur.

When there is amblyopia, symptoms that are caused by a pathologic deviation can be lessened if the amblyopic eye is primarily affected and increased when it is the nonamblyopic eye.

Motility

Most pathologic deviations are paralytic or paretic. The term *paretic* will be used here to indicate all ocular deviations that are caused by the malfunction of one or more of the extrinsic ocular muscles. Such deviations are noncomitant, and the motility test is therefore an important part of the investigation. The eye movements are observed as the eyes follow a fixation target moved in different directions of gaze in and beyond the limits of the binocular field of fixation.

A small light or penlight is a very suitable target for the patient to follow, and observation of the corneal reflex will assist precise judgment of the eye movements. The binocular field can be thought of as an area 50 cm (20 inches) square at a distance of 50 cm in front of the patient's face. If the fixation target is moved outside this area, fixation will not be possible with one of the two eyes, since the target always will be obscured by the patient's brow or nose for one eye. Any diplopia of the penlight target must occur within the area of the binocular motor field (some patients may report doubling of the general field outside this area, even when fixation of the penlight with one of the eyes has been lost). Patients are asked to follow the moving light outside the binocular field into the extremes of gaze. They are asked to report any doubling of the fixation light. The practitioner observes the eyes, noting whether both are following smoothly, whether there is a corresponding lid movement accompanying vertical eye movements, and whether there is a restriction or overshooting of one eye in a particular direction of gaze. In elderly patients, there is often a bilateral restriction, particularly upwards; that is, the eyes do not move as far as they do in younger patients. When the eyes follow the light out of the binocular part of the field, one eye will continue to fix the light, and the other normally will undertake movement similar in degree and direction. In noncomitant deviations, the patient may report diplopia in the binocular field, and the restriction of movement becomes more obvious to the practitioner as the fixation light moves toward the extremes of the monocular field of fixation.

In one simple and quick routine (Pickwell 1981), the penlight first is held centrally so that the eyes are in the primary position and fixation can be checked in both eyes. If the observer sits directly behind the light, the corneal reflections of the light should appear symmetrical in the pupils and slightly nasal for a normal angle kappa. The penlight then is moved downward and back to the horizontal center of the field on the median line. The lid signs can be checked when this is being done (to be discussed later). The light then is moved into the right extreme of the top of the field and slowly across the upper part of the field to the extreme left. This horizontal movement is repeated across the horizontal center of the field and again at the lower extremities. The horizontal movement across the top of the field allows the actions of the elevator muscles to be checked. The movement across the center of the field allows any abnormality of the lateral and medial recti muscles to be detected, and the movement across the bottom of the field should reveal any anomalies of the depressors. If an abnormality is seen, the likely cause can be determined from an analysis of the restrictions with respect to the actions of the individual muscles (Pickwell, 1974).

The medial and lateral recti muscles are simple adductors and abductors, respectively, so when the eyes move to the left or right across the center of the field, they do so mainly by the action of these four muscles (two in each orbit). Movements to the right should be executed by the right lateral rectus and left medial rectus. If the right eye does not move adequately in this direction, there probably is a lateral rectus (or sixth nerve) palsy.

In people with no paresis but normal binocular vision, the elevator muscles are the superior rectus and the inferior oblique in each orbit. Their anatomic features are such that the line of action of these two muscles lies in two different vertical planes that intersect medially to the plane containing the center of rotation of the eye. This is shown in Figure 3.1, in which *ab* represents the plane containing the superior rectus, and *cd* represents the plane containing the inferior oblique. The right eye is shown in the primary position. As the superior rectus muscle is attached to the eye slightly above the limbus at *a,* and its line of action is in a direction a little nasal to the center of rotation *(R),* it will have secondary actions of adduction and intorsion, as well as its primary action of elevation. The inferior oblique is attached to the back of the eye, and its line of pull passes under the eye and is again nasal to the center of rotation. From the primary position, therefore, its secondary functions — abduction and extorsion — will be opposed to those of the superior rectus, but its primary function will be elevation. The primary and

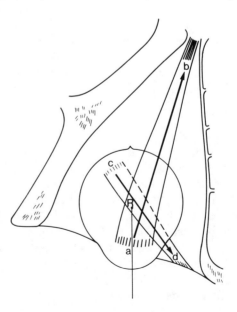

Figure 3.1 Patient's right orbit showing the planes of the actions of the superior rectus *(ab)* and the inferior oblique *(cd)* muscles relative to the eye's center of rotation *(R).*

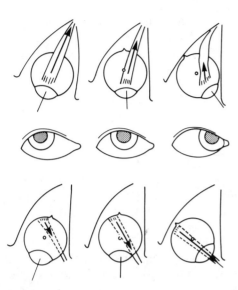

Figure 3.2 Actions of the elevator muscles, the superior rectus, and the inferior oblique. (Left) The eye is in the abducted position. The upper figure shows the superior rectus pulling over the center of rotation and having its maximum elevating power with no secondary actions. The lower figure shows the inferior oblique pulling at an oblique angle to the visual line and having little power as an elevator, but greater secondary action. (Center) Both muscles are contributing to elevation. (Right) The eye is in the adducted position. The ability of the superior rectus to elevate the eye has declined in the upper figure. The lower figure shows the inferior oblique muscle in the position of maximum power as an elevator, with minimum secondary action.

secondary actions of these muscles can be seen to arise from the anatomic fact that their lines of actions pass medial to the eye's center of rotation.

Figure 3.2 shows the lines of pull as the eyes move across the top of the motor field. When the eye is turned out (abducted), elevation is maintained by the superior rectus, because in this position, its line of pull will have been carried more nearly over the center of rotation. In this position, it will have the greatest advantage as an elevator. However, the inferior oblique will be pulling nearly at right angles to the line of sight, and, therefore, it will have little ability as an elevator in this position; it will have become primarily an extortor. It also can be seen from Figure 3.2 that when the eye turns inward (is adducted), the mechanical advantage of the superior rectus to maintain elevation of the eye will decline, and the inferior oblique will increase its ability to maintain elevation. Elevation is maintained by the superior rectus when the eye is turned out by both elevators when fixing directly above the primary position, and by the inferior oblique when turned in. In other words, one elevator gradually takes over from the other as the eye moves across the top of the motor field (Pickwell, 1974).

A similar analysis of the depressor muscles can be made. This is illustrated for normal binocular vision in Figure 3.3. Depression of the eyes is maintained by the inferior rectus when the eyes are turned outward, by both muscles when fixing in the median plane, and by the superior oblique when turned inward.

It follows from this that an inability of one eye to maintain elevation or depression when turned outward is most likely to be caused by an anomaly of the superior or inferior rectus muscle. An inability to maintain elevation or depression when abducted is caused by an anomaly of one of the oblique muscles. Difficulty in elevation or depression when fixing in the median plane is likely to indicate a malfunction of several muscles or some more general orbital anomaly.

The motility test is the only clinical method of detecting noncomitancy objectively in routine eye examination. Small deviations of an eye in a tertitary position are not easy to see. Observation of the corneal reflection makes them easier to detect. Also, the eye's position is compared with the lid positions. The lid openings are not symmetrical, but the position of one eye during dextroversion can be compared with the other eye on levoversion. Fortunately, underaction of a muscle often is accompanied by an overaction of the contralateral synergic muscle, and this exaggerates the angle and assists detection.

Patients with active pathology will nearly always have diplopia. The exception is when a pathologic cause occurs in a patient who has had a long-standing squint, deep amblyopia in one eye, or both. Where there has been no previous squint, very small degrees of diplopia can be appreciated by the patient, making diagnosis more certain. The subjective analysis of the oculomotor deviation can be assisted by the use of red-green diplopia goggles.

The usual elderly patient suffering from sudden diplopia will be mentally alert and can readily appreciate small degrees of diplopia when wearing red-green goggles and also can appreciate and report changes in the magnitude of the diplopia as fixation is changed into the different fields of gaze. This subjective evaluation is more sensitive and quicker than the objective observation of restrictions in ocular movements when the patient is mentally alert. If the fixation target is a streak of light rather than just a spot, the patient can report whether the target tilts as the gaze is changed. This helps differentiate between an involvement of one of the oblique muscles and an involvement of one of the vertically acting recti. (The fixation light can be changed most easily to streak by using a Maddox rod before one eye instead of the red-green goggles.)

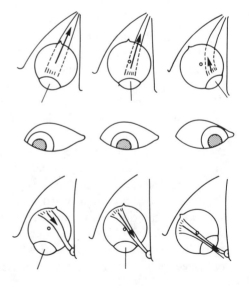

Figure 3.3 Relative actions of the inferior rectus and superior oblique muscles as the eye moves across the bottom of the motor field in the positions shown (Center). The power of the inferior rectus to depress the eye is maximum when the eye is turned outward and the muscle pulls over the center of rotation, and minimum when the eye is turned inward (Top). The lower figures show the increase of the power of the superior oblique to depress the eye as it moves in the same direction from the abducted to the adducted position.

Where it is appropriate to monitor any change in a noncomitant deviation, a quantitative analysis can be made. All methods of recording the actual amount of noncomitancy rely on measurements of the subjective diplopia in different parts of the field. The Hess screen or one of its modifications is the most appropriate method for doing this.

Lid Signs

Abnormalities of the lids sometimes may indicate the presence of noncomitant deviations in elderly people. The width of the lid openings should be observed with the eyes in the primary position and during the motility test.

Lid Openings in the Primary Position

Compare the right and left palpebral fissures. The depth can be judged by comparing the amount of the limbus visible through the fissure. In elderly patients, less of the upper part of the limbus is seen with the eyes in the primary position. An abnormally wide fissure (Dalrymple's sign of thyrotoxicosis) may be accompanied by hypophoria or hypotropia, which increases on elevation of the eyes. A hypotropic position of one eye may be revealed by pseudoptosis; the upper lid is slightly lower as the eye is turned down. Ptosis may be a sign of third nerve palsy.

Lid Openings during the Motility Test

A failure of the upper lid to follow downward movements of the eyes (von Graefe's sign) also may be present in thyroid conditions.

Abnormal Head Postures

In elderly patients, a habitual abnormal head posture can be present in a number of circumstances, which vary from unilateral deafness to oculomotor anomalies. Recently acquired abnormal head position is significant in diagnosing paretic oculomotor conditions. Abnormal head postures also can be caused by a recession of the near point of convergence, out-of-date spectacle corrections, or restrictions of the field of view in one or both eyes.

As a response to an oculomotor anomaly, an abnormal head posture is an attempt to compensate for the binocular vision difficulty by holding the head in a position that gives more comfortable single vision. It therefore indicates that binocular vision is possible in at least part of the motor field. It may be adopted in the early stages of a paresis, when there is still binocular vision in one direction of gaze. With other patients, no such compensation is possible, and diplopia is present in all directions from the dramatic onset of the disease. Sometimes an abnormal head posture will be adopted as the paresis diminishes. The patient then may cease to complain of diplopia.

Sometimes an abnormal head posture can be used to compensate for congenital conditions throughout life; in elderly patients, however, the head tends to straighten, and this gives rise to intermittent diplopia. Old photographs of the patient will show if there had been an abnormal head position for most of the patient's life (Hugonnier and Hugonnier 1969).

An unusual head position may be thought of as having one or more components:

1. *Facial turn to the left or right.* By itself, such a habitual turn may accompany an anomaly of a medial or lateral rectus muscle. For example, diplopia may be avoided in right lateral rectus palsy by turning the face to the right so that contraction of the right lateral rectus muscle is not necessary.

2. *Lowered or raised chin.* This may occur in the A or V syndromes, which are congenital deviations. A raising or lowering of the chin, however, may accompany other components of the abnormal head positions that are caused by paresis.

3. *Head tilt.* If binocular vision is present in only part of the motor field, the head tilt may make it easier to avoid diplopia or extend the area of single vision. The head tilt usually is combined with a facial turn and a raised or lowered chin. The direction of the tilt may be determined by the interests of leveling the diplopic images to assist fusion or by the attempt to compensate for the loss of cyclorotation of one eye if there is paresis of one of the oblique muscles.

Localization Disturbances

The localization of objects in space is determined by a combination of two visual mechanisms: sensory retinal localization and the motor system. The position of the image on the retina determines the direction in which it will be perceived (its visual location). Because the eyes and the head can move, the brain must take these movements into account in localizing objects in space. Disturbances of localization can occur in either the retinal or motor aspects of the combined system. Eccentric fixation will disturb the retinal system, and past pointing may occur. Also, if the eyes do not move correctly in response to the nerve impulses sent out from the brain, as in paretic squint, the motor system will be disturbed. The patient will not be able to locate things correctly and will have difficulty moving about. This will be more marked if the unaffected eye is covered or closed.

The past pointing test may be used to demonstrate these motor disturbances. It is applied monocularly to each eye in turn. The past pointing will be most marked in the eye with the affected muscles. The degree of past pointing will increase in the direction of gaze of the primary action of the affected muscle, and it will not occur in the opposite direction of gaze. The test can be made more effective by holding a card horizontally at the level of the patient's upper lip. A small object is placed on the far edge of the card, and the patient is asked to point with a finger under the card to the position directly below where the object is perceived to be. The card occludes the patient's hand from view and insures that the location of the object is determined only by the motor system. The patient's head is kept still while the object is moved across the field, and the patient is required to locate it with the eyes in different directions of gaze.

EXTERNAL EXAMINATION AND OPHTHALMOSCOPY

The general appearance of the patient may show an obvious squint. Scars or asymmetries of the orbital region may indicate a previous injury. Eye signs of systemic disease may be present; for example, there may be exophthalmos, ciliary injection, or ptosis. The internal examination of the eyes also may reveal signs of vascular or metabolic disease, which may be accompanied by a noncomitant deviation and therefore help confirm the diagnosis that medical help is needed.

EVALUATION

Having carried out full optometric examination that gives special emphasis to the aspects previously discussed, it is necessary to assess the results. No one clinical procedure will indicate in every case that a binocular vision anomaly involving the oculomotor system is pathologic. In some cases, it will be very easy to decide, but in others, a careful evaluation of all the clinical findings will be necessary. The practitioner needs to look at all the results of all the tests undertaken and ask, "What does it all add up to?" A sudden onset of diplopia in elderly patients can have a number of nonpathologic causes that have created the decompensation of the binocular vision. An adverse change in visual working conditions, the need for up-to-date spectacle correction, worry and anxiety, and old age itself can all cause a long-standing heterophoria to become decompensated. It would be wrong, however, to attribute all decompensated heterophoria to these causes without carefully considering the possibility of pathology.

Similarly, noncomitancy can be long-standing and not the result of active pathology. Where it exists, careful evaluation is required in the interests of the patients' getting the sort of care they need. A summary of the factors that will help assess noncomitancy deviations is given in Table 3.1.

POSSIBLE CAUSES OF BINOCULAR PATHOLOGY

In deciding if a patient with a noncomitant deviation requires immediate medical investigation, it is often helpful to be aware of the conditions that can cause ocular paresis and the other signs and symptoms that may accompany them. In the elderly patient, a very large number of conditions may have paretic

Table 3.1 Comparison of long-standing noncomitant deviations with those of likely pathologic cause

Factor	Signs of Long-standing or Congenital Deviations	Signs of Deviations of Likely Pathologic Cause
Diplopia	Unusual	Always present in at least one direction of gaze
Onset	Usually gradual; the patient may not know when	Sudden and distressing
Amblyopia	Often present	Very unlikely
Comitancy	Increases with time; becomes nearly comitant	Always noncomitant
Abnormal head posture	Slight, but persists on covering the paretic eye	More marked; patient aware of it; disappears on covering the paretic eye
Past pointing	Absent	Present
Other symptoms	Unlikely	May be present because of the primary cause

deviations as part of their characteristics. These include infections of the nervous system, metabolic disorders, vascular lesions, neoplasms, and toxic conditions. Some of the conditions that most commonly occur with older patients and can present ocular palsy as an early sign follow. The signs and symptoms that also could be present in these conditions also are summarized, as these can help diagnose the deviation as being of recent pathologic cause. These conditions also are reviewed in other chapters.

Diabetes

A high percentage of ocular palsy is found in diabetic patients. It usually affects the third cranial nerve and sometimes may include pupillary anomalies. In older patients, the onset is usually gradual.

In addition to the diplopia, general symptoms may include generalized headache, increased thirst and urination, increased appetite with loss of weight, constipation, and boils or other skin conditions. When diabetes occurs in older patients, it is more frequent in overweight women.

Thyrotoxicosis

Thyrotoxicosis can occur with muscle palsy but without the exophthalmos. There usually is difficulty in elevation of the eyes, and more than one muscle is involved. A contracture of the inferior rectus is most frequent; this may give a clinical picture of a palsy of the superior rectus muscle.

General signs and symptoms may include exophthalmos (resulting from the enlargement of the muscle tissue in the orbit), von Graefe's sign, retraction of the upper lid, infrequent blinking, conjunctival injection, and vertical diplopia. It occurs more in older females and may be accompanied by increased appetite with loss of weight, clammy hands, and tremor of the outstretched hand and arm.

Hypertension

The chances of high blood pressure's being accompanied by ocular palsy increase with age as the blood supply to the cranial nerves becomes involved. Hypertension is the cause of about 10% of muscle palsy in older patients. There usually are fundus signs of the vascular changes. General symptoms may include headache that is present early in the day, dizziness, breathlessness, and ringing in the ears.

These are perhaps the three most common underlying causes of pathologic deviations in elderly people. It must be remembered, however, that other conditions may give incomitant deviations. Another aspect that may help diagnosis is the recognition of particular palsies.

Fourth Nerve, or Superior Oblique Palsy

Fourth nerve, or superior oblique palsy, is most common as a congential palsy or as a result of an accident, but it may occur after an intercranial vascular accident. Diplopia will be greatest when the patient is looking down and in or when reading.

Sixth Nerve, or Lateral Rectus, Palsy

The long intracranial nerve path of the sixth nerve makes it particularly susceptible to the sort of lesions that occur in later life. Because of the close association of the seventh cranial nerve in the midbrain, the facial muscles also may be involved.

Third Nerve Palsy, or Ophthalmoplegia

If the extrinsic ocular muscles are involved, the condition is known as *external ophthalmoplegia;* it is called *complete oculomotor palsy* if all are involved. Paresis of the ciliary muscles and sphincter of the iris is known as *internal ophthalmoplegia,* and when both internal and external muscles are affected, there is *total ophthalmoplegia.* In the latter case, there will be a divergent squint with the eyes slightly depressed, as well as a loss of accommodation and pupil action. Other accompanying symptoms can include headache, a tremor of contralateral limbs resulting from the involvement of the red nucleus where the third nerve fibers pass, and the other symptoms that may be present in diabetes.

Gaze Palsies

Gaze palsies occur because of lesions in the frontal motor center, gaze centers in the pons, or the interconnecting pathways. There is seldom diplopia, but the eyes move together in most directions of gaze. In one direction, however, the eyes cannot move reflexly to take up fixation, or more rarely, they cannot follow a moving target (pursuit palsy). In lateral gaze palsy, the two eyes do not move beyond the midline. In vertical gaze palsy, movements above the horizontal are restricted, or there is no movement at all; rarely, there is no downward movement.

REPORTING AND REFERRAL

It is first essential to decide if the oculomotor anomaly is likely to have a contributory cause that requires medical attention. From the discussion so far, it is clear that the clinical procedures, the history, and the symptoms may cause the practitioner to suspect that pathology is present. Further questioning of the patient may reveal signs and symptoms of general bodily conditions that the patient has not previously mentioned. This is particularly true in the early stages when intermittent diplopia is the patient's main reason for consultation, and the other symptoms have not yet become a very major cause of concern to the patient. In such cases, the patient may have a heterophoria rather than an actual squint. However, during the examination, it may be found that the binocular vision is very unstable and likely to break down into a squint if some slight impediment is applied. For example, a septum that dissociates the center of the field, as in the Turville infinity balance method, sometimes will cause binocular vision to break down. Fixation disparity may be present and may increase if the patient's eyes are not in the primary position. The patient can be asked to report any fixation disparity with a Disparometer or Mallett Fixation Disparity unit with the head in the primary position and then with the head tilted so that the eyes are moved into a tertiary position relative to the orbits. Another useful procedure is to repeat the cover test with the eyes looking in different directions of gaze. A failure of the normal heterophoria recovery movement in one direction of gaze can give a useful indication of noncomitant heterophoria. However, it must be remembered that if this test is applied while the patient is wearing a correction for anisometropia, the differential prismatic effect will change the apparent degree of heterophoria, but not just in one direction of gaze.

If a pathologic cause is suspected, referral needs to be considered, along with whether to refer the patient to a general medical practitioner, an ophthalmologist, or a neurologist. If the patient is under the care of a general physician, a report of the optometrist's examination should go to the physician, particularly when the coordination of the patient's health care is being undertaken through such a general medical practitioner, as is the case in many countries. The report should include the diagnosis made or suspected and the ocular signs and symptoms that have led to this conclusion. This will enable the doctor to know where to begin the medical investigation or whether to refer the patient on to a specialist colleague. When a vascular accident or other urgent problem is apparent, the patient should be referred straight to the appropriate specialist, and a copy of the report sent to the general practitioner.

Patients with general bodily conditions also may require optometric care of some kind. Usually, elderly patients require at least a pair of reading glasses. These may require some prism relief in the case of small or intermittent deviations. However, this may be only a temporary measure, as the primary condition may improve; as the condition responds to treatment or to time, it is to be hoped that the binocular problem also will be alleviated. When optometric treatment of any kind is given or considered, it is useful to mention this in the report to the medical advisor.

In some cases, the patient's general condition already may be receiving medical attention. For example, this is often the case with vascular conditions in elderly patients. When this is the case, the optometric care usually can proceed, and the ocular deviation be reported to the medical practitioner so that this development can be taken into account in the general health care of the patient. This is particularly true of those cases in which the binocular anomaly is in its early stages. As mentioned earlier, other cases are more likely to have a dramatic onset of diplopia and other marked symptoms of the primary condition, which takes them to a medical practitioner in the first place rather than to the optometrist.

The possibility of detecting a pathologic deviation in its early stages should be a primary concern of optometrists in respect to elderly patients with heterophoria or intermittent squint. This possibility must always be kept in mind, and the optometric examination must include the necessary clinical procedures to diagnose deviations with a primary cause that indicates the patient requires medical attention.

REFERENCES

1. Duke-Elder, S. *System of Ophthalmology:* 6. Ocular Motility and Strabismus. London: Kimpton, 1973.
2. Hugonnier, R., and S.C. Hugonnier. *Strabismus, Heterophoria and Ocular Motor Paralysis.* Translated by S. Veronneau-Troutman. St. Louis: CV Mosby, 1969.
3. Pickwell, L.D. "Analysing Eye Movements." *Aust. Optom.* (May 1974): 154–158.
4. Pickwell, L.D. Incomitant Deviations: 2. *Optician* (April 24, 1981):11–15.

SUGGESTED READINGS

1. Ball, G.V. *Symptoms in Eye Examination.* London: Butterworth Scientific, 1982.
2. Burian, H.M., and G.K. von Noorden. *Binocular Vision and Ocular Motility.* St. Louis: CV Mosby, 1974.
3. Moses, R.A. *Adler's Physiology of the Eye: Clinical Application.* St. Louis: CV Mosby, 1981.
4. Pickwell, L.D. "Basic Clinical Concepts in Binocular Vision: Incomitant Deviations." *Optician* (March 27, April 24, May 22, June 26, 1981).

4

Ocular Disease in the Elderly

David D. Michaels

Each age has its virtues and its defects, its chores and its delights. The defects, unhappily, multiply disproportionately as we grow older. A dismal list of cumulative incapacities fills the geriatric literature. We progress, according to the latest statistics, in ever-increasing numbers toward second childhood. We are embalmed from birth, it seems, by the genetic limits of our protoplasm. If, therefore, little can be said for old age, even less can be asserted for the alternative. We cling to our universe for fear of finding something worse; however poor may be the start, few are anxious to depart.

AGING: A PERSPECTIVE

What is aging? Decay of the flesh, loss of vital substance, entropy, the victory of catabolism over anabolism. It is the stage when other people look old who have reached our age. It is wisdom without tranquility, compassion without passion. All definitions incorporate the element of time; every night we are poorer by a day. Aging is universal, progressive, inescapable, mainly intrinsic, and generally deleterious. It is evolution's way of getting rid of the superfluous. Its features, after centuries of inquiry, continue to attract because of our awe of life and fear of death. The chronicle of the care of the elderly is the history of civilization.

What causes aging? Theories of aging are rather vague. Most concentrate on the genetic apparatus, the intercellular substance, and the noxious effects of the environment. Cellular hypofunction is illustrated by a decline in DNA and RNA synthesis. A hereditary influence on life expectancy is demonstrable by twin and familial studies. Sustained sublethal injury leads to intracellular inclusions of glycogen, complex lipids, and pigments. Intercellular accumulations of amyloid are seen in aging tissues. Some tissues grow old as a direct result of wear and tear, evident in teeth, bone, cartilage, and joints.

Is aging inevitable? Current evidence suggests that it is. The life span of normal human cells (in contrast to malignant ones) is only about 50 doublings before they are no longer capable of replication. Nor does transplanting the cell into a fresh environment alter these limits. Not only do genetic factors regulate life cycle, they also affect how and to what degree a cell responds to injury. For example, patients with xeroderma pigmentosa have a genetically determined enzyme deficiency that prevents repair of DNA in squamous epithelium after ultraviolet exposure.

Is aging a disease? Normal aging affects all body functions, and it is difficult to separate the physiologic from the pathologic. Ischemia, for example, increases the rate of anaerobic glycolysis, causing a sodium-potassium imbalance that leads to intracellular edema and eventual death. The same effect can be produced by trauma, infection, toxins, and metabolic disorders. The similarity of the biochemical and structural end result — whatever the cause of cellular injury — has been termed the final common path. Aging and disease are but collateral channels to this terminal goal.

Can aging be prevented? From a therapeutic point of view, differences between normal aging and disease are largely irrelevant. If the loss of immunologic and hormonal mechanisms reduces the body's ability to repair itself, such deficiencies can be medically replaced, toxic agents can be removed, infections can be combated, and harmful radiations can be filtered. In fact, the increased longevity we enjoy today is largely the result of intervention at the environmental level. No one knows what controlled genetic manipulations hold for the future. In the meanwhile, many complications of aging can be postponed to achieve that contentment which is the nectar, if not the spice, of life.

THE AGING EYE

Senescence is inevitable, but not identical, for everyone; the strands of life unravel at different rates for the eye as well as other organ systems. Ocular morphologic changes are usually bilateral; often symmetrical; and, although not constant, fairly typical. Functional visual deficits exhibit a spectrum ranging from those that restrict daily activities to some that can be demonstrated only in the laboratory. These changes deserve close scrutiny, for they place the ophthalmic diseases of later life in proper perspective.

The enophthalmos of aging is more apparent than real. Although orbital fat may shrink and fascial connections loosen, the primary factor is flaccidity of the lids. Older people exhibit a decrease in appositional tension between the eyeball and the ease with which the lid may be lifted off the globe. With advancing age, the lateral canthus drifts inward, shortening the palpebral aperture. The increased flaccidity of the lower lid may result in an inward flip (senile entropion) or an outward sag (senile ectropion). Vertical dimensions of the palpebral aperture also diminish due to reduced function of the levator and sagging skin. Flaccid lids may not adequately support a hard contact lens and make its removal from the eye more difficult.

In older eyes, the distance between preseptal and pretarsal portions of the orbicularis is reduced; hence, the force exerted on the lacrimal fascia is diminished. Failure of the lacrimal pump coupled with displacement of the lacrimal punctum results in epiphora. Since tear production decreases with age, the older eye cries less but waters more.

The skin of the lids, like skin elsewhere, dries out from loss of oily secretions. The hair grays, and eyebrows and lashes thin out. The dermis becomes dehydrated and loses its elasticity and vascularity. Atrophy of subcutaneous fat leads to wrinkling and deepens the lid folds. Sagging skin may rest on the lashes to produce pseudoptosis. Orbital fat prolapses to form the typical bulge at the inner half of the upper lid. Freckles and lentigo are common, and the skin itself acquires a yellow tinge. Melanophore migration sometimes involves both lids and resembles ecchymosis. Baggy lower lids may represent not only relaxed tissue, but accumulation of fluid from cardiac or renal failure. Benign tumors such as papillomas, xanthelasma, and keratoses are common in the elderly. Cosmetic surgery may be indicated in the eternal struggle to remain young or, at least look young.

The aging conjunctiva becomes thinner, more friable and acquires a yellow color. Loss of transparancy results from hyaline and fatty changes. Hyaline degeneration refers to the deposition of a homogeneous eosinophilic material — either within cells or in the interstitial spaces — probably from excess glyco-proteins. Fatty deposits probably are derived from damaged tissues. Two common conjunctival lesions in the aged are pingueculae and pterygiums. A pinguecula is a small, yellowish, elevated mass in the interpalpebral fissure and represents degenerated collagen fibers. Pterygiums are probably further progressions to form the characteristic triangular fold of tissue that invades the cornea. The prevalence of these lesions in the exposed areas of the bulbar conjunctivae supports the concept of an external irritant. Areas of keratinization produce the pearly appearance of Bitot's spots and may result not only from malnutrition, but also from chronic exposure, as in lagophthalmos and exophthalmos. Inspissated concretions in the upper tarsus can feel like a foreign body.

Tear production diminishes with age and can be recognized by a smaller-than-normal tear film meniscus and a positive Schirmer test (less than 15 mm wetting). The normal tear film is composed of an outer lipid layer, a middle aqueous layer, and an inner mucin layer. The lipid layer prevents evaporation, and the mucin layer aids in maintaining adhesion to the corneal epithelium. Each of the three layers may be selectively involved by disease. Aqueous deficiency is most common and is termed *keratitis sicca* (as contrasted to Sjögren syndrome, characterized by dry eyes, xerostomia, and rheumatoid arthritis). The effect of the aqueous deficiency on the cornea include desiccation, dry spots (dellen), erosions, neovascularization, and scarring. Tear deficiency may preclude satisfactory adjustment to contact lenses. Recent evidence suggests that excess tear evaporation plays a significant role in dry eye syndromes.

Aging changes in the cornea include stippling of Bowman's membrane (crocodile shagreen), destruction of Bowman's membrane near the limbus (white limbus girdle), excrescences on Descemet's membrane (Hassall-Henle bodies), and arcus senilis. Hassall-Henle bodies appear as dark holes in the endothelium when observed by specular reflection with the biomicroscope. Annular accumulations of lipids in the peripheral cornea produce the arcus senilis, which may be complete or incomplete. The cause is probably local, induced by sclerosis of the perilimbal vascular plexus. The fatty deposits are separated from the limbus by a characteristic clear interval. Optical changes in the aging cornea consist of increased light scatter and an overall flattening, most marked in the vertical meridian.

The sclera becomes more transparent and yellowish with age, due to dehydration and lipid deposits. The yellow color should not be confused with jaundice. Local areas of excessive translucency (hyaline plaques) may be mistaken for tumors or inflammation. Intrascleral nerve loops are sometimes misdiagnosed as melanomas. Increased scleral rigidity with age has clinical application in interpreting Schiøtz tonometry and tonography.

The anterior chamber becomes progressively shallower with age due to growth of the crystalline lens. The potential risks of angle closure following mydriatics therefore increase, and a flashlight estimate of chamber depth should be made before drugs are instilled. Increased hyalinization of the trabeculae, changes in the trabecular ground substance, and loss of endothelial lining cells make the older eye more susceptible to glaucoma. There is no definite evidence, however, that aqueous outflow decreases with age in normal eyes.

Atrophic changes in the iris are evident as depigmentation, pigment migration, and opacification of the supporting tissue. Surface markings and crypts may be obliterated, resulting in partial color change. The collagen fibers aggregate and hyalinize, so tissue elasticity decreases. The pupil therefore becomes more rigid and does not dilate as readily in the dark. Liberated pigment is carried by aqueous convection currents and deposited on the posterior corneal surface (Krukenberg's spindle), on the lens, and in the lower portion of the chamber angle.

Failure of the pupil to dilate well is one factor in the complaint of poor night vision by older people. Contributing to the pathophysiology are reduced retinal illumination, crystalline lens discoloration and opacification, increased light scatter, uncorrected senile myopia, and a slower rate of dark adaptation. Changes in adaptation are probably the result of slower photoreceptor processing and nerve conduction, but the exact cause is not known. Increased reaction time and perceptual delays perhaps also play a role.

The ciliary muscle atrophies with age, but this does not appear to contribute to presbyopia, and the AC/A ratio does not increase. Thus, phorias tend to shift to an exo rather than an eso direction. An eso shift would represent increased ciliary effort to drive the accommodative mechanism. Interestingly, the circular part of the ciliary muscle undergoes marked degeneration, whereas the longitudinal fiber bundles that attach to the scleral spur remain practically unchanged.

Morphologically, the ciliary processes become hyalinized, and these areas may contain granular calcium deposits. The thickness of the external limiting membrane increases with age, and the blood vessels undergo sclerosis and eventual obliteration. Aqueous secretion diminishes somewhat in older eyes.

The crystalline lens continues its growth throughout life, although the rate slows with age. Sclerosis of the lens substance and decreased elasticity of its capsule are the main factors causing loss of accommodation. Progressive lens surface flattening is compensated by compaction of the nucleus, so no significant change in refraction occurs. Perhaps most remarkable is that these changes occur in all lens meridians symmetrically and in both eyes simultaneously.

Cataract is superimposed on the normal aging of the lens, and, indeed, differences may be imperceptible in early stages. Among well-established age changes are an increased proportion of insoluble proteins, yellow discoloration, and increased lens weight. Biochemical alterations reflect a progressive decrease in metabolic activity. Yellowing represents an oxidation byproduct — perhaps of tryptophan and tyrosine — in which ultraviolet exposure may play a role. Lens fluorescense is also greater. Lens weight increases three times or more from birth to old age.

Age changes of the vitreous consist of liquefaction, cavitation, shrinkage, and detachments. Fibrillar aggregates may cast a shadow on the retina if the pupil is small and become visible as muscae volitantes. Contraction of the vitreous gel with a separation of solid and liquid components is termed *syneresis*. This may occur 10 to 20 years earlier in myopic eyes.

The choroid is the vascular and pigmented tunic of the eye. Blood vessels reach it from both anterior and posterior vessels and nourish the outer half of the retina and all of the fovea. The thickness of the choroid gradually diminishes with age due to arteriolar sclerosis, even in the absence of systemic vascular disease. Atrophic changes are particularly prominent around the optic disc (senile peripapillary atrophy). Diffuse attenuation of pigment occurs regularly with age and gives the senescent fundus its tessellated appearance.

The retina is the central nervous system outpost of the brain. Since it cannot regenerate, retinal disorders are always sight threatening. The aging retina becomes thinner due to loss of neural cells. In the periphery, actual spaces appear, which may coalesce to form vacuoles (peripheral cystic degeneration). Lipofuscin, the degradation product of photoreceptor discs, accumulates in pigment epithelial cells and displaces melanin. The glistening ophthalmoscopic reflexes of the youthful fundus disappear, and the foveal reflex is lost. Degenerative changes in the optic nerve include corpora amylacea and arenacea. These basophilic staining bodies are visible only on histologic specimens and have no clinical significance.

Our list of changes peculiar to each ocular tissue would tend to suggest that the older eye does not see because nothing is as it used to be. In fact, visual function remains remarkably efficient in the absence of disease. Acuity declines very little, visual fields remain full, ocular motility stays brisk, and night vision is only slightly impaired. Of course, there are annoyances, fortunately mostly minor. We must learn to put up with presbyopia and bifocals, with color deficiencies under reduced illumination and fluorescent lights, with spots and dots in our visual field, and with assorted cosmetic blemishes. Overall, however, if work is less fun and fun is more work, we must blame ourselves rather than our eyes.

CLINICAL EVALUATION OF THE AGED EYE

Examination of the aged eye does not differ in essentials from any other eye, except it takes more time, more tact, and more patience. It takes more time, because older people frequently have many nonspecific complaints, poorly expressed and sequentially muddled. Some symptoms may go unreported because of memory loss, fear, or indifference. It takes more tact, because, in the nature of things, some senescent diseases are not only chronic, but irreparable. Clinicians must suppress their own feelings of impotence and stress the positive aspects. It takes more patience, because the aged eye often suffers multiple defects that must be sorted out. For example, a person with reduced acuity may have some corneal endothelial changes, some lens vacuoles, some macular pigment dispersion, some amblyopia, and some misplaced spectacles. These causes must be partitioned, since each can contribute to the decreased vision, which may not even be the chief complaint.

Older patients should never be treated condescendingly, called by their first name, or addressed by fatuous words of endearment. It gives me great pleasure to converse with the aged, wrote Plato, they have been over the road that all of us must travel, and know where it is rough and difficult, and where it is level and easy.

To define an illness, goes the proverb, don't ask the doctor — ask the patient. Expert diagnosticians consistently emphasize listening to patients for they are telling you the diagnosis. But listening must be analytic to develop the sequence of the disease process, and it must be informed to group the findings into recognizable syndromes. Psychogenic complaints are not unusual and often represent attempts to gain attention, affection, or respect. The office visit can be a major event in the life of the elderly, and the clinician should seize this opportunity to bolster their confidence and dignity.

Much information can be obtained by simple observation — indeed, as soon as the patient walks into the room. Skin color and texture, posture and gait, cranial and facial features, ptosis and ectropion, head tilt and strabismus — all have diagnostic meaning to the alert examiner. A shrewd guess of the life course can be made by comparing apparent and stated age. Old photographs are sometimes helpful to separate acute from chronic afflictions.

Of all the criteria of visual performance, acuity is the simplest, the most widely used, and the most clinically rewarding. It is true that the Snellen chart is poorly standardized and poorly calibrated, and the test is sometimes poorly administered. But it is surprisingly accurate, and it has maintained that reputation after a century of practical use. The responses of patients with scotomas, hemianopia, amblyopia, latent nystagmus, ptosis, myopia, and presbyopia — although not diagnostic — are highly suggestive. Some lens opacities interfere with acuity more in dim light; some, more in bright light. Subcapsular opacities tend to compromise near vision more than distance vision. The decreased acuity of macular edema may be accompanied by metamorphopsia; that of corneal edema, by halos and coronas. Of course, all this information will be missed if the acuity examination is delegated to an assistant.

The absence of light perception is a serious diagnosis and carries with it many therapeutic limitations. Patients tend to confabulate invisible targets because hope springs eternal, and surgical procedures to restore function will be disappointing for all concerned if light perception is absent. The diagnosis, therefore, should be made not only on the basis of subjective responses, but on objective evidence of an amaurotic pupil.

Contrast sensitivity is a new method of evaluating acuity. Unlike high-contrast optotypes, gratings can be adjusted spatially and temporally to analyze high- and low-frequency loss. But, the tests take more time and are not easily understood by older patients. Clinical correlations with disease also have not been established. Contrast sensitivity, like standard acuity, is influenced by refractive errors. Moreover, no optical aids are available to correct low-frequency loss.

The aging crystalline lens creates the effect of looking through a yellow filter. Although color discrimination is not seriously affected, aging of the lens sometimes leads to peculiar responses in duochrome refractive tests. More important, by checking color vision for each eye separately, one occasionally can pick up supporting evidence for macular or optic nerve disease.

Vision takes time, a factor usually ignored in practice, not because it is irrelevant, but because there are no convenient clinical tests to measure it. Dynamic visual acuity, flicker fusion frequency, perceptual span, reaction time, light adaptation, and masking are examples of theoretically important, but clinically unexplored functions. Exceptions are the time delay in optic nerve conduction manifest as the Marcus Gunn pupil or the analogous Pulfrich phenomenon, the time delay of glare recovery in macular disease, and the focusing inertia patients complain of in early presbyopia.

In contrast to central acuity, perimetry measures the peripheral field of vision. Ideally, every patient should have fields recorded, but this is not always practical. Perimetry is indicated, however, in any elderly patient who gives headache as a primary complaint; who reports flashes, floaters, or curtains in the field of vision; who has episodes of transient visual loss or transient refractive changes; who exhibits personality and cognitive changes, diplopia, or other neuro-ophthalmic signs and symptoms; whose visual deficit cannot be explained by external or ophthalmoscopic findings; and whose intraocular tensions are outside the normal range. Although different parts of the visual field interact to function as a whole, it is useful to separate the central and more peripheral fields. Each can be studied independently by tangent screen and perimeter. Central fields should be done with optical correction; peripheral fields without spectacles. One may need larger-than-average targets for older patients; stimulus size should also be commensurate with available vision. Central fields find the greatest utility in detecting early glaucomatous damage; peripheral fields, in detecting neuro-ophthalmic disorders. Central fields are usually unrewarding in the very old, those with poor vision, and aphakics. In unreliable or bedridden patients, a good confrontation field will identify any significant hemianopia or quadrantic defect. The double-finger counting technique provides rapid information with minimal effort.

Senescent changes in isopter dimensions are common and mostly artifacts due to poor or unsteady fixation, slow reaction time, limited attention span, large nose, overhanging brow, sagging lids, or thick spectacle frames. Another common error in glaucoma follow-ups is to attribute progressive field loss to poor pressure control when increasing lens opacities are actually responsible. To guard against this, fields should be periodically repeated with the pupil dilated. Computerized perimetry is a continuously evolving refinement. Data storage allows comparison of successive fields in the same patient and simultaneous comparison to normals.

The pupil is of signal importance not only in neuro-ophthalmic diseases, but also in the evaluation of any eye with media opacities. If the fundus cannot be seen, one can still formulate an estimate of retinal integrity by noting whether the consensual reflex is present in the other eye.

Pupillary reflexes (direct and consensual) should be obtained with a good light. The best near reflex target is the patient's own finger. Responses are graded from 1 + to 4 +. Anisocoria can be detected only if the eyes are inspected in both dim and bright light. A spurious anisocoria results from a bound-down pupil following an old injury or uveitis. In Horner's syndrome, the abnormal pupil is miotic; in Adie's syndrome, the abnormal pupil is mydriatic. A blind eye still exhibits a near and consensual reflex. Light-near dissociation is not always luetic; more common causes are pituitary lesions, myotonic dystrophy, Adie's syndrome, and aberrant regeneration of the third nerve. The afferent pupillary defect (Marcus Gunn pupil) is best elicited with the swinging flashlight test. Shining the light from one eye to the other, one sees a pupil dilation instead of constriction – an apparent paradoxical reaction. The significance of the Marcus Gunn pupil is that it practically always means a conduction defect in the optic nerve. Macular disease, media opacities, and amblyopia do not cause afferent pupil defects. A fixed dilated pupil is usually caused by drugs or by third nerve palsy or compression. Myopathies never involve the pupil.

Intraocular tensions should be obtained in every older patient at every routine examination. Applanation tonometry is preferred over Schiøtz, because it is not influenced by ocular rigidity. At any ocular pressure level, however, the risks of glaucomatous damage increase with age. The debate whether ophthalmoscopy or perimetry detects the earliest glaucoma changes ignores the fact that the two methods are complementary, not exclusive. Selective perimetry may save time by concentrating on paracentral scotomas and nasal steps.

Biomicroscopy is a unique method of ophthalmic examination not duplicated by any other technique. It affords visibility of anatomic details not only magnified, but in depth and stereoscopically. It serves as a guide in diagnosis, prognosis, and treatment. The cornea, anterior chamber, iris, and crystalline lens of the aged eye deserve obvious attention and are best evaluated with the biomicroscope. Vitreous prolapse and adhesions may follow lens dislocation or cataract extraction. Iris atrophy, discoloration, adhesions, ruptures, nodules, new vessels, and tumors are readily seen. The classification of senile cataracts is based on slit lamp appearance. The location and fixation of intraocular implants can only be studied biomicroscopically. For general examination, the low power

($10 \times$ to $12 \times$) is most useful. Methods of illumination include diffuse, focal, scatter, retroillumination, indirect, specular, and tangential. Switching from one technique to the other, coupled with oscillations of the beam, becomes automatic after some practice.

Loss of corneal luster is common in older eyes. Sometimes it simply represents a tear deficiency, but in many cases it reflects pathologic surface changes. These might include epithelial edema, erosions, dry spots, scars, infiltrates, tumors, dystrophies, foreign deposits, and neovascularization. Simple flashlight inspection, therefore, can reveal a great deal about the state of corneal health. Corneal curvature can be further documented by keratometry coupled with photographic keratoscopy. Such measurements are useful in following postsurgical healing, fitting contact lenses, analyzing corneal molding by a contact lens or pterygium, or modifying curvature by radial incisions and wedge resections.

Fundus details are best analyzed with direct and indirect ophthalmoscopy. Both methods are based on illuminating the patient's fundus and observing this area with an appropriate optical system. The direct method uses the optics of the patient's eye to obtain a real image; in the indirect method, the reflected rays are focused by the condensing lens to produce an inverted aerial image. Magnification is inversely proportional to the power of the condensing lens. The usual magnification obtained by the direct method is about $15 \times$; with the indirect, about $3 \times$. The field of view is thus about 2 disc diameters with the direct technique and 8 disc diameters with the indirect. The direct method can be compared to the high power and the indirect to the low power of the microscope. The indirect method is indispensable for observation of peripheral degenerative changes common in the elderly. A third method of examination is fundus biomicroscopy with a preset Hruby or contact lens. This technique combines the optical advantage of the slit beam with the magnification of the biomicroscope and might be compared to the oil-immersion power of the microscope. The Hruby lens needs no topical anesthetic; contact lenses require both topical anesthesia and gonioscopic solution. Several wide-angle contact lenses (for example, Panfunduscope) are now available, that give an excellent overall view of the fundus almost up to the ora serrata without mirrors or scleral depression. Subtle vitreous changes can be observed, including cells, cavities, and detachments. Fundus areas of elevation and depression are seen in optic sections, and hemorrhages, exudates, and pigments can be localized in depth. Optic disc imaging with electronic optical instruments and laser scanning are recent advances in diagnostic techniques.

Fundus features of the aged eye that deserve special emphasis are those related to diseases common in later life — namely, the optic disc changes of glaucoma and ischemic neuropathies, the vascular changes of hypertension and arteriosclerosis, diabetic retinopathy in all its variations, macular degeneration, peripheral retinal degenerations, retinal detachment, and the normal aging changes of the choroid and retina previously described.

The integrity of macular function is frequently compromised in the elderly, and the diagnosis may not be obvious from ophthalmoscopic inspection, even under high magnification. A few simple tests are available, however, that can help localize disease to this area. The Amsler grid is a self-administered tangent screen test confined to the central 20 degrees. A reasonably intelligent patient can be instructed to report any distortions in the grid. The test is especially applicable in serous macular detachments and also can be used to follow the progress of the disorder by giving the patient some graph paper for home use. The photo-stress test is a measure of macular glare recovery. One compares the time it takes, after exposure to a strong light, for each eye to recover the maximum acuity of which it is capable. In macular disease, recovery time is significantly prolonged, presumably because photopigment regeneration is delayed. Neutral density filters can differentiate between organic and functional amblyopia. The filter reduces acuity more severely in macular and optic nerve disease than in functional amblyopia.

In contrast to macular disease, optic neuritis causes a decrease in vision characterized by a central scotoma, sometimes a generalized field reduction, defective color vision, and a normal photostress test. In comparing brightness, the patient may report that it appears reduced on the side of the neuritis. This is the subjective analogue of the Marcus Gunn pupil. The swinging flashlight test is, of course, positive in neuritis and normal in macular disease. Red-free ophthal-moscopy may also reveal nerve fiber dropout, atrophy of the disc, and fewer disc capillaries. If the retina is also involved (neuroretinitis), there may be papillitis and perifoveal exudates.

Gonioscopy is indicated in the initial work-up of every glaucoma patient. It differentiates open- from closed-angle mechanisms, the treatment for each of which is fundamentally different. The most popular technique utilizes the biomicroscope and a mirrored contact lens applied to the topically anesthetized eye. The mirror makes an angle of 64 degrees so that the lower chamber angle is seen when the mirror is placed above. Slit lamp magnification of $16 \times$ to $20 \times$ is most suitable, and both broad and narrow beams help define the configuration of the angle. The goniolens is then rotated to study the angle circumferentially. The angle is classified from Grade IV to Grade 0, the latter representing a closed angle. Peripheral anterior synechiae may also block aqueous outflow and can result from uveitis, trauma, previous angle closure, and intraocular surgery. Thus, a combined mechanism may result from a flat chamber following a procedure for open-angle glaucoma. One can observe the presence of new vessels, blood, pigment, tumor cells, and foreign bodies. Congenital adhesions are present in iridocorneal dysgenesis syndromes.

Refraction of the elderly patient proceeds at a more leisurely pace with more tolerance for indecision. Refractive errors are the most common cause of blurred vision, and their rehabilitation has probably added as much to the quality of life and extended its usefulness as any advance in biology. But ametropia and presbyopia also occur in diseased eyes, and it is not unusual to confuse blurred vision with loss of vision. Even patients with cataract or macular disease can often have useful vision restored by proper refraction with or without low-vision aids. The examination of such combined disorders may require stronger light, higher contrasts, and nearer test distances.

Transient refractive changes can only be detected by repeated examination. They may result from drugs used topically or systemically, lens swelling from electrolyte imbalances, and corneal edema from endothelial decompensation or contact lens overwear. Fluctuating ametropia may also occur in retinal edema, with orbital masses and following ophthalmic surgical procedures.

Binocular motility disturbances may result from progressive loss of accommodative vergence in presbyopia. The increased exophoria in cases of fusional deficits may cause intermittent diplopia. Convergence insufficiency is not unusual and may require reducing the add, or utilizing base-in prisms. The latter can sometimes be achieved by spectacle lens decentration or separate reading glasses. Aniseikonia can become symptomatic when unilateral lens swelling induces sudden anisometropia. Such optical incongruities may interfere with stereopsis. Patients wearing aphakic spectacles seldom achieve true binocularity, though they may not complain. Aphakic contact lenses cause about a 6% image disparity, and the binocular potential is somewhat better, but unpredictable. Best results are reached with intraocular implants. Vertigo and spatial distortions are not uncommon complaints in uninitiated bifocal wearers. Aphakic spectacles also cause field restrictions, ring and roving scotomas, and magnification and prismatic displacements with consequent eye-head and eye-hand incoordination and lack of confidence. Unilateral blindness results in sensory exotropia.

Monocular diplopia is a fairly common complaint in the elderly. The usual cause is an improperly positioned bifocal seg. Another common mechanism is a lens vacuole or cleft that acts as a beam splitter. This can be confirmed with a card or pinhole. Other causes are tear film debris, corneal irregularities, oily topical medications, and macular edema.

It may perhaps be useful to summarize this section on examination by re-emphasizing some clinical points. Unlike pathology textbooks, patients seldom present with the names of their disease. Diagnosis proceeds from signs and symptoms, not the other way around. Moreover, textbook descriptions tend to emphasize advanced, or at least typical, features of disease, whereas in practice one often deals with minimal signs. Classic patterns of disease are also altered in the elderly because of greater response variability and concurrent illnesses. Older patients may forget or mix up therapeutic admonitions and instructions. Finally, compliance in diagnostic tests is seldom perfect; hence, cross-checks should be incorporated in the examination to confirm validity.

AGE-RELATED OCULAR DISEASE: TOPICAL ASPECTS

One advantage of aging is that it need not be repeated. But this is not true for diseases. For example, clinical manifestations of retinitis pigmentosa, keratoconus, migraine, diabetes, and multiple sclerosis may recur and progress in later life. It follows that not only are the elderly prone to diseases of old age, but also to the aggregate effects of illnesses whose onset is earlier and that may even be congenital. Although we consider only some age-related diseases, this pathologic background must always be remembered in the differential diagnosis. In all instances, moreover, vision-threatening conditions get priority. Obviously, it is also more important to identify disorders for which effective treatment is available. Thus, papilledema is a critical diagnosis; recognition of optic atrophy can be placed on the back burner. Fortunately, medical and surgical therapy is constantly evolving; many diseases for which no treatment was available only a few years ago can now be controlled or even cured.

Orbital Diseases

Cardinal features of orbital disease are proptosis, ptosis, pain, pulsation, and restricted ocular motility. Other manifestations include choroidal wrinkling and transient hyperopia from pressure on the globe. Neuropathies or myopathies cause diplopia. Trigeminal involvement produces corneal and periorbital anesthesia. Lacrimal complications lead to tear deficiency. Pressure on the optic nerve may cause blindness; extension into the cranial cavity may cause death.

In evaluating orbital disorders, one notes rate of onset, progression, and systemic features of endocrine disease. In addition to inspection, palpation, compression, auscultation, visual fields, forced ductions, plain X-ray, and biopsy, a variety of specialized diagnostic techniques are now available. These include tomography, ultrasonography, venography, arteriography, pneumography, and contrast injections into orbital soft tissues. Computerized tomography and magnetic resonance (MR) imaging have revolutionized noninvasive methods of visualizing orbital tissues; natural high-density differences allow clear distinctions between fat, nerves, muscles, and vessels. MR angiography is a technique for visualizing blood flow.

The most prominent presenting feature of orbital disease is proptosis (or exophthalmos). It may be unilateral or bilateral, and globe displacement may be axial or eccentric. Quantitative measurement with a Hertel-type exophthalmometer document progression and help rule out enophthalmos on the opposite side or an apparent proptosis due to lid retraction. In recording such measurements, one should specify both the degree of protrusion and the interorbital distance, making due allowance for facial asymmetry and parallax. The differential diagnosis usually centers around endocrine exophthalmos, inflammation, pseudotumor, vascular anomalies, true neoplasms, and trauma (for example, hematomas and foreign bodies). Since neoplasms may be primary, metastatic, or involve the orbit by extension from adjacent areas, neurologic, ears, nose, and throat (ENT) and general medical evaluation are often necessary. Laboratory tests for thyroid function, blood dyscrasias, sarcoidosis, diabetes, lues, and systemic infections are part of the work-up.

Infection (cellulitis) causes rapidly developing proptosis with swelling, redness, pain, tenderness, lid edema, chemosis, fever, and leukocytosis. The source may be a foreign body, adjacent sinuses, the eye or its adnexa, or a systemic infection. Chronic cellulitis can occur with dacryoadenitis (Mikulicz syndrome), sarcoidosis, tuberculosis, or lues. An important cause to recognize (because it is potentially lethal) is mucormycosis. This fungus infection occurs in debilitated or diabetic patients, or following cancer chemotherapy. The infection starts in the nose and spreads rapidly as a black gangrenous mass through the soft tissue. Thrombophlebitis and cavernous sinus thrombosis may develop with alarming speed.

Pseudotumor is a nonspecific, chronic inflammatory process that mimics neoplasms. Unlike true tumors, the inflammation eventually involves both sides, some signs of inflammation may be found, there are usually no bone erosions, and it tends to respond to steroids. Indolent inflammation may involve the superior orbital fissure and produce a painful ophthalmoplegia (Tolosa-Hunt syndrome).

Vascular anomalies such as carotid-cavernous fistula or aneurysms exhibit pulsation, and the patient may complain of a bruit. Pulsations also occur because of defects in the orbital roof or angioma and may vary with head position.

Endocrine exophthalmos is considered in a subsequent section. It is important to point out, however, that although this is a systemic illness, the exophthalmos is often unilateral. Eye signs can occur in the absence of obvious thyroid dysfunction.

Orbital tumors in the elderly may be benign or malignant. These include hemangiomas, lymphomas, neuromas, carcinomas, and meningiomas. The diagnosis depends on clinical features and biopsy. X-ray changes in the optic canal may explain compressive optic neuropathy. A- and B-scan ultrasonography can often identify the size, location, configuration, and density of the lesion.

Trauma to the orbit can occur at any age. Like the proverbial broken egg, a fractured orbit is hard to put together again. Deformity, muscle entrapment, persistent diplopia, neural involvement, and enophthalmos are major complications of blow-out fractures of the orbital floor. Optic nerve function must be carefully monitored. Proper surgical repair, properly performed, can usually, but not always, restore normal function.

Diseases of the Lids

Patients with lid disorders may complain of pain, red eyes, itching, tearing, dryness, a sleepy sensation, swelling, tics, and cosmetic deformity. Common lid disorders in the elderly include inflammation, skin problems, ectropion and entropion, ptosis and pseudoptosis, anomalies of lid closure, trauma, and neoplasms.

Examination of the lids includes inspection of the skin, lashes, caruncles, puncta, and eyebrows; palpation for cysts and tumors; compression to determine Meibomian secretions and lacrimal sac regurgitation; evaluation of lid-globe apposition; and estimates of levator and orbicularis function. Since the posterior layer of the lids is continuous with the globe, inflammation of one affects the other, as in allergic dermatoconjunctivitis. The lids also participate in generalized skin diseases such as atopic dermatitis, in metabolic disorders such as diabetes, in collagen diseases such as disseminated lupus, in myopathies such as myasthenia, and in neurologic afflictions such as parkinsonism.

Infection of the lid margin (blepharitis) is common in the elderly and is usually associated with seborrhea of the eyebrows, skin of the nose, cheeks, and scalp. It is a chronic, annoying, sometimes disabling, often disfiguring disorder. The lid margins are red, thickened, may develop ectropion, and dusted by fine dandruff-like flakes. Scarring may result from the lashes rubbing against the cornea. Secondary staphylococcus infections cause styes, ulceration, chalazia, and abscesses. The patient complains of itching; burning; scratching; tearing; and intolerance to light, smoke, and dust. The wrinkled skin, especially at the canthi, predisposes to retention of moisture and tears, causing cracking and further irritation. All this is often complicated by allergic reactions to a variety of prescribed medications and assorted home remedies. This may include steroids used for long periods, causing iatrogenic glaucoma, cataract, superinfection, or reactivation of herpetic ulcers. An often overlooked cause is rosacea; hence, all patients with blepharitis should have their facial skin evaluated.

Allergies result from local interaction of antibodies and antigens, causing release of chemical mediators that act on blood vessels to produce vasodilation and attract additional cells capable of responding to the foreign intruder. Clinical signs and symptoms are lid edema, redness, swelling, itching, eruptions, scaling, eczema, crusting, and lichenification. Of particular importance in the elderly is contact dermatitis caused by drugs, chemicals, cosmetics, and other substances applied to the skin surface. Atopic eczema is caused by pollens, dust, animal substances, and bacterial products in patients predisposed to hay fever and asthma. Finally, some reactions are not allergic, but are direct toxic effects of drugs such as atropine, eserine, phospholine iodide, and assorted antibiotics.

Skin disorders frequently involve the lids of the elderly. Xanthelasma is a yellowish lipoidal degenerative condition typically presenting as a discrete, slightly elevated mass, often symmetrical, near the inner angle. It grows slowly and requires excision only for cosmetic reasons. Large defects may need skin grafting. Papillomas are elevated, localized, warty lesions that should not be confused with infectious verrucae found in the young. Senile keratoses are flat, irregular, slightly brownish lesions, presumably due to long exposure to the sun, and important because they are potentially malignant. Lentigines are senile freckles commonly known as liver spots, though they have nothing to do with liver function. Seborrheic keratoses are elevated, fleshy papules having a stuck-on appearance with a characteristic greasy scale resembling candle wax drippings. Small cysts or milia have an easily recognizable, pearly white appearance; clear cysts of occluded sweat glands disappear when punctured. The eyelids may be involved in psoriasis, pseudoxanthoma elasticum, acne rosacea, and sebaceous adenomas of the face. Senile pruritus from dry, brittle skin is a common complaint that often persists despite all local treatment.

Laxity of the lid margins may lead to eversion or ectropion. Chronic ectropion causes thickening of the lid margins, epiphora, excoriation of the skin, and exposure keratitis. The degree of laxity can be estimated by the force required to pull the lower lid away from the globe. Senile flaccidity is the most common cause of ectropion. In contrast, loose tissue may cause the border of the tarsus to swing in, giving rise to senile (spastic) entropion. The chief symptoms are due to the constant rubbing of the lashes against the cornea, which produces a painful keratopathy. Both ectropion and entropion can be corrected by relatively simple surgical procedures.

Ptosis (blepharoptosis) may be congenital or acquired. The acquired forms can be neurogenic, myogenic, inflammatory, mechanical, or spurious (pseudoptosis). Neurogenic ptosis is seen in oculomotor nerve palsy and Horner's syndrome; myogenic ptosis, in senile loss of levator tone, progressive external ophthalmoplegia, and myasthenia; inflammatory ptosis, in chronic lid edema; mechanical ptosis in lid tumors and scarring; and pseudoptosis, in phthisis and dermatochalasis. In evaluating ptosis, measurements are obtained of the vertical diameter of the palpebral aperture in the primary position, and in up- and down-gaze. The presence of Bell's phenomenon should be noted. A Tensilon test is indicated in a patient with ptosis and diplopia. Photographs are useful to document progression.

Anomalies of lid closure interfere with the tear film and may fail to protect the eye, particularly during sleep. A common cause in the aged is Bell's palsy due to inflammation of the facial nerve in the stylomastoid foramen. Although spontaneous resolution is the rule, a tarsorrhaphy may be needed to protect the cornea in the meanwhile. Orbicularis weakness associated with trigeminal anesthesia, hearing loss, and sixth nerve palsy should lead to intensive investigation for acoustic neuroma.

Blepharospasm is not unusual with a corneal foreign body, keratitis, uveitis, or any condition associated with intense photophobia. It is also a sequel to facial nerve palsy or stroke. It sometimes appears as an isolated, presumably psychogenic phenomenon for which no cause can be discovered. Some of these patients eventually manifest signs of parkinsonism.

Lid lacerations require prompt treatment if they are not to result in corneal exposure, deformity, and disfigurement. The most important part of examining a traumatized lid is to check the eyeball for wounds or foreign bodies. Contusion injuries often cause massive hematomas, which may make examination of the globe difficult without special retractors. Orbital and skull fractures must always be considered. Thermal, radiation, and chemical injuries will require special attention.

The most common malignant lesion of the lid is the basal cell carcinoma. Other neoplasms such as squamous cell carcinoma, adenoacanthoma, cancerous melanosis, and melanoma are rare. In examining a lid lesion, one evaluates size, shape, color, consistency, degree of elevation, ulceration, surrounding hyperemia, location, draining lymph nodes, and associated lesions elsewhere on the skin. The typical basal cell lesion occurs in the lower lid or inner canthus. It presents as a nodule with a central necrotic ulcer that has rolled, raised, pearly borders. Early lesions are nodular without ulcers; atypical lesions may be diffuse, multicentric, or even pigmented. Basal cell carcinomas are slowly progressive and do not metastasize. The diagnosis is established by biopsy.

Diseases of the Conjunctiva

Many factors that normally protect the eye from infection and injury are absent or diminished in the elderly: the flushing action of sufficient tears, the bactericidal action of lysozyme, the mechanical barrier of normal blinking, and the presence of unimpaired immune mechanisms.

The causes of conjunctival disease are numerous: infectious, allergic, toxic, mechanical, traumatic, metabolic, degenerative, vascular, and neoplastic. Symptoms and signs might include hyperemia, exudates, scratchy or burning sensations, tearing, and chemosis. Symptoms may be out of proportion to apparent severity of disease. Pain, photophobia, and decreased vision occur if the cornea is involved; itching, if there is an allergic component.

Evaluation should include a thorough history with respect to acute or chronic onset, the use of drugs or home remedies, predisposition to atopy and blephorrhea, and exposure to either environmental toxins or allergens. A sequential plan of examination is helpful: periorbital skin, lids, lashes, tear film debris, tear break-up time, draining lymph nodes, bulbar and tarsal conjunctiva proper, sclera, cornea, and the remainder of the anterior segment. Specific features of conjunctivitis might include type of exudate, petechiae, membranes and pseudomembranes, granulomas, pigmentation, corneal staining, infiltrates, or neovascularization. The type of conjunctival reaction — papillary or follicular — is most important. Finally, one evaluates the lacrimal sac as a source of infection. Scrapings, culture, and biopsy may be required for a definitive diagnosis.

Bacteria may involve the eye in several ways; they may grow upon the surface and cause damage by liberating exotoxin, they may invade the epithelium, they may grow beneath the epithelium and proliferate in the subepithelial stroma, or they may produce inflammation from a distance by an allergic mechanism. Viruses cause damage within the cell, cause proliferative changes in other cells, or act as antigens. The conjunctival response to infection may be categorized into two broad types: papillary and follicular. Papillae are tufts of new capillaries that rise perpendicularly in the tarsal conjunctiva. Their diameter is about 0.1 mm, and they are separated by colorless, threadlike spaces. Papillae are therefore the direct result of vascular irritation. Follicles represent a lymphoid hyperplasia of the adenoid layer of the tarsal conjunctiva. They are directly proportional to the degree of inflammation. The follicles consist of a dense collection of mononuclear cells separated by clear areas. They are several times larger than papillae and appear as translucent, hemispheric protuberances. Small vessels may climb over their surface but do not appear in the center, as in papillae. While both papillae and follicles are nonspecific and may occur together, the follicular response predominates in viral and toxic disorders.

A common cause of catarrhal conjunctivitis in the elderly is *Staphylococcus* infection. The conjunctiva is edematous and hyperemic, and the papillary response gives it a velvety appearance. Hyperacute infections, as seen in children, are uncommon in adults. The usual symptoms are tearing, discharge, and irritation. Both eyes are generally involved. Lower corneal ulceration is common and may represent a reaction to exotoxins, though this is in dispute. Seborrhea predisposes the eye to chronic infection. Chronic irritation and maceration of the outer canthi may resemble angular conjunctivitis caused by *Moraxella*. Gram-negative infections occur in elderly debilitated individuals, not infrequently from chronic dacryocystitis or contaminated contact lenses.

In contrast to bacterial infections, viruses produce a follicular reaction and regional lymphadenopathy. Corneal involvement is common and often characteristic. The most important viral infection from an epidermiologic viewpoint is adenovirus (epidemic) conjunctivitis. This disease is now endemic, as well as intermittently epidemic. There is marked hyperemia; a follicular reaction; lymphadenopathy; hemorrhages; lid edema; and, in severe cases, pseudomembranes. The clinical picture may resemble an injury. One week after onset, the cornea may show superficial punctate erosions producing a foreign body sensation and photophobia. In about half the cases, this is followed by subepithelial, nonstaining corneal infiltrates that reduce vision and may last for months. The smear/scraping shows predominately lymphocytes. There is no satisfactory treatment for this infection. Recognizing it is important because it can be transmitted by fingers or instruments to one's own eye and to the eyes of other patients. Care should therefore be taken to examine these eyes with a cotton applicator, and hands should be frequently and thoroughly washed.

Toxic follicular conjunctivitis is caused mainly by miotics such as eserine and antiviral agents such as idoxuridine. Occasionally, molluscum contagiosum may shed toxic material into the conjunctival sac and produce a follicular reaction. These conditions are chronic as long as the inducing agent persists. The smear shows as lymphocytic rather than the eosinophilic reaction found in allergy. If chronic corneal involvement occurs, it may result in pannus and scarring.

Not every red eye is caused by infection. Conjunctival congestion can also result from air pollution, ultraviolet exposure, alcohol, and lack of sleep. Passive congestion may be caused by venous obstruction from orbital tumors or dysthyroid ophthalmopathy, as well as by hyperviscosity syndromes such as multiple myeloma. Cavernous sinus fistulas and carotid stenosis produce active congestion. In uveal and scleral disease, the deeper vascular networks are involved, and these may be mistaken for conjunctival vessels.

Allergic conjunctivitis is generally characterized by itching, occasionally burning, and eosinophils in the smear. There is a watery discharge, redness, and papillary reaction, and this may be accompanied by an eczematous skin response. Two major types of allergic mechanisms are recognized: the immediate immunoglobulin-mediated response and the delayed cell-mediated response. The immediate reaction might be caused by grasses, pollens, dust, or similar allergens in predisposed (often atopic) individuals with a family history of allergy and other allergic symptoms such as hay fever, hives, or asthma. The delayed response is commonly precipitated by drugs, chemicals, cosmetics, or even eyeglasses in patients who have no atopic history but may report previous contact with the offending agent. A variant of this is the giant papillary conjunctivitis in response to a foreign body such as contact lenses. Giant papillae are not lymphoid tissue and rather resemble those seen in children with vernal catarrh.

Injuries to the conjunctiva are common and may be mechanical or chemical. Foreign bodies lodged in the fornix can easily be overlooked; even contact lenses have been "lost" in the upper fornix. It is most important to estimate the speed of a particle that struck the eye. Drilling, nailing, and similar activities may allow perforation of the globe; this is not likely with something that "blows" into the eye. If, in addition, there is a conjunctival laceration, soft tissue X-rays and exploration may be advisable.

Chemical burns can be industrial, agricultural, or from the use of household agents. Alkali burns are especially dangerous, because they do not delimit themselves. If the cornea is involved, hospitalization and intensive therapy may prevent permanent scarring. Finally, mild and often unrecognized injuries can cause subconjunctival hemorrhages that, though asymptomatic, greatly alarm the patient. The condition is benign and resolves within a few days. Repeated hemorrhages, however, should trigger an evaluation of drug use and hemotologic disorders.

Diseases of the Cornea

The cardinal features of corneal disease are pain, photophobia, lacrimation, and impaired vision. Pain from corneal disease may be described as sandy, scratchy, burning, or gritty. True photophobia is ocular pain induced or exacerbated by light. It differs from dazzling or glare, in which discomfort results from excessive illumination. Lacrimation is a reflex response to trigeminal stimulation. Impaired vision follows excessive light scatter, clouding of the stroma, epithelial edema, and scarring. Corneal disease in the elderly may result from infections, toxins, metabolic changes, tear deficiency, exposure, trigeminal involvement, trauma, degenerations, and neoplasms.

Corneal examination is best done with the biomicroscope. One notes shape; size; curvature; thickness; luster; opacities; infiltrates; vesicles; ulcers; filaments; pannus; neovascularization; pigmentation; edema; keratic precipitates; hypopyon; blood staining; and involvement of adjacent sclera, conjunctiva, and lids. Corneal sensitivity is checked with a wisp of cotton. Staining characteristics are helpful. Fluorescein stains the stroma where epithelial cells are absent. Rose bengal stains devitalized epithelial cells themselves. The staining pattern may suggest a possible mechanism: linear in abrasions, dendritic in herpes, 3 and 9 o'clock with hard contact lenses, filamentary for keratitis sicca, punctate for many viral diseases, geographic in drug reactions, craterlike in ulcers, involving aqueous in perforating wounds, vesicular in bullous keratopathy, and stippled with topic anesthetics or contact lens overwear. The staining distribution is also helpful: lower cornea in *Staphylococcus* infections and exposure keratopathy and upper cornea in trachoma, verruca, or a foreign body under the lid.

Corneal ulcers are uncommon but may become an emergency in older patients who are diabetic, debilitated, or immune suppressed. Failure to find and treat the cause may lead to corneal scarring at best, or perforation and endophthalmitis at worse. Pyogenic ulcers are gray with poorly defined margins, and there may be iritis, hypopyon, and intense cirumcorneal injection. Fungus ulcers have feathery edges and may have satellite lesions. Smears and cultures are mandatory; they are the only ways to identify the specific organism.

Herpes simplex viruses are a leading cause of corneal disease. The epidemiology is worldwide, and people seem to be the only natural reservoir. Two viral types are recognized; Type I is responsible for ocular and skin infections, while Type II causes neonatal and genital disease. In adults, the ocular disease usually causes dendritic ulcers confined to the corneal epithelium. Attacks may be recurrent, so a history of prior eye or skin lesions is important. In early stages or as a recurrence variant, the infection may present as a superficial punctate keratitis or a localized stromal edema with or without epithelial involvement. The reason for the dendritic pattern is not known. A number of trigger mechanisms may lead to recurrence: fever, sunburn, mechanical trauma, contact lenses, emotional stress, and topical steroids. Stromal disease may be accompanied by iritis and elevated intraocular pressure. In some cases it results in a permanent discoid opacity.

Herpes zoster is caused by the same virus that causes chickenpox but has serious implications in the elderly. First, it often occurs in patients who may have underlying malignancy; second, it can produce severe uveitis, as well as keratitis; third, the corneal lesion may be confused with herpes simplex; and fourth, long after cutaneous lesions heal, neuralgic pains may persist and last for months and even years.

Toxic disorders of the cornea may follow the use of antimalarial drugs such as chloroquine, which produce a characteristic whorllike pattern; hyphema with elevated intraocular tension, which produces blood staining; the use of silver preparations, which cause argyrosis; and retained iron foreign bodies, which cause siderosis. Corneal changes also occur in disorders of fat, protein, copper, and calcium metabolism. Thus, the Kayser-Fleischer ring is pathognomonic of Wilson's disease.

Disorders of the mechanisms that maintain normal corneal deturgescence alter optical homogeneity and therefore transparency. The marked affinity of the cornea for water is counteracted by an active metabolic pump within endothelial cells. Thus, endothelial disease (from dystrophy, trauma, or improper irrigating solutions during intraocular surgery), elevated intraocular pressure, or severe hypotony cause corneal edema. On the epithelial side, water may enter the stroma if the epithelial barrier is broken, the tear film loses its isotonicity, or there is chronic anoxia. Since the cornea swells perpendicular to its surface, edema can be quantified by measuring thickness (pachometry). Biomicroscopically, edema is evident as vertical striae; folds or breaks in Descemet's membrane; increased relucency; and, eventually, by epithelial vacuolization, cysts, and erosions. An important example of endothelial disease is cornea guttata. This is an extension of the process of Hassall-Henle body formation on Descemet's membrane. As the endothelial cells are stretched over these excrescences, they become thinned and eventually disappear with endothelial pump decompensation. Water from the aqueous enters the stroma and percolates into and between epithelial cells. The swollen epithelial cells form vesicles, which burst to cause painful erosions, photophobia, and visual impairment. At this stage, the clinical picture resembles that of any other bullous keratopathy. Causes might include glaucoma, keratonconus, mechanical trauma, inflammation, vitreous touch syndromes, corneal graft failure, and contact lens overwear.

Dry eye syndromes are an important cause of disability in the elderly. Tear volume is reduced, and so is the force and completeness of blinking. This is frequently complicated by lid-cornea incongruities (ectropion, trichiasis, pterygiums, contact lenses, lid margin hypertrophy), or orbicularis weakness. Finally, corneal sensitivity may be decreased. The problem, therefore, is not only that the patient has a dry eye, but that he or she does not blink normally in response to the dryness. This results in dry spots (dellen), which may progress to erosion and ulceration. Symptoms include irritation, foreign body sensation, intolerance to dust and smoke, and, occasionally, excessive tearing. Biomicroscopy reveals an irregular tear meniscus containing mucous debris, corneal filaments, punctate staining in the lower half of the cornea, a rapid tear breakup time (less than 10 seconds), and a positive Schirmer test. In some cases, the clinical picture resembles papillary conjunctivitis.

Exposure keratopathy is a variant of dry eye syndromes in which, because of proptosis or lagophthalmos, the cornea is inadequately protected from tear evaporation. When exposure is coupled to loss of corneal sensitivity, trophic effects can quickly lead to disaster (neuroparalytic keratopathy).

Corneal injuries are common; some causes are abrasions, foreign bodies, chemicals, ultraviolet exposure, and contact lens overwear. Most heal uneventfully and, if not too deep, without significant scarring. In some cases, however, the patient suffers recurrent erosions that present a clinical challenge. In this condition, the epithelium repeatedly breaks down following some minor injury such as a fingernail scratch. Strangely, the recurrence is sometimes at a site different from that of the initial surgery. The clinical picture is characteristic and the diagnosis can almost be made from the history. The patient, weeks or months after the original injury has healed, notes a sudden, sharp pain in the eye on awakening associated with all the other features of an abrasion. The pathology is not clearly understood but is apparently related to some defect in basement membrane synthesis, which holds epithelial cells to the underlying Bowman's membrane.

Corneal neoplasms are rare. Important in the elderly are papillomas, Bowen's disease, and melanomas. Bowen's disease generally occurs at the limbus as an elevated, highly vascularized, gelatinous tissue. Biopsy confirms diagnosis.

The normal cornea is avascular and this protects it from immune mechanisms. Pathologic neovascularization diminishes this isolation and makes prognosis of keratoplasty less favorable. Indications for corneal grafting might include keratoconus, advanced corneal guttata (Fuchs' dystrophy), dense corneal scars, trauma, degenerative ulcers, and neoplasms. Grafts may be total or partial and are designed to achieve optical and/or therapeutic goals. Risks are warranted only when vision is considerably impaired.

Diseases of the Lens

Cataracts are naturally a major topic in any discussion of ocular disease in the aged. The histopathology, despite multivaried clinical appearance, is remarkably uniform: degeneration and atrophy of epithelium, water clefts in the cortex, lens fiber fragmentation, and deposits of crystals such as calcium and cholesterol. Whatever the means, the symptomatic end is equally simple: progressive visual impairment. The rate of progression can be months to years. Patients should therefore be reassured that one or two opacities do not require immediate or even eventual surgery.

The causes of cataract can be congenital, toxic, metabolic, traumatic, or senescent. Although our discussion will be limited only to the last, other causes should be kept in mind in the differential diagnosis. For example, diabetes may induce a specific type of cataract, but also predisposes to ordinary senile cataracts at an earlier age.

The lens has a high potassium and low sodium concentration, which is maintained by active epithelial pumps. Glucose diffuses into the lens and is metabolized by anaerobic glycolysis and, to a limited extent, by aerobic Krebs cycle enzymes. A pentose shunt and sorbitol path is implicated in diabetic cataracts. The lens also contains large amounts of ascorbic acid, glutathione, inositol, and taurine. The biochemistry of cataract is complex, and the causes of opacities remain elusive. In some cases, an understanding of biochemical mechanism has proved of great value (for example, in galactosemia, renal failure, and drug-induced cataracts). As for senile cataract, however, neither cause nor prevention is known, and the only effective treatment is surgical. Fortunately, cataract extraction is progressively safer and effective. Even aphakia is no longer inevitable, as intraocular lenses have become practical alternatives to contact lenses and spectacles.

Senile cataract is the most common disorder of the crystalline lens. The opacities may be classified as cortical, subcortical, and nuclear. In advanced stages, these coalesce. Cortical cataracts are characterized by translucent grayish spokes, flakes, and dots arranged radially. Subcapsular opacities usually involve the posterior poles and appear as irregular granules, vacuoles, and crystals of various colors. Nuclear cataracts are an exaggeration of the yellow aging change and may cause a myopic shift in refraction, due to swelling. Although senile cataract is a bilateral disorder, it is usually asymmetric; one eye may be involved months to years before the other.

In evaluating visual disability from a cataract, the usual distance acuity test is insufficient. Some cataracts interfere more with far vision; others, with near vision. Glare may also be more incapacitating outdoors. A cleft or vacuole can cause monocular diplopia. Lens swelling produces transient refractive changes, and the patient may even be able to read without glasses. Sequential spectacle changes may restore useful vision for a time. A record of such refractive changes is most helpful in choosing proper intraocular lens power.

The presence of a cataract does not preclude other disorders. Many concurrent causes of poor vision are common in this age group. The differential diagnosis would certainly include corneal disease; macular degeneration; optic neuropathy; amblyopia; glaucoma; diabetic retinopathy; and, occasionally, psychogenic factors. In most cases these can be ruled out by history, tonometry, perimetry, and careful ophthalmoscopy. Indirect ophthalmoscopy often allows visualization of the fundus despite lens opacities. One can also formulate an estimate by comparing the patient's acuity with the clarity that the fundus can be seen. Nevertheless, sometimes the cataract is so dense that fundus visualization is not possible. Several tests are available to bypass the opacities, thus allowing some judgment of retinal function. Such tests also apply to opacities from an opaque cornea, vitreous membranes, or vitreous hemorrhage. No matter how dense the cataract, the patient should be able to see light, one color, and shadow movements. Light projection can be faulty in vitreous hemorrhage where no image is produced because of diffusion. With cataracts, however, projection generally is accurate. Pupillary reflexes are normal with cataracts. Shadow recognition may permit a simple hand confrontation field. Entopic visualization of retinal vessels or of leukocytes against a blue field is reassuring, but it may be absent if light is greatly diffused. Bright flash eletroretinography and visual-evoked potentials are sometimes useful. Ultrasonography can provide information about the vitreous cavity and retinal detachments. Laser interference fringes are a new method, useful if available.

The decision to operate for cataracts is based on three questions: What is the patient's disability? Will the operation reduce this disability? And, what are the risks of adding to the disability? The primary indication is when patients can no longer carry out activities important to them. This will depend on age, occupation, driving, avocation, mental status, whether they must care for themselves, and so on. It follows that cataract surgery is sometimes necessary on an eye that is not in perfect health, in patients who are not in the peak of condition. Balancing risks and rewards is, of course, the essence of surgical judgment. The choice between a visual result that may not be ideal versus a procedure that is never totally innocuous is always an individual matter. Results must be calculated not by what is taken, but by what is left.

Surgical planning naturally includes considerations regarding acceptability of spectacle correction, feasibility of contact lens wear, or advisability of an intraocular implant. Each has advantages and disadvantages that vary for different patients. Indication would certainly change for someone who has only one eye, a retinal detachment, poorly controlled glaucoma, repeated episodes of uveitis, or chronic tear deficiency.

Evaluation of the recently operated eye must consider the coherence of the wound, the functions of the anterior segment, the clarity of the optical media, and the integrity of the macula and optic nerve. Thus, corneal curvature fluctuates during the healing period, the aqueous may be filled with protein and red cells, the iris is somewhat inflamed, the vitreous may be prolapsed, the choroid may be detached, the macula may be edematous, and intraocular tension may fluctuate.

Distinguishing the normal from the pathologic and deciding what, when, and how to treat are responsibilities the surgeon is committed to when undertaking to perform the procedure.

Several postoperative complications require immediate surgical or medical attention. These include loss of the anterior chamber, particularly if the corneal endothelium contacts an intraocular implant; wound leakage, which sets the stage for ciliochoroidal detachment; hypotony and potential infection; epithelial downgrowth; pupillary block glaucoma; vitreous touch syndromes; endothelial decompensation and corneal edema; implant dislocation; the "ugh" syndrome of pseudophakia (uveitis, glaucoma, and hyphema); ischemic optic neuropathy; endophalmitis; cystoid macular edema; and retinal detachment. The differential diagnosis of these and related conditions requires experienced judgment, since the welfare of the eye hangs in the balance. In addition, a number of elective procedures are sometimes indicated to improve the visual result. For example, careful keratometric monitoring of corneal wound healing may require cutting or adding sutures or wedge resections to reduce or eliminate astigmatism. Retained lens material or posterior capsular opacification can be treated with lasers.

Cystoid macular edema is a condition of unknown etiology that is, unfortunately, a common complication of cataract surgery. Typically, one to three months after surgery, acuity decreases several lines and the eye becomes irritable and photophobic with circumcorneal injection. Ophthalmoscopy may show little, or there may be some yellow deposits and cysts in the macula. The cystoid spaces are best seen with fluorescein angiography, which demonstrates the characteristic honeycomb leakage. Despite the extensive macular pathology, acuity is surprisingly good, and functional recovery is common. The pathogenesis remains obscure. Vitreous traction has been implicated but does not seem to be a major cause. Permanent macular degeneration may follow persistent edema.

Cataract extraction nowadays is commonly followed by an intraocular implant. The postoperative refraction of such eyes deserves special mention. First, there are considerably more reflections, which makes retinoscopy difficult. These reflections occur because the crystalline lens with its lamellar structure has been replaced by a homogeneous plastic. Second, healing of the corneal incision takes several weeks, with considerable variability in refraction findings (particularly astigmatism). Third, the pupil of eyes supporting an iris-clip pseudophakos must not be dilated, as dislocation may result. Fourth, the refractive power of the eye is often deliberately altered either toward emmetropia or iseikonia, depending on estimated future status of the opposite eye. This, fifth, makes binocular vision possible in a high percentage of cases, so analysis of fusion and binocular reflexes requires attention.

Optical correction of aphakia may involve spectacles or contact lenses. Spectacles may be spheric or aspheric; glass or plastic; full-field or lenticular; with round, flat top, or multifocal segs. Contact lenses may be hard or soft; daily or extended wear; of high or low water content; single vision or bifocal; and with variable oxygen transmission. The clinician should be aware of the indications and contraindications for each that will best suit the visual needs of the patient.

Many optical problems remain unresolved, including lens design, the need for ultraviolet protection, and how to reestablish iseikonia with the phakic eye.

Diseases of the Uveal Tract

Although uveitis is common, its prevalence decreases with age. It may be classified as anterior or posterior. The division into granulomatous and nongranulomatous may be confusing, since the two forms are not the result of different causes and may, in fact, appear sequentially. Uveitis in the aged might be associated with surgical trauma, hypersensitivity to drugs or crystalline lens material, reactions to degeneration products in chronically sick eyes, intraocular tumors, systemic infections, severe ischemia, herpes zoster ophthalmicus, and intraocular foreign bodies.

The signs and symptoms of anterior uveitis are rather typical. Pain results from irritation of the ciliary nerves and is referred to the eye or periorbital area. It is aggravated by light and pressure. Pain and photophobia are more severe in acute than in chronic iridocylitis. Tearing is a minor feature and is secondary to reflex irritation of the corneal and ciliary nerves. Circumcorneal injection differs from conjunctival hyperemia by its violet hue and the fact that the vessels do not blanch with topical vasoconstrictors. Blurred vision may be due to ciliary spasm, exudation into the anterior chamber, or macular edema. Prolonged inflammation may result in pigment deposits and fibrous proliferation from the iris onto the lens capsule. This and an associated glaucoma with corneal edema further blurs vision. Keratitis can result from extension of inflammation into the peripheral cornea from the limbal circulation or through damaged endothelium. This may result in band keratopathy, which is characterized by a progressive superficial deposition of calcium across the central cornea. Persistent corneal edema is usually followed by pannus and neovascularization. Keratic precipitates are deposits of inflammatory cells on the corneal endothelium. They may vary in size, number, and disposition, depending on the aqueous current and composition. Thus, aqueous containing fibrin and large amounts of protein circulates poorly and traps the cells so that they cannot adhere to the cornea. Macrophages tend to form larger precipitates (mutton fat keratic precipitates), whereas lymphocytes and plasma cells tend to be white and smaller and are typical of nongranulomatous uveitis. Aqueous flare is a Tyndall phenomenon and represents disease activity. It is due to protein in the aqueous and is readily detected by the narrow slit of the biomicroscope in a dark room. Various cells may appear in the slit lamp beam, including inflammatory cells, macrophages, pigment cells, and granules. They originate from adjacent tissue or from capillaries. The number of cells per field is graded like the aqueous flare. Precipitates may be found in the chamber angle and on the surface of the iris (Koeppe's and Busacca's nodules). Aqueous containing much fibrin may clot, or in some cases, an inflammatory exudate forms in the floor of the chamber (hypopyon).

Bleeding into the anterior chamber is not unusual in traumatic or herpetic uveitis. Iris atrophy results from prolonged inflammation. The loss of pigment is especially evident in heterochromic cyclitis. Synechiae in the chamber angle are detected by gonioscopy. Cataracts may result from the toxic effects of uveal inflammation (complicated cataracts). Hypotony is characteristic of active uveitis; late glaucoma is a complication.

The signs and symptoms of posterior uveitis are also characteristic. Vitreous opacities are inflammatory cells, red blood cells, tissue cells, and debris, best seen with fundus biomicroscopy and retroillumination. Vitreous exudate produces a positive Tyndall phenomenon. If the vitreous is detached, a flare still appears in the retrovitreal space. Vitreous detachment is due to liquefaction and shrinkage. With vitreous collapse, a ring floater may be visible to the patient, representing previous attachment to the optic disc. Retinal edema is common in posterior uveitis and, if the macula is involved, causes reduced vision. Prolonged macular edema leads to cystic changes and permanent loss of central vision. Disc edema is usually transitory and is the result of irritation, particularly when the inflammatory process is nearby (for example, Jensen's juxtapapillary choroiditis). Active chorioretinal lesions appear gray or white and vary in size, shape, depth, and outline. Poorly defined edges indicate infiltration. Deeper lesions are obscured by overlying tissue, and associated vitreous haze is less marked. Satellite lesions may appear in the vicinity of older, healed areas. Retinal detachment follows serious exudation, but holes are generally absent. Perivasculitis may occur from cellular infiltration or by retrograde inflammation into the perivascular spaces. Exudates, bleeding, and occlusion are secondary complications. Visual disturbances are often associated with photopsia, metamorphopsia, and scotomas.

Serous choroidal detachment is a complication of intraocular and retinal detachment surgery. The combination of trauma and hypotony causes an abnormal aqueous flow into the space between the ciliochoroid and sclera. The result is a dramatic ophthalmoscopic picture of a large, dark bulge protruding into the vitreous, which may be mistaken for a tumor or retinal detachment. Central vision is usually unaffected unless the posterior fundus is involved, but some pain is common. The effusion tends to subside after one or two weeks. The most serious complication is a flat anterior chamber, which, if there is an intraocular implant, becomes a surgical emergency.

Choroidal melanomas are the most important malignant intraocular tumors of the elderly. Approximately half of all uveal melanomas occur in the fifth and sixth decades of life. The chief symptom is a change in visual acuity, and this depends on tumor size and position and associated retinal detachment. Scotomas may be interpreted as blurred vision. Macular edema may cause metamorphopsia. Pain and redness are uncommon. The chief sign is the discovery of a mass in the fundus. Appearance can vary from a small, flat lesion resembling a nevus to a large, protuberant mass that invades the retina and vitreous. Retinal detachment invariably occurs, which may make visualization of the underlying solid tumor difficult. Pigmentation can vary greatly and may be absent. The differential diagnosis, because nevi and melanocytomas, includes metastatic neoplasms, hemangiomas, and disciform degeneration. Since so much depends on a proper diagnosis, patients exhibiting a suspected mass in the fundus must be referred to an ophthalmologist who has experience with gradations of appearance and malignancy and who can promptly initiate ancillary diagnostic tests.

Diseases of the Retina

Retinal disease is a dominant cause of visual disability in the elderly. It is also a topic of extraordinary interest for several reasons. First, one can usually relate visual impairment to the ophthalmoscopic picture. Second, the histologic substrate can often be deduced from fundus appearance. Third, recent advances such as fluorescein angiography and electrophysiologic tests have clarified the basis for both pathologic and clinical findings. And, fourth, new therapeutic techniques such as photocoagulation, vitrectomy, and retinal microsurgery have brought about exciting changes in prognosis.

Despite its histologic and functional complexity, most diseases produce rather stereotyped retinal changes. These include edema, infarcts, exudates, hemorrhages, pigment dispersion, vascular changes, atrophy, deposits of foreign cells or material, cysts, holes, breaks, schisis, and detachments. In interpreting retinal lesions, one notes size, shape, location, color, border, depth, effect on adjacent tissue, translucency, and elevation.

Retinal edema may be localized or general, chronic or evanescent. The retina appears boggy, pale red or white, and more or less thickened. Color changes are most evident when contrasted to a normal area. The cherry red macular spot of central retinal artery occlusion is a classic example. Macular edema is suggested by a loss of transparency, thickening of Henle's layer, and distortion of the narrow beam of the slit lamp on the fundus biomicroscopy. The patient may report metamorphopsia.

Infarcts, or cotton wool spots, are sometimes called "soft exudates." They are white, fluffy, located mostly in the posterior pole, invariably superficial (that is, they often cover retinal vessels), and do not stain with fluorescein. Histopathologically, infarcts represent focal swelling of nerve fibers (cytoid bodies).

Exudates (also called hard exudates) are yellow to white lesions with sharp margins that are most abundant in the posterior poles. Occasionally, they are arranged in a circinate or star-shaped pattern. They occur in the middle retinal layers and consist of fatty material. Hard exudates should be differentiated from drusen of Bruch's membrane. The latter are not associated with retinopathy and may fluoresce, whereas exudates obscure background choroidal fluorescence. Hemorrhages may be subretinal, intraretinal, or preretinal. Subretinal blood has a gray green color. Intraretinal hemorrhages are punctate or rounded when in the deeper layers and flame shaped when in the nerve fiber layer. Preretinal blood tends to form large masses and may have a fluid level. Extensive retinal hemorrhages are usually the result of venous congestion. Hemorrhages with a white center (Roth spots) occur in leukemia and endocarditis. Vitreous hemorrhage may result from breaks in proliferating new vessels or from a retinal tear and detachment. Even vitreous hemorrhage should be assumed to hide a retinal detachment in older people until proved otherwise.

Pigment dispersion is a reaction to injury and may represent pigment epithelium cell migration or loss, or phagocytosis. Although nonspecific, the pigment distribution sometimes presents as a diagnostic pattern as in retinitis pigmentosa. Vascular changes consist of alterations in the pattern, reflexes, diameters, and crossings of retinal arteries and veins. Narrowing, tortuosity, congestion, sheathing, obstruction, vascular shunts, and new vessels are adaptations to pressure changes, ischemia, and infection. Atrophy refers to loss of cells or diminution of cell size. Repair may be complete or incomplete, resulting in holes, cysts, or glial proliferation. If pigment epithelium and choroid are absent, the white sclera is visible. Areas of atrophy frequently are surrounded by pigmented margins, which distinguish them from colobomatas.

Foreign cells are illustrated by metastatic tumors; foreign material is usually endogenous and might include cholesterol, hemosiderin, melanin, and lipoids. Bright, scintillating spots overlying an artery are atheromatous emboli. Breaks in Bruch's membrane are illustrated by angioid streaks, lacquer cracks, and traumatic ruptures. Schisis represents splitting within the retina, usually from merging of cystic areas. Detachments represent a splitting between the neural and pigment epithelial layers. Fluid or vessels may cause pigment epithelium to detach from Bruch's membrane.

In evaluating retinal lesion one may make use of shadowing, parallax, focusing the ophthalmoscope, red-free light, and observing what structures overlie or are in turn obscured by it. The depth of the lesion may also be evident from limitations imposed by surrounding tissue, as in flame-shaped hemorrhages and macular star exudates. The slit beam of fundus biomicroscopy confirms elevations or depressions.

Fluorescein angiography has greatly aided the interpretation of fundus pathology and made purely descriptive discussions in older textbooks obsolete. Intravenous injection of fluorescein allows observation of ocular circulation and adequacy of blood-aqueous barriers. A permanent record is obtained by sequential photography. Normally, fluorescein does not stain the retina, because retinal vessels and pigment epithelium have tight junctions that act as barriers. Fluorescein does escape from normal choriocapillaries (background fluorescence). Detachment of pigment epithelium allows dye to puddle in the involved area. Areas where pigment is lost act as windows to the underlying choroidal fluorescence (window defects). Blood and exudates in the retina obscure background fluorescence. Damaged retinal vessels leak dye into the retina proper. Fluorescein angiography might be indicated in diabetes, macular edema, nonrhegmatogenous detachments, disciform degeneration, vascular occlusion syndromes, sickle cell disease, presumed histoplasmosis, and whenever neovascularization is suspected.

Macular degeneration is by far the most important retinal disease in the aged. The average age of onset is 65, and the second eye is generally involved within four years. Loss of central vision results from exudative detachment of pigment epithelium, choroidal neovascularization and hemorrhage, and geographic atrophy of the pigment epithelium. Although the disease is primarily an aging phenomenon, a hereditary dystrophy may also be implicated. We have already seen that there is progressive loss of choroidal capillaries with age. Secondary changes develop in Bruch's membrane, characterized by drusen and irregular pigment changes. Drusen usually increase in size and number and may cause minor visual loss. This may be followed by direct progression to geographic atrophy, or there may be intermediate stages of serous detachment. Thinning of the retina may result in a macular hole. In another form of this disease, there is an ingrowth of fibrovascular tissue from the choroid through breaks in Bruch's membrane. The presence of new vessels is suggested by clinical observation of a yellow to gray circular patch, subretinal pigment, and a ring of hemorrhage or exudates. Rupture and bleeding of these new vessels causes sudden, total loss of central vision. Repair may be followed by a disciform atrophic scar that varies in color from white to brown or even black. Further hemorrhages may occur at the margins of the disciform lesion. Current interest centers around photocoagulating leaking vessels, providing the branches are sufficiently distant from the fovea.

A number of other conditions may be associated with neovascularization in the elderly. In degenerative myopia, hemorrhage with pigmentary and atrophic scarring results in Fuchs' spot. Drusen of the optic nerve may be associated with macular edema. Angioid streaks represent breaks in Bruch's membrane through which choroidal vessels can gain access to the retina.

Occlusive disease of the retinal circulation may involve either arteries or veins. Central artery occlusion is the most dramatic, the most sudden, and the most catastrophic of all ocular diseases. There may be a history of previous transient ischemic attacks. The cause can be thrombotic or embolic. Most, but not all, patients have accompanying systemic vascular disorders (carotid atheromas, giant cell arteritis, valvular heart disease, hypertension, or diabetes). Branch retinal artery occlusion usually involves the temporal vessels, and visual loss depends on macular involvement. Central retinal vein obstruction is also a disease of older people with a peak incidence in the sixth decade. The pathogenesis remains unknown, but concomitant arterial disease and local thrombotic factors are implicated. Inflammatory causes are unusual. The clinical picture in central retinal vein obstruction is a sudden, painless decrease of vision, but not as profound as with arterial occlusion. The ophthalmoscopic picture of massive hemorrhages with dilated vessels is characteristic. Pathologic changes are due to hemorrhagic infarction with destruction of neural elements. The most dreaded complication is neovascular glaucoma, which begins about three months later. The relation between preexisting glaucoma and vein obstruction dictates a careful work-up in the opposite eye. Branch vein obstruction is much more common than central vein obstruction and usually involves the superior temporal vessel (two-thirds of cases) or the inferior temporal vessel (one-third of cases). The patient may describe acuity loss or distorted vision. If the macula is not involved, there may be no symptoms. The ophthalmoscopic picture is a segmental area of hemorrhages and exudates.

Flashes and floaters are common complaints of the elderly. They may represent only innocuous muscae volitantes, but also can be precursors of serious vitreoretinal disease. Floaters are usually vitreous opacities or aggregates: the closer they are to the retina, the more obvious the shadow they cast. When the pupil is small, as in reading outdoors, the opacity is more likely to block the light and become visible. Movement depends on the fluidity of the vitreous. Traction on the retina or bumping of detached vitreous against the retina causes flashes, often compared to lightning streaks. They differ from the scintillating scotomas of migraine, which are uninfluenced by eye movements. The incidence of retinal complications in patients complaining of flashes and floaters is 10% to 15%. It follows that separating the innocuous from the pathologic requires meticulous examination with the indirect ophthalmoscope, fundus biomicroscope, and perimeter.

Retinal detachment is a serious and complex disease that may occur with (rhegmatogenous) or without breaks. Most rhegmatogenous forms begin in the peripheral retina. Predisposing peripheral degenerations that may lead to holes are lattice degeneration, zonular traction tufts, and degenerative retinoschisis. The retinal break connects the vitreous cavity to the subretinal space. Symptoms include blurred vision, flashes, floaters, and a curtain of visual loss corresponding to the detached area. Ophthalmoscopy reveals the typical gray membrane with folds or bulla when highly elevated. Aphakia and myopia predispose to retinal detachment, probably on the basis of vitreous detachment and traction. The importance of identifying and localizing breaks is that these are surgically treatable lesions. An adhesive chorioretinitis surrounding the break is created by heat, cold, or photocoagulation to reduce the risk of fluid undermining the retina.

In general, untreated rhegmatogenous detachments are progressive and spread from ora to disc. They usually have regular convex borders with pigment lines at stationary edges. In contrast, nonrhegmatogenous detachments tend to be confined to either the peripheral or central fundus, with irregular, sometimes concave borders and no pigment lines. Peripheral cystoid degeneration has a characteristic stippled appearance and does not progress. Retinoschisis tends to be circular, without folds, and does not undulate with movement. Areas of retinal edema are shallow, nonprogressive, with irregular borders that gradually regress. Exudative detachments from tumors and inflammation show gravitation of fluid, fluid shifts, and a bullous configuration. Tractional detachments occur in proliferative diabetic retinopathy, lattice degeneration, chorioretinitis, trauma, aphakia, and following the use of strong miotics. The combination of rhegmatogenous and traction detachments may result in massive vitreous retraction with a crumpled retina and star folds. Complications of surgical repair of retinal detachment include uveitis, glaucoma, cataracts, hazy media, preretinal membranes, and refractive changes.

Preretinal macular gliosis is a disorder of older eyes characterized by a membrane on the surface of the retina. There may be preexisting retinal disease, or the condition may be primary. The ophthalmoscope reveals traction lines, vascular tortuosity, and a cellophane appearance. Posterior vitreous detachment is common. The pathology is migration of glial cells through breaks in the internal limiting membrane. The usual predisposing causes of preretinal membranes are retinal detachment, diabetic retinopathy, retinal vein obstruction, inflammation, and photocoagulation.

Diseases of the Optic Nerve

Diseases of the optic nerve may be inflammatory, compressive, vascular, infiltrative, degenerative, toxic, or traumatic.

Inflammation of the optic nerve, characterized by hyperemia, edema, and cells in the vitreous, may accompany any inflammatory process of the retina. When inflammation affects the nerve head, the term papillitis expresses the ophthalmoscopic appearance. If the retro-ocular portion of the nerve is involved, the disc appears normal, and diagnosis depends on acuity, fields, pupil signs, and color or brightness comparison. The differential diagnosis of papillitis includes edema, high refractive errors, drusen, tilted-disc syndrome, myelinated nerve fibers, and preretinal gliosis. Although demyelinating diseases rarely start in later life, the residua of previous episodes may be visible as optic atrophy.

Disc edema, as contrasted to papilledema, is the result of local ocular disease. There is progressive visual loss, an afferent pupillary sign, color defects, and field changes if conduction is compromised. Disc edema can be unilateral, whereas edema from raised intracranial pressure is always bilateral, although it may be asymmetric (for example, if there is prior optic atrophy on one side). Unilateral disc edema may be found in orbital disease, optic nerve tumors, uveitis, periphlebitis, intraocular tumors, papillitis, occlusive disease of retinal veins, hypotension following intraocular surgery, drusen, ischemic neuropathies, and accelerated hypertension. The pathophysiology may involve neural elements (axon transport block), neurological elements (for example, drusen), and vascular components (for example, central retinal vein obstruction or ischemic neuropathies). Fluorescein angiography and ultrasonography can be helpful in the differential diagnosis. Papilledema is discussed under neuro-ophthalmic disorders.

Low-tension glaucoma refers to a disorder characterized by normal intraocular pressures, normal diurnal pressure curves, and normal tonography, yet complicated by progressive glaucomatous-type field loss and disc cupping. The mechanism apparently is some imbalance in ocular pulse volume and systemic blood pressure. The disease is difficult to treat and may involve central fixation much earlier than ordinary open-angle glaucoma. A more common disorder of the optic nerve–characterized by pathologic cupping and sector field defects, but which is not progressive–is shock optic neuropathy. The mechanism is some hemodynamic crisis such as cardiac failure or acute blood loss in an older patient. Overcontrol of hypertension may result in decreased perfusion pressure and nerve damage.

Ischemic optic neuropathy is primarily a disease of the elderly, with a peak incidence in the sixth decade. There is sudden loss of vision in one eye and practically no visual recovery. The ophthalmoscope reveals a pallid disc edema. Perimetry shows a typical altitudinal defect, although isolated central scotomas are also found. The nerve gradually becomes atrophic. A recurrent attack in the same eye is very rare, but months to years later a similar, often symmetrical attack occurs in the opposite eye. The second eye may be involved in one-third of cases, and in one-half of these within 6 months. Disc edema in the second eye, coupled with atrophy in the other, may be confused with a Foster-Kennedy syndrome. The pathology is an ischemic infarction of the prelaminar portion of the optic nerve. Associated diseases commonly found in these patients include hypertension, diabetes, arteriosclerotic heart disease, and cerebrovascular disease, but the relation, if any, remains unclear. There is no satisfactory treatment for this disorder. The differential diagnosis includes mainly two other entities: hypertensive optic neuropathy and temporal arteritis, both of which are treatable. These are discussed under systemic disorders.

Toxic optic neuropathies present as painless, bilateral, progressive loss of visual acuity. Visual fields may show a central or caecocentral scotoma with sloping margins. Among the causes implicated are malnutrition, pernicious anemia, tobacco or alcohol toxicity, heavy metals, chemicals such as methanol and benzene, and assorted drugs (ethambutol, isoniazid, streptomycin, chloramphenicol, quinine, penicillamine, Antabuse [disulfiram, Wyeth-Ayerst Laboratories, Philadelphia, PA], vitamin A excess, steroids, and cancer chemotherapy). The importance of recognizing these disorders is that the damage is potentially reversible if nutritional deficiencies are replaced or toxins removed.

Optic atrophy in the elderly entails a difficult differential diagnosis. Care must be taken not to call every pale disc atrophic unless there is confirmatory acuity and visual field evidence. The most common cause is glaucoma, followed by vascular, demyelinating, compressive, and traumatic disorders. Drusen of the disc may give it a pale appearance.

Injuries to the optic nerve may occur at any age and can be direct or indirect. Direct injuries are caused by sharp instruments and missiles. Indirect avulsions and fractures are generally the result of head trauma. Visual loss is immediate and often complete. Pupillary signs are positive. X-ray evidence is often nonconclusive. The mechanism of indirect injury is probably on a concussion basis, with contusion and edema of the nerve tissue, interruption of its vascular supply, or an actual tear.

Glaucoma

Glaucoma is a leading cause of blindness throughout the world. Since the incidence of elevated intraocular pressure and the susceptibility of optic nerve damage increases with age, early recognition is a fundamental responsibility in the care of the elderly.

Glaucoma refers to a group of diseases characterized by elevated intraocular pressure, which, if sustained, causes progressive optic nerve damage. Two broad categories are recognized, based on whether the anterior chamber angle is open or narrow. In addition, glaucoma may be classified as primary or secondary. Primary glaucomas are probably genetically influenced, although the exact cause is unknown. Secondary glaucomas are the result of some prior or concurrent ocular abnormality or trauma. Secondary glaucomas may have open angles (as in steroid-induced pressure rise) or closed angles (for example, those induced by a swollen cataractous lens). Space precludes discussion of these many entities which encompass a vast and detailed literature. This section is limited to primary open-angle glaucoma and, specifically, to its early recognition.

Patients with primary open-angle glaucoma have no symptoms, and the condition is almost invariably discovered by checking intraocular tensions on routine examination. It is generally possible to distinguish three groups on the initial office visit: normal, glaucoma suspects, and those with definite glaucomatous disease. In the first group are those with normal discs, normal fields, and an intraocular tension under 21 mm Hg. In the second group are those whose tension is above 21 mm Hg and who will therefore require further investigation. In the third group are those whose tension is obviously abnormal (say, over 30 mm Hg) or where the diagnosis is already established. The third group also includes those who have ophthalmoscopic or visual field changes consistent with glaucoma even though intraocular pressure appears to be within normal limits. Our emphasis will be on the second group.

At what pressure level does one become suspicious? Although there is no absolute value, 21 mm Hg applanation is widely accepted. After the sixth decade, 23 mm Hg might be considered the upper limit of normal. Care must be taken to avoid tonometric artifacts such as incomplete patient relaxation, incorrect instrument calibration, corneal edema, and postural effects.

What factors increase the risks of glaucoma? Several conditions are recognized as predisposing eyes to optic nerve damage: a family history of glaucoma, advanced age, myopia, previous retinal vein occlusion, pressure rise induced by steroids, diabetes, pseudoexfoliation of the lens capsule, evidence of prior uveitis, albinism, postoperative complications such as vitreous loss, and vascular crises such as changes in blood pressure or blood volume.

How does one detect the earliest features of glaucomatous damage? The two primary techniques are ophthalmoscopy of the optic disc and perimetry. While optic disc cupping is highly correlated with field changes, the relation is by no means absolute. Older patients tend to demonstrate field loss before disc changes; hence, the two techniques complement each other. Moreover, field changes are unequivocal, whereas disc anomalies are more open to interpretation. Finally, ophthalmoscopy is objective, whereas perimetry is a psycho-physical measurement.

What are the earliest optic disc changes in glaucoma? The best way to detect early disc changes is with fundus biomicroscopy. The second best way is with the narrow beam of the direct ophthalmoscope. In evaluating appearance with respect to glaucoma, the most important factor is the size of the optic cup compared with the size of the entire nerve head (cup/disc ratio). This comparison is usually made in the horizontal meridian, although it can be made in any direction. An asymmetric cup/disc ratio found by comparing one eye to the other is also highly suspicious. Although the size of the cup can be defined by color change, the configuration is more important. These estimates should be made (and recorded) on every patient to gain familiarity with normal variations. The cup is usually centrally located; extension to the disc margin–especially above, below, and temporally–is highly suspicious. The depth of the excavation will determine how much blood vessels are pushed aside (bayonet appearance) as they climb up the cup. Patients with such symptoms are likely to have advanced rather than early field defects. Small, flame-shaped hemorrhages may be found near or crossing the disc margin. Other patterns of abnormal cupping such as ovalization, saucerization, temporal unfolding, polar notching, and increased translucency of the neural rim have also been described. Glaucomatous changes must always be interpreted in light of many normal disc variations. A drawing or photograph is of great help in documenting progression.

What are the earliest field changes in glaucoma? The most important is the nerve fiber bundle defect although it is not pathognomonic; ischemic neuropathies, branch vessel occlusion, neuritis, drusen, and even chiasmal lesions can produce them. In early stages, nerve fiber damage can cause small paracentral and arcuate scotomas; later, nasal steps and sector-shaped defects. These are best demonstrated by tangent screen examination with emphasis on the innermost 30 degrees. In advanced glaucoma, the perimeter can record progressive, overall, concentric contraction, which eventually results in a temporal island of vision and culminates in total blindness. Automated instruments can be programmed to search for early features of glaucoma, but they require an alert and cooperative patient. These desirable characteristics are not always available in the older population.

Eyes that have suspicious pressures but no field or disc defect always present a challenge. One must balance potential visual damage months or years down the line, with the inconvenience, side effects, and expense of lifelong treatment. Obviously, the higher the pressure, the greater is the risk of eventual damage. In the context of this chapter, moreover, the older the patient, the greater the risk.

AGE-RELATED OCULAR DISEASE: SYSTEMIC ASPECTS

To the poet, the eyes are the windows of the soul, but to the physician–whatever the specialty–the eyes provide a glimpse into the state of general health or disease. A corollary is that when the eye specialist refers a patient to a medical colleague, the latter naturally assumes that purely ocular disease has been ruled out. Thus, the neurologist, asked to evaluate a patient with suspected optic neuropathy, is likely to proceed on the basis that visual loss is not caused by amblyopia, refractive error, or macular disease.

Arteriosclerosis

The cardiovascular system undergoes significant changes with age. Cardiac output decreases almost linearly after the third decade. Systolic blood pressure rises because of loss of recoil of larger arteries; diastolic pressure rises because of increased peripheral resistance. Arterial walls undergo a symmetrical increase in intimal thickness. Lipid infiltration — mainly cholesterol ester and phospholipid — progressively increases with age, even in the absence of disease. These diffuse age changes differ from the focal raised fibromuscular plaques that characterize atherosclerosis. Atherosclerosis involves mainly the intimal layers of major vessels, including coronary and cerebral arteries. Arteriolosclerosis is characterized by hyaline and degenerative changes in the media and intima of small arteries and arterioles, usually the result of hypertension. In severe hypertension, there may be actual necrosis of the vessel wall. Arteriosclerosis is a generic term for thickening or hardening of any arterial wall.

The most significant effect of arteriosclerosis is narrowing of the vascular lumen, thus reducing blood flow to the tissues (ischemia). In addition to arteriosclerosis, narrowing or obstruction can result from thrombosis, embolism, spasm, inflammation, or mechanical compression. Thrombosis refers to an intraluminal obstruction formed from elements of circulating blood; an embolus is an abnormal mass of undissolved material carried in the bloodstream. The main factors in thrombosis are changes in the vessel wall, blood stasis, and altered blood coagulability. Emboli may be atheromatous plaques, detached thrombi, tumor cells, fat, gas, or foreign bodies. Spasm is rare, except in severe hypertension. Inflammatory obstruction is exemplified by syphilis and polyarteritis. Mechanical compression might be caused by tumors, hematomas, and displaced bone fractures. Unlike arterial thrombosis, which often is based on atherosclerosis, venous thrombosis is usually precipitated by blood stasis and, in the case of retinal veins, compression by a crossing artery.

Normal retinal vessels are actually invisible; what is seen ophthalmoscopically are blood columns. When the walls become opacified — usually by arteriolosclerosis — there is a change in color, and stripelike densities may appear along the vessel surface. Colors have been compared to copper or, in more advanced stages, to silver wire. These changes do not imply vascular obstruction, which is more closely related to the width of the light reflex along the surface of the blood column. In contrast, yellowish stripes along the sides of a vessel — called perivascular sheathing — are due to exudation into the surrounding spaces. Perivascular sheathing is characteristically seen along veins in papilledema and along arteries in hypertension. Sclerosis may also result in generalized narrowing, so the normal two-to-three ratio of arteries to veins is altered.

The retinal arteries lie mainly in the nerve fiber and ganglion cell layer. At its entrance within the nerve, the central artery has several layers of smooth muscle; this decreases to two or three at the equator. An anatomic peculiarity is that arteries and veins share a common adventitial coat; hence, one can be compressed by the other (arteriovenous nicking). Branch retinal vein obstruction is most commonly due to this mechanism, and it increases in frequency with age. More rarely, occlusion is the result of stagnation and primary thrombus formation or of intrinsic venous disease. In the acute stage, the ophthalmoscopic picture has been described as if one had stroked the involved retinal area with red paint because of the massive hemorrhages. In the chronic stage, one sees retinal edema, serous detachment, vessel collaterals, exudates, microaneurysms, and neovascularization. Visual loss is due to macular edema and vitreous hemorrhage. Central retinal vein occlusion has the same pathogenesis, but the entire retina is involved because of compression at the lamina cribrosa. Macular edema always occurs. The most serious complications are vitreous hemorrhage and neovascular glaucoma.

Branch retinal artery occlusion is usually the result of embolization. Cotton wool spots appear in the region of nonperfusion and may last for days or weeks. In hypertension, occlusion may be due to focal arteriolar necrosis. The occlusions seen in collagen diseases are probably on a hypertensive basis. Central retinal artery obstruction is usually due to atheromatous changes but may be caused by emboli or hemorrhages beneath the atheromas. Rarer causes are arteritis and trauma. The clinical picture is a white, edematous retina with a cherry-red macular spot and narrowed arteries. The cherry-red spot differs from lipoidoses, where the macula actually contains material deposited in ganglion cells. A wider area of perfusion may be observed with a patent cilioretinal artery. Central retinal artery occlusion causes total visual loss without recovery. The scotoma of branch artery occlusion is confined to the involved area. Involvement of the opposite eye, fortunately, is rare. Obstruction of small vessels behind the lamina cribrosa may give rise to ischemic optic neuropathy. Arcuate scotomas of vascular occlusion may be centered on the disc rather than on the macula, as they are in neurologic disorders.

Hypertension

Hypertension is a disorder characterized by sustained elevated blood pressure (arbitrarily defined as exceeding 160/95 mm Hg at rest). In most cases, the cause is unknown (essential hypertension). Hypertension is said to enter the accelerated phase when retinal hemorrhages and exudates develop — irrespective of the absolute blood pressure level, although this is often above 200/140 mm Hg. Age, race, sex, smoking, serum cholesterol levels, glucose intolerance, weight, and renal factors modify the prognosis for the disease. Young untreated hypertensives have a poorer life expectancy than the aged; conversely, accelerated artherosclerosis invariably accompanies hypertension.

The ophthalmic manifestations of hypertension can be classified in various ways, the most popular of which is the Keith-Wagener. It recognizes four stages of progressive severity (see Table 4.1). In fact, there is probably a qualitative change between the early and later stages. Only about 1% of hypertensive

Table 4.1 Keith-Wagener classification of hypertension

Grade 1: Mild narrowing or sclerosis of retinal vessels
Grade 2: Focal constrictions, arteriovenous nicking
Grade 3: Cotton wool spots, hemorrhages, retinal edema
Grade 4: Papilledema

patients develop the malignant phase; even with the advent of effective therapy, only half of these survive for more than 5 years.

The diagnosis of hypertension is made with a blood pressure cuff, not an ophthalmoscope. Nevertheless, fundus changes provide clues to severity and progression, particularly when the disease enters the accelerated stage. These include linear or flame-shaped hemorrhages, cotton wool spots, hard exudates, and blot hemorrhages. Of course, exudates and hemorrhages are found in diseases other than hypertension; hence, the association between these and general medical features (for example, high blood pressure, dyspnea, proteinuria, and chest and cardiac findings) is crucial. Unusual but known mechanisms of hypertension must be ruled out (for example, pheochromocytoma, Cushing syndrome, renal disease, aldosternomism, oral contraceptives, and coarctation). "Unilateral" hypertension fundus changes may occur in patients with stenosis of the carotid system, which maintains lower pressures on that side.

The pathophysiology of vascular changes can be studied in experimental hypertension followed by fluorescein angiography. Recall that the retinal circulation is controlled by autoregulation, which permits a nearly constant blood flow over a wide range of perfusion pressures (that is, mean arterial pressure minus intraocular pressure). A rapid rise in arterial pressure causes vasoconstriction; the precapillary arterioles become occluded and eventually necrose. The vessel loses its ability to remain constricted, and a dilation and plasma leakage follow. Fluorescein demonstrates this breakdown of the blood-retinal barrier. Further leakage into the vessel wall causes capillary occlusion, retinal edema, cotton wool spots, and hemorrhages. The presence of arteriosclerosis modifies the response of retinal arterioles to pressure changes. This is probably the reason for focal constriction.

The malignant phase of hypertension is characterized by retinal and disc edema, in addition to exudates and hemorrhages. The pathology is fibrinoid necrosis of the arterioles. The patient may complain of headaches, shortness of breath, and blurred vision, and there may be signs and symptoms of renal failure. Papilledema is due to accumulated cotton wool spots at the disc rather than hypertensive encephalopathy, although axoplasmic transport block may occur in both. Prolonged disc edema may result in atrophy. Hypertensive optic neuropathy must be distinguished from ischemic neuropathy and the neuropathy associated with temporal arteritis.

Diabetes

The incidence of diabetes in the United States is estimated at almost 5% of the population. About three-fourths of the patients first diagnosed under age 29 eventually develop retinopathy. About 10% to 18% of those with retinopathy progress to the proliferative stage. Diabetes, therefore, is, or soon will be, the leading cause of blindness in the United States.

Diabetes is a disease that gets more complex with every advance in metabolic and biochemical research. For our purposes, it may be defined as a hormone-induced metabolic abnormality involving carbohydrate, fat, protein, and insulin utilization. Long-term complications are the result of microvascular lesions demonstrable by electron microscopy. The classic symptoms of diabetes are polyuria, polydipsia, and polyphagia. Weakness, weight loss, recurrent infections, ulceration of the extremities, and neuropathies are other features of progression. Two distinct forms of the disease are recognized: juvenile-onset (insulin dependent) and maturity onset (noninsulin dependent). Juvenile-onset diabetes can progress rapidly to ketoacidosis, lethargy, and coma. It is difficult to control, and death may result from cardiovascular or renal failure. However, juvenile-onset diabetes, which used to be the equivalent of a death sentence, is now well controlled by insulin and dietary management. Most juvenile diabetics survive to old age. Adult-onset diabetes can usually be managed by diet and oral hypoglycemic agents. For every symptomatic diabetic patient, however, there is probably another without symptoms but abnormal blood glucose tolerance (preclinical diabetes). Obesity, advancing age, and a family history of diabetes are predisposing factors.

Ophthalmic complications of diabetes are partly metabolic (crystalline lens swelling and cataracts), but mostly vascular (diabetic retinopathy). Although the vascular changes are mainly evident in the fundus, they also may involve conjunctiva, iris, choroid, ciliary body, and nerves (diabetic neuropathy). Diabetic fundus changes may be classified into background retinopathy (in which the pathology is essentially within the retina) and proliferative retinopathy (in which the changes extend over the retinal surface and into the vitreous).

Probably the earliest change in diabetic retinopathy is increased capillary permeability. This has been demonstrated by an elegant technique that measures small amounts of fluorescein in the vitreous. Leakage can be demonstrated within 6 months after onset, even in those without clinically recognizable retinopathy.

Although fundus changes in diabetes are not characteristic, they are generally so typical that the diagnosis can be suspected without difficulty. Mild background retinopathy is characterized by microaneurysms and punctate hemorrhages in the posterior pole, particularly in the region temporal to the macula. The arrangement is haphazard, but occasionally they border an area of soft exudate. Cotton wool spots gradually become more numerous but are less white and less opaque than those seen in hypertension. Microaneurysms are much more numerous than one suspects from ophthalmoscopic observation. This has been repeatedly demonstrated by fluorescein angiography. Microaneurysms are round, range in size from 15 μ to 50 μ, and vary in color from venous to arterial blood. Histopathologically, they are seen chiefly on the venous side of the capillary and represent bulges due to a selective loss of mural pericytes. Some aneurysms become hyalinized, and their lumens are lined with degenerated endothelial cells. The cause remains unclear; weakness of the wall, traction, and abortive new vessel formation have all been postulated. Aneurysms differ from blot hemorrhages in that the latter are absorbed and disappear. Capillary closure with areas of nonperfusion persists after the associated cotton wool spot is absorbed. Shunt vessels, connecting arterioles to venules, appear. Damaged vessel walls take up fluorescein. Venous changes include dilatation, tortuosity, beading, and sheathing, and arteriosclerotic changes are accelerated. Hard exudates appear as yellow to white lesions that may coalesce or form a circinate or star pattern around the macula. The visual prognosis is poor if a ring is formed around the macula or hard exudates encroach on the fovea. Hard exudates may improve with time. The most common cause of poor vision, however, is macular edema. It tends to be symmetric, progressive, and surrounded by an area of nonperfusion larger than normal. Edema is the result of abnormal vascular permeability. If the site of leakage can be identified — and it is some distance from the fovea — photocoagulation may help. Long-standing edema, macular hemorrhage, holes or membranes have a poor outlook.

Proliferative diabetic retinopathy is characterized by the formation of new vessels, which may develop either on the disc or in the periphery. New disc vessels have a poorer prognosis, because they tend to bleed into the vitreous. The pathophysiology of new vessel formation is unknown, but ischemia and anoxia are undoubtedly major factors. The vessels are accompanied by a thin film of fibrous tissue that runs across the retinal surface and through the internal limiting membrane. Hemorrhage and retinal detachment result from vitreous contracture. This form of vitreous collapse differs from the normal aging process in being more gradual and incomplete. Traction and epiretinal membranes may respond to vitrectomy and retinal microsurgery, in which epiretinal membranes are actually peeled off the surface with specially designed instruments.

New iris vessels may involve the angle and produce neovascular glaucoma. The mechanism is unknown, is presumably anoxia, and the prognosis is poor. Other causes of neovascular glaucoma must be kept in mind: retinal vein occlusion, central retinal artery occlusion, malignant melanoma, and retinal detachment. Recurrent anterior chamber hemorrhages progressively compromise aqueous outflow. These eyes respond poorly to miotics, carbonic anhydrase inhibitors, or surgery. Laser photocoagulation holds some promise for controlling this serious disease.

Diabetic neuropathy may affect any part of the nervous system. It presents most commonly as a peripheral neuropathy. Symptoms are palsies, paresthesias, numbness, and pain. Diabetic neuropathy may involve any of the ocular motor nerves (painful ophthalmoplegia); hence, diplopia may be the presenting symptom. Pathologically, there is small-vessel occlusion with local demyelination, but recovery within weeks to months is the rule. Aberrant regeneration does not occur, and the pupil is spared. Differential diagnosis includes trauma, tumor, aneurysm, migraine, and increased intracranial pressure. Decompensated strabismus is an unlikely cause.

Giant Cell Arteritis

Giant cell arteritis (temporal arteritis, cranial arteritis, polymyalgia rheumatica) is an inflammatory disease of arteries in older people. The etiology is unknown, but both humoral and cellular immune reactions to elastic arterial tissue have been postulated. Any large- or medium-sized artery may be involved, and there is a predilection for extracranial vessels. The peak incidence is in the 60- to 75-year range. Both sexes are affected, with a slight predominance in women. The disease is not rare; about 1.7% of 889 postmortem cases where temporal artery sections were taken. Familial associations are uncommon, but there is a geographic preference for northern climates. The condition is uncommon in blacks.

The importance of recognizing this disease is that it is potentially blinding for both eyes consecutively, it may be fatal, and treatment is available that may avoid these complications.

Systemic symptoms include headache; malaise; low-grade fever; scalp tenderness; jaw claudication; arthralgias and myalgias; anorexia; weight loss; depression; and tenderness of the course of the temporal arteries, which may feel thickened.

Ophthalmic findings include a sudden, transient loss of vision (amaurosis fugax) that may persist for minutes to hours. This may be followed by unilateral blindness, which may be partial or complete. The pathology is an ischemic optic neuropathy. The opposite eye may be involved within a week or months later. If untreated, 65% of patients develop bilateral disease, and almost one-third of these are totally blind. Ophthalmoplegia with ptosis or other extraocular muscle palsy occurs in 5% of the patients. More rarely, presenting findings are central artery occlusion or anterior segment ischemia with neovascular glaucoma. Ophthalmoscopy shows a pale (not hyperemic), swollen disc. Disc edema may be minimal, but the margins are blurred, and a few hemorrhages may be seen. The arterioles of the affected eye are narrowed and often show focal constrictions. The visual deficit is generally out of proportion to the mild disc changes. After about a week, disc edema disappears, and the optic nerve gradually becomes pale. The narrowed arteries persist, and no improvement in vision is to be expected.

The most significant laboratory findings are an elevated erythrocyte sedimentation rate (ESR) — usually exceeding 50 mm per hour by the Westergren method — and a positive temporal artery biopsy. The histopathology shows the occluded lumen and multiple giant cells. Prompt recognition and initiation of steroid therapy may prevent loss of vision. If ischemia is complete, treatment may prevent loss of the opposite eye. The patient should be warned that treatment is not invariably effective. The management of this disease is best undertaken as a joint effort between ophthalmologist and internist.

Cranial arteritis should be distinguished from ischemic and hypertensive optic neuropathy. In classic ischemic neuropathy, no treatment is effective. In hypertensive neuropathy, reduction of blood pressure is indicated. Neither condition shows an elevated ESR, and both tend to occur in a somewhat younger age group (late middle life). Low-tension glaucoma and shock optic neuropathy must also be kept in mind.

Transient Ischemic Attacks

Transient ischemic attacks (TIAs) are fleeting episodes of focal neurologic deficits lasting minutes to hours. An attack that lasts longer than 24 hours is treated as a completed stroke, and it is in the prevention of stroke that the recognition of transient attacks is important.

The pathogenesis of ischemic attacks is complex and varied. Causes might include stenosis of the carotid and vertebrobasilar systems, embolism (atheromatous, platelet, or myxomatous), decreased cardiac output (from failure, arrhythmias, dehydration, anemia, or overcontrol of hypertension), compression of vessels in the neck, hypoglycemia, hypercoagulation states, cranial arteritis, migraine, and reverse flow in cerebral vessels (for example, steal syndromes). Snapping mitral valve syndrome has recently been implicated as a source of emboli.

Clinical features depend on whether the carotid (anterior) or vertebrobasilar (posterior) distribution is involved. The importance of this differentiation is that carotid disease is potentially subject to surgical treatment, whereas the posterior distribution is usually not.

Signs and symptoms of carotid system disease include monoparesis, hemiparesis, hemiparesthesias, and contralateral visual loss. Vertebrobasilar diseases produce brain stem symptoms, including monoparesis, alternate-side paresis, facial numbness on one side and motor loss on the other, diplopia, dysarthria, vertigo, drop attacks, and dysphagia. Loss of consciousness, confusion, amnesia, and tonic-clonic activity are not usually due to transient ischemic attacks, and the practitioner should suspect mass lesions.

Examination might include testing the blood pressure in each arm, auscultation of carotids, determining the pulse rate, palpation of temporal arteries, taking the temperature of limbs, and looking for signs of congestive failure. Compression of neck vessels is never done as a provocative test. The laboratory work-up might include a complete blood count (CBC), urinalysis, electrocardiogram, serology, echocardiogram, lipid profile, sedimentation rate, glucose tolerance, chest X-ray for cardiac configuration, skull films, brain scan, and arteriography if the patient's condition permits.

Ophthalmic manifestations occur in 40% of patients with carotid disease and are the result of transient hypoxia of the retina rather than of the higher visual pathway. Monocular visual loss is therefore more common than transient episodes of hemianopia. Amaurosis fugax may be described by the patient as blur-outs, gray-outs, visual field contractions, a curtain or window shade phenomenon, or a cloud or mist in the field of vision. If one has a chance to observe the patient during the attack, one may observe nonreactive pupils; narrowed retinal arteries; perhaps an embolus at the bifurcation of an artery; and, occasionally, a Horner syndrome. Cotton wool spots and hemorrhages are features of retinal ischemia. Two types of emboli are commonly seen: orange, scintillating cholesterol flakes (Hollenhorst's plaques) and dull white platelet emboli.

Ophthalmic signs of vertebrobasilar insufficiency may include transient visual loss, but this tends to be mild and is often unreported. Oculomotor palsies, including nystagmus, are important eye symptoms. Attacks may be precipitated by turning the head to one side or using one arm. Diplopia is uncommon with carotid insufficiency.

Ophthalmodynamometry is a noninvasive, but not totally innocuous, procedure. If performed incorrectly, it may result in severe ischemia or even central retinal artery occlusion. Several techniques are available: compression, suction, oculoplethysmography, Doppler flow sonography studies, and oculocerebrovasculometry. The principle involves elevation of intraocular pressure with a tension-recording instrument while observing the pulsation of the central retinal artery ophthalmoscopically. Carotid stenosis must exceed 50% to become hemodynamically significant. Observation of diastolic pressure is safer than increasing tension to the point of total collapse of the artery. Diagnosis is based on noting a pressure difference of the two sides.

The significance of emboli in producing transient episodes of visual loss is apparently related to fragmentation and dissolution of plugs on the one hand and passage to smaller vessel branches on the other. Another mechanism appears to be a transient circulatory arrest within the eye followed by reactive vasodilation. In some cases, no emboli are found, and the mechanism may be transient optic nerve ischemia.

The time sequence has some diagnostic value. Vascular ischemic attacks last 5 to 15 minutes and are unilateral. Attacks lasting seconds, occurring in both eyes, and repeated many times during the day may be due to chronic papilledema. Migraine attacks may be accompanied by photopsias and headache and can last up to 30 minutes. Very short episodes that alternate from one eye to the other may be hysterical. In auscultating the carotid system, a pediatric bell endpiece should be placed over the angle of the jaw, the middle of the neck, and the heart. The absence of a bruit can mean either normal flow, less than 50% stenosis, or total stenosis.

Thyroid Ophthalmopathy

Thyroid ophthalmopathy can be discussed equally well under neuro-ophthalmic disorders, because eye manifestations are often independent of the endocrine course, motility disorders are a common presenting complaint, and the chief visual risk of the disease is compression of the optic nerve.

Graves' disease may occur at any age but is most common in the fourth decade. It has a greater prevalence in women and in those who have other autoimmune disorders. The etiology is unknown; an imbalance in the homeostatic mechanism between thyroid secretion and tissue utilization is postulated, possibly because of the presence in plasma of an abnormal thyroid stimulator. Clinical manifestations of hyperthyroidism include goiter, weight loss, fine tremor, nervousness, excessive sweating and heat intolerance, palpitations, arrhythmias, tachycardia, and cardiac failure.

Ophthalmic features include a characteristic frightened appearance because or proptosis and lid retraction, lid lag on downgaze, infrequent blinking, convergence insufficiency, and restriction of ocular movements (exophthalmic opthalmoplegia). In rapidly progressive exophthalmos, there is chemosis, conjunctival injection, corneal exposure with ulceration, and optic nerve compression leading to atrophy. The proptosis is usually bilateral, but it may be unilateral. The differential diagnosis includes orbital masses, hemorrhage, vascular malfunctions, inflammation, uremia, and Cushing's syndrome. The pathology is characterized by an inflammatory infiltrate of orbital contents with water, connective tissue, lymphocytes, plasma cells, and mast cells. Infiltration of extraocular muscles may simulate tumors on computerized tomography and is responsible for the ophthalmoplegia. Neural and myopathic ophthalmoplegias may be confused with this. Lid retraction and lid lag are important signs and are attributed to excessive innervation of Müller's muscle. If the levator muscle is infiltrated, exposure keratopathy is possible. Bell's phenomenon should be checked. Other causes of lid retraction are uncommon (aberrant third nerve regeneration, pineal tumors, myotonic dystrophy, and ptosis on the opposite side).

The most common motility disorder is a double elevator palsy (an old orbital floor fracture should be considered). Forced ductions may help identify mechanical restrictions. The most serious complication is optic nerve compression. Danger signals are a central scotoma, color defects, afferent pupil sign, and disc edema. Such findings require emergency decompression of the orbit to save vision.

The course of the disease is unpredictable; ophthalmopathy may progress despite resolution of hyperthyroidism, and radioiodine therapy may in fact aggravate it. After reaching a plateau, the eye findings may subside spontaneously, with variable recovery.

Neuro-ophthalmic Disorders

Neurologic diagnosis is thrice unique; it logically follows anatomy, requires minimal equipment, and demands the most systematized reasoning. A practical plan of examination consists of an appropriate history, a specific workup, and pertinent laboratory tests. If a diagnosis is still found wanting, either Nature cures the patient, or autopsy reveals the exact pathology.

The history is fundamental, because many neurologic symptoms have no physical manifestations (for example, headache, pain, photopsias, parethesias, or obscurations). We must rely on patients to tell us what they see or feel, or, indeed, if they can see at all. Moreover, the history is not only a diagnostic, but a therapeutic, tool.

Diminished smell, hearing and sight contribute to sensory deprivation in the elderly. Hearing loss (presbycusis) increases with age and is usually sensorineural. Speech sounds become distorted and unintelligible, although patients know when they are being spoken to. People with hearing loss naturally must rely more on visual cues; hence, concurrent visual impairmant greatly compounds the sense of isolation.

Dizziness is a common complaint of older patients. True vertigo is characterized by a sensation of motion or rotation, either of self or the environment. It is often accompanied by nausea and blurred vision, hearing loss, tinnitus, and nystagmus, perhaps aggravated by head turning and upright posture. True vertigo should be differentiated from lightheadedness, faintness, nervousness, or spatial disorientation precipitated by new glasses. Labyrinth disease is the most common cause of vertigo. Meniere's disease on the other hand is an endolymphatic hydrops characterized by vertigo, unilateral fluctuating sensorineural deafness, and tinnitus. Toxic labyrinthitis may follow the use of drugs (streptomycin, sedatives, phenytoin, or diuretics), heavy metals, or alcohol. Common motion sickness may be precipitated by sudden movements of the head in the elderly. Lesions of the vestibular nuclei cause severe vertigo and may result from demyelinating disease, vascular insufficiency, tumors, and edema. Central vertigo is usually associated with headaches, diplopia, vomiting, and elevated intracranial pressure. Vertigo may be a prodrome of migraine, epilepsy, or TIAs. Vertigo associated with facial, trigeminal, and auditory signs may be due to acoustic neuromas.

Trigeminal nerve disease can be caused by aneurysm; mass lesions; inflammation of the orbital apex, the superior orbital fissure, the cavernous sinus, or the gasserian ganglion outside the brain stem, or within the brain stem. The chief ocular symptom is corneal anesthesia. Local corneal anesthesia also occurs with herpes simplex infection and following a variety of intraocular surgical procedures. The combination of facial nerve palsy, insufficient tear production, and corneal anesthesia is part of the cerebellopontile angle tumor syndrome. Trigeminal neuralgia is a disease of older people characterized by attacks of intense pain in the distribution of any of the three branches of the ganglion; its cause is unknown. Surgical relief may be complicated by corneal anesthesia. Neuroparalytic keratitis may result in perforation in a matter of days unless the cornea is properly protected.

Headaches are probably universal, but the patient who presents with headache as the chief complaint deserves special attention. Since physical signs are usually absent, a meticulous history is essential. The key question is: In what way are these headaches different from those you usually experience? Any headache of sudden onset, incapacitating severity, or increasing frequency or duration that is not relieved by previously successful therapy or that is accompanied by focal neurologic signs or mood changes should have an ophthalmic work-up, including pupil evaluation, intraocular tension, funduscopy, visual field, blood pressure, carotid auscultation, temporal artery palpation, and whatever laboratory tests are indicated by the examination. As a checklist, headaches may be conveniently classified as vascular (including migraine), muscle contraction, traction, inflammatory, and psychogenic (especially depression).

About 60% of patients with brain tumors complain of headaches. The pain may be dull, intermittent, and interrupt sleep. It is often made worse by factors that increase intracranial pressure (coughing, stooping, or straining). Mass lesions in the elderly may include abscess, aneurysm, and tumor. The tumors are frequently metastatic and may be symptomatic before the primary lesion. The diagnosis of mass lesions depends on correlating signs and symptoms with neuroradiologic findings. The most common symptoms are headache, seizures, personality changes, and motor and speech disturbances. Diagnosis has been markedly facilitated by computerized tomography (over 90% detection by this method). Angiography is indicated in planning surgery.

The chief ophthalmoscopic sign of increased intracranial pressure is papilledema. Its features include the loss of a previously noted venous pulse, hyperemia, blurring of the disc margin, venous congestion, peripapillary edema with concentric traction lines, and hemorrhages. Filling in of the physiologic cup is not a reliable sign, and an enlargement of the blind spot is of no help except in following the course of the disease. In contrast to optic neuritis, the vision is generally good, there is no Marcus Gunn pupil, no inflammatory cells in the vitreous, and no pain upon eye movement. Color vision is not affected. Patients with increased intracranial pressure are often ill, with nausea, vomiting, headaches, and even fluctuating levels of consciousness. In chronic papilledema, there may be transient obscurations of vision. When conduction in the nerve is compromised, the signs and symptoms of neuritis appear. Funny-looking discs may be confused with papilledema. These include congenital anomalies, staphylomas, hyperopia, and optic nerve drusen. Drusen are often familial, are rare in blacks, and have an incidence of almost 0.5%. Disc margins may be blurred with a scalloped contour. Drusen tend toward a yellow translucent color and may be elevated several diopters. Buried drusen are invisible but become more superficial with age. Occasionally, they erode peripapillary capillaries (causing hemorrhages) or compress optic nerve fibers (causing atrophy). Optic nerve drusen can be associated with any ocular disease, including papilledema.

Perimetry plays a major role in neuro-ophthalmic diagnosis because of the long course of visual sensory fibers from one end of the skull to the other. The concept of the field as an island of vision in a sea of blindness is useful in understanding that the field can be approached from the side (kinetic perimetry) and from above (static perimetry). The use of targets of different sizes (or differing luminances and colors) is termed *quantitative perimetry*. The problem is that it also takes a quantity of time, but the temptation to omit or postpone the test must be resisted. As regards automated instruments, Traquair's admonition–that visual fields are tested by the perimetrist, not the perimeter–should be kept in mind. At least two isopters are always plotted to confirm validity and reliability. In many disorders, field defects are the only clue to the presence of disease. Unilateral field abnormalities suggest a careful search for defects in the "normal" eye, for bilaterality is not always symmetrical. A bilateral anomaly usually places the problem in the chiasma or beyond. Recall that lesions of the optic tract and anterior radiation tend to be incongruous, whereas posterior lesions are congruous; this rule is of no value once the hemianopia is complete.

Acquired diplopia is a serious, potentially life-threatening symptom in the elderly. The causes may be traumatic, infectious, vascular, metabolic, or neoplastic. In a certain proportion of cases, no cause can be discovered. True diplopia can be distinguished from monocular diplopia by asking the patient to close one eye. Neural disorders can be differentiated from mechanical restrictions by forced duction tests; from myopathies by lack of innervational pattern; and from strabismus by history, old photographs, and presence of amblyopia. Diagnosis is based on accompanying features, and in this way the disease generally can be traced to the orbit, the orbital apex, the cranial cavity, or the brain stem. For example, a painful sixth nerve palsy associated with a hearing loss on the same side may suggest Gradenigo syndrome or an angle tumor. Bilateral sixth nerve palsies with papilledema suggest intracranial pathology. Isolated fourth nerve palsies are often traumatic. Third nerve palsies may result from aneurysm, diabetes, migraine, and tumors. Aberrant regeneration is found after aneurysm and trauma, rarely with tumors, and never with infarcts or diabetes. Multinerve involvement is often neoplastic. Lesions of the base of the brain may show visual field defects or other signs of vascular insufficiency. Supranuclear palsies are characterized by disturbances of saccadic, pursuit, vergence, or vestibular eye movement systems; diplopia is rare. Brain stem lesions often involve adjacent nerves (facial, auditory, vestibular, or trigeminal), the pupils, and the medial longitudinal fasciculus. Unlike strabismus in the young, diagnosis is simplified by the absence of suppression, anomalous correspondence, and eccentric fixation. The work-up should include specification of the timing, direction, and magnitude of the deviation in different cardinal positions. Note head tilt, ptosis, proptosis, pupil involvement, visual field defects, lid retraction, papilledema, orbital and carotid bruits, tenderness of temporal arteries, facial and auditory nerve function, corneal sensation, mechanical restriction, periorbital anesthesia, nystagmus, blood pressure, and evidence of aberrant regeneration. Pertinent laboratory tests, in addition to radiologic investigations, might include blood sugar level, sedimentation rate, serology, and hematocrit. When indicated, Tensilon test, angiography, lumbar puncture, biopsy, and neurosurgical consultation are helpful.

Transient diplopia occurs in multiple sclerosis, vertebrobasilar insufficiency, epilepsy, myasthenia, parkinsonism, minor strokes, phoria decompensation, and intermittent squint. The presence of a head tilt means fusion is present in some directions of gaze. Mechanical mechanisms of diplopia have no neural pattern. Peripheral neuropathies may involve any nerve branch.

Involvement of the extrapyramidal system is common in the aged, evident as rigidity, hypokinesia, flexed posture, and tremor. The tremor exists at rest, is coarse, and is aggravated by voluntary movements and stress. In contrast, the tremor of parkinsonism exists at rest but subsides on willed movements. In its fully developed form, the clinical picture of paralysis agitans is highly characteristic: stooped posture, stiffness, slow movements, fixed facial expression, festinating gait, and no sensory changes. Postencephalitic parkinsonism may be indistinguishable from the primary disease. Drug-induced parkinsonism should be ruled out. Disturbances of vertical gaze and lid movement, oculogyric crises, and blepharospasm are the usual ophthalmic findings.

Myasthenia gravis is a muscular disease that can occur at any age and in both sexes. In males, the peak incidence is in the sixth and seventh decade. The mechanism appears to be an increase in circulating antibodies to acetylocholine receptors on an autoimmune basis. Pathologically, muscles are infiltrated with small, round cells. Ophthalmic findings occur early because of the high nerve-to-muscle ratio of extraocular muscles. Clinically, the onset is chronic, and often insidious. Bilateral ptosis or other extraocular muscle weakness occurs in 90% of cases. Weakness progresses with exercise or during the day. Pupils are never affected. Choking and food aspiration may be due to weakness of palatal muscles, and the voice may have a nasal quality. Infections, large meals, and alcohol aggravate the symptoms. The incidence of thyroid disease, arthritis, and cancer is higher in these patients. Diagnosis is based on the history and the improvement of muscle function with the edrophonium test.

Joint and muscular disease in the elderly frequently is treated with corticosteroids. Steroid-induced glaucoma and cataracts, therefore, deserve special mention. Tonometry will reveal a rise in pressure, and funduscopy may show disc changes. The crystalline lens often exhibits posterior capsular opacities, and the patient may complain of glare, halos, and monocular diplopia. A disproportionate loss of reading vision compared with distance vision can be misinterpreted as progressive presbyopia. Finally, the presenting complaint may be a red eye due to bacterial, fungal or herpetic infection exacerbated by steroids.

The clinical syndrome of dementia is characterized by deficits of memory, judgment, language, and other cognitive functions, as well as changes in personality and behavior. The causes are varied; some are treatable, such as drug reactions, metabolic dysfunctions, infections, trauma, nutritional deficiencies, or benign neoplasms. Unfortunately, the most frequent causes of dementia are progressive, despite symptomatic treatment. These include Alzheimer's disease and multi-infarct dementia. Alzheimer's disease is a senile dementia of unknown etiology; its diagnosis is based largely on exclusion. Current research focuses on correcting possible neurotransmitter imbalances and preserving the function of surviving neurons. Treatment is symptomatic. Multi-infarct dementia may occur after repeated cerebrovascular accidents, and the diagnosis is based on a history of recurrent strokes. Dementia must be differentiated from functional and emotional disturbances. Apathetic patients may fail to respond to questions regarding orientation in time, place, and events. Loss of remote memory carries a more grave prognosis than loss of recent memory. All organic brain syndromes have a functional overlay, because patients react emotionally when aware of intellectual deterioration.

CARE OF THE ELDERLY: A SUMMARY

Older people are more fragile than their younger counterparts. Relatively trivial breakdowns in homeostasis can have irreversible and fatal consequences. Nevertheless, clinicians are sometimes "turned off" by the elderly. Several reasons require careful, introspective analysis. First, the tradition of health care savors the instant gratification of rapid and complete cures. In diseases of old age, we must settle for short-term gains instead of long-term satisfaction. Second, clinicians may have difficulty extrapolating from their own anticipated reactions to the actual responses of the elderly. Habits and attitudes are more rigid; they tend to resist change and hold tenaciously to their limitations. Third, emotional response to physical illness in the elderly is often colored by fears of death, isolation, pain, and blindness. The therapeutic value of communicated understanding is lost if one provides reassurance on matters that the patient is not concerned about. Such failures can only be avoided by listening to the patient carefully. Fourth, depression is the most frequent functional psychiatric disorder of the elderly. It is hard to praise life when life abandons us. Depression, in contrast to grief reactions, is accompanied by diminished self-esteem and overwhelming guilt. It is difficult to empathize with depressed people because of their intense self-preoccupation. Fifth, hearing loss, slow reaction time, and apathy make examination more difficult. This may result in misinterpretations or even omitting important tests. The solution is to allow more time, and, if necessary, repeat the office visit. Sixth, the elderly often misunderstand the proper use of medications or fail to comply with directions because of economic and transportation problems. One therefore should question patients about the use and abuse of drugs, especially when multiple prescriptions are involved (as they frequently are). Seventh, drug interactions and the prolonged use of sedatives, tranquilizers, or alcohol may not only produce organic syndromes, but change previously controlled diseases such as glaucoma and diabetes. Eighth, older people may ignore or suppress important symptoms either from fear, a sense of inevitability, or depressed responsiveness. Such symptoms must be actively sought to avoid their being overlooked. Ninth, loss of appetite, indifference, lack of companionship, and economic factors make the elderly the most common undernourished segment of the population. This can alter wound healing, predispose to infection, and modify expected responses to therapy. Tenth, the clinician should make sure that incentives and means are available for periodic reexaminations and follow-ups.

To acknowledge senescence, however, is not to predict senility, although the terms are often used interchangeably in clinical parlance. Intelligence, in fact, is seldom impaired, and learning ability, in the absence of disease, is undiminished. The person who is too old to learn was probably always too old to learn.

Because the number of elderly people is increasing, the prevalance of visual impairment is growing. The major challenge of the future is to balance the services the elderly need against the availability and appropriateness of the services they receive. The best must sometimes yield to the best obtainable, but excellence cannot be bought by expediency. The notion that health care can be provided to the elderly (or anyone else) only on the basis of cost effectiveness substitutes economic policy for clinical judgment, platitudes for empathy, and "cases" for patients. Demographic studies that focus exclusively on common disorders are of little help to the patient with a rare disease or the symptomatic patient with no disease. In a free society, the individual must always remain the end and not the means to a better future.

This chapter has, of necessity, emphasized the constraints of age; little was said of its possibilities. But there is health as well as disease, pleasure as well as pain, growth as well as decay, life as well as death. The rules for caring for the old, it seems to me, are also good rules for growing old: To do what we can, the best we can, while we can.

SUGGESTED READINGS
General Texts

1. Apple, D.J. *Clinicopathologic Correlation of Ocular Disease.* St. Louis: C.V. Mosby, 1978.
2. Duane, T. *Clinical Ophthalmology.* New York: Harper & Row, 1980.
3. Duke-Elder, S. *System of Ophthalmology,* 15 vols. St. Louis: C.V. Mosby, 1956–1976.
4. *Harrison's Principles of Internal Medicine.* New York: McGraw-Hill, 1980.
5. Havener, W.H. *Synopsis of Ophthalmology.* St. Louis: C.V. Mosby, 1979.
6. Newell, F.W., and J.T. Ernest. *Ophthalmology: Principles and Concepts.* St. Louis: C.V. Mosby, 1978.
7. Vaughan D., and T. Asbury. *General Ophthalmology.* Los Altos: Lange, 1980.

Special Texts

1. Beard, C. *Ptosis.* St. Louis: C.V. Mosby, 1976.
2. Blodi, F.C., et al. *Stereoscopic Manual of the Ocular Fundus in Local and Systemic Disease.* St. Louis: C.V. Mosby, 1964–1979.
3. Cogan, D.G. *Ophthalmic Manifestations of Systemic Vascular Disease.* Philadelphia: W.B. Saunders, 1974.
4. Cogan, D.G. *Neurology of Ocular Muscles.* Ann Arbor: Thomas Press, 1978.
5. Fedukowicz, H.B. *External Infections of the Eye.* New York: Appleton-Century-Crofts, 1978.
6. Friedlaender, M.H. *Allergy and Immunology of the Eye.* New York: Harper & Row, 1979.
7. Gass, J.D.M. *Macular Diseases.* St. Louis: C.V. Mosby, 1977.
8. Harrington, D.O. *The Visual Fields.* St. Louis: C.V. Mosby, 1976.
9. Jaffe, N.S. *Cataract Surgery and Its Complications.* St. Louis: C.V. Mosby, 1976.
10. Jones, I.S. *Diseases of the Orbit.* New York: Harper & Row, 1979.
11. Keeney, A.H. *Ocular Examination.* St. Louis: C.V. Mosby, 1976.
12. Kolker, A.E., and J. Hetherington. *Becker-Shaffer's Diagnosis and Therapy of the Glaucomas.* St. Louis: C.V. Mosby, 1976.
13. L'Esperance, F.A. *Current Diagnosis and Management of Chorioretinal Diseases.* St. Louis: C.V. Mosby, 1977.
14. Mausolf, F.A., ed. *The Eye and Systemic Disease.* St. Louis: C.V. Mosby, 1975.
15. Michaels, D.D. *Visual Optics and Refraction.* St. Louis: C.V. Mosby, 1985.
16. Paton, D., and M.F. Goldberg. *Management of Ocular Injuries.* Philadelphia: W.B. Saunders, 1976.
17. Reese, A.B. *Tumors of the Eye.* New York: Harper & Row, 1976.
18. Reichel, W., ed. *Clinical Aspects of Aging.* Baltimore: Williams & Wilkins, 1978.
19. Sekuler, R., et al., (eds.). *Aging and Human Visual Function.* New York: Liss, 1982.

20. Steinberg, F.U., (ed.). *Cowdry's The Care of the Geriatric Patient.* St. Louis: C.V. Mosby, 1976.
21. Straatsma, B.R., et al. (eds.). *The Retina.* Berkeley: The University of California Press, 1970.
22. Tolentino, F.I., et al. *Vitreoretinal Disorders.* Philadelphia: W.B. Saunders, 1976.
23. Wise, G.N. et al. *The Retinal Circulation.* New York: Harper & Row, 1971.
24. Yanoff, M., and B.S. Fine. *Ocular Pathology.* New York: Harper & Row, 1975.
25. Zinn, K.M., and M.F. Marmor. *The Retinal Pigment Epithelium.* Cambridge: Harvard University Press, 1979.

Additional References

1. Ai, E., and W.R. Freeman. "New Developments in Retinal Disease." *Ophthalmol. Clin. North Am.* 2, no. 3, Philadelphia: W.B. Saunders, 1990.
2. Berkow, J.W., et al. "*Fluorescein Angiography.*" *Am. Acad. Ophthalmol. Monogr.,* 1991.
3. Bressler, N.M., et al. "Age Related Macular Degeneration." *Surv. Ophthalmol.,* 32 (1988): 375–412.
4. Cibis, G.W., and M.S. Mancillas. "Contrast Sensitivity." *Curr. Opinion Ophthalmol.,* 2 (1991): 81–84.
5. Coles, W.H. *Ophthalmology.* Baltimore: Williams & Wilkins, 1989.
6. Davson, H. *Physiology of the Eye.* New York: Pergamon Press, 1990.
7. Easty, D.L. *Virus Diseases of the Eye.* Chicago: YearBook Publishers, 1985.
8. Enoch, J.M. "The Design of an Instrument for Evaluation of Vision Before, During, and After Refractive Surgery." *Lasers and Light in Ophthalmol.* 4 (1991): 111–119.
9. Frisen, L. *Clinical Tests of Vision.* New York: Raven Press, 1990.
10. Gold, D.H. (ed.). "Systemic Associations of Ocular Disorders." *Int. Ophthalmol. Clin.* 31 (1991): 31.
11. Hedges, T.R. *Consultation in Ophthalmology.* Philadelphia: B.C. Decker, 1987.
12. McCrary, J.A. "Magnetic Resonance Imaging Applications in Ophthalmology." Int. Ophthalmol. Clin., (1991); 31: 101–115.
13. Puliafito, C.A. "Lasers, Light Hazards and the Clinician." *Ophthalmology,* 98 (1991): 565–566.
14. Tomey, K.F., and Traverso, C.E. "The Glaucomas in Aphakia and Pseudophakia." Surv. Ophthalmol., (1991): 36: 79–112.
15. Walsh, T.J. "Visual Fields." Am. Acad. Ophthalmol. Monogr., 1990.

5

Pharmacologic Aspects of Aging

Siret D. Jaanus

It has been estimated that patients over the age of 65 years receive approximately 35% of all prescription medications in the United States (Baum et al., 1981). About 40% of the elderly need at least one drug a day to be able to pursue the activities of daily living (Lamy, 1980). Not only are the elderly prescribed more medications than other age groups, they are also the major consumers of nonprescription (OTC) drugs. Studies also indicate that the use of drugs in this age group is associated with significant medication errors (Schwartz et al., 1962; Tobias, 1988; Buecchler and Malloy, 1989). Table 5.1 lists the drugs most often prescribed for the geriatric population. Among these are cardiac drugs, including the antihypertensives, antihyperlipidemics, and the nonsteroidal anti-inflammatory drugs (NSAIDs). The use of the NSAIDs in particular, increases with advancing age (Lamy, 1986).

The incidence of adverse drug reactions also increases with age. It has been estimated that it is three times more common in the 70 to 90 year old age group (Jernigan, 1984). In addition, under-recognition of adverse effects by geriatric patients (Klein et al., 1984) and the potential for clinically important interaction between drugs taken (for example, drug-drug interactions and their interaction with coexisting medical conditions, that is, drug-disease interactions) appears to be greater in the elderly (Ouslander, 1981). Prevention of drug reactions requires understanding of both the physiologic changes that take place in the aging patient, as well as the pharmacologic characteristics and disposition of drugs that tend to cause reactions. An awareness of pharmacologic principles, as they relate to geriatric drug effects, is of importance to the eye care practitioner to both help prevent as well as minimize age-related adverse drug effects.

PHARMACOKINETIC AND PHARMACODYNAMIC FACTORS
Absorption

Clinical studies generally have failed to demonstrate age-related effects in drug absorption from the gastrointestinal tract for most drugs tested (Goldberg

Table 5.1 Drugs most frequently prescribed for the geriatric population*

Aspirin and other nonsteroidal anti-inflammatory agents
Antianginals
Antihyperlipidemics
Antihypertensives
Beta-receptor blocking agents
Calcium channel blocking agents
Cardiac glycosides
Diuretics
Potassium supplements
Vitamin B

* Listed in alphabetical order.

and Roberts, 1983). Although elevations in gastric pH, decreased gastric emptying, and impaired intestinal motility are found in the elderly, drugs whose absorption is pH-dependent, such as digoxin (Lanoxin, Burroughs Wellcome, Research Triangle Park, NC), for example, do not exhibit changes in total bioavailability. The lack of effect of age on drug absorption may be related to the fact that most drug absorption is passive and dependent on drug concentration gradients. However, studies do suggest that agents absorbed by active transport mechanisms, such as calcium, organic iron, and certain vitamins, are absorbed to a lesser extent in the elderly (Bhanthumnarin and Schuster, 1977; Greenblatt et al., 1982). Disease conditions, presence or absence of food, and concurrent use of drugs are most likely more important factors in drug absorption than is age.

Distribution

Following absorption, the distribution of drugs in the body depends on body composition, plasma protein binding, and blood flow to the organs. Body weight generally decreases and body composition, particularly adipose and muscle tissue mass, changes with age. The percent of body weight contributed by fat increases from 18% to 36% in men and 33% to 45% in women. Lean body mass decreases (Novak, 1972). Total body water also decreases with age between the ages of 30 and 80 years by 18.3% in men and 13.4% in women (Lamy, 1980). These factors can alter the volume of drug distribution in the elderly. Fat-soluble drugs, such as the barbiturates (phenobarbital), benzodiazepines (diazepam), and the phenothiazines (chlorpromazine) may be stored in fatty tissue to a greater extent in the elderly, who may exhibit undesirable effects at the usually prescribed dosages because of longer half-lives of drug elimination (Trounce, 1975). Conversely, the volume of distribution of water-soluble drugs, such as ethanol, digoxin, and cimetidine, is smaller, but initial plasma concentrations can be high, leading to unexpected adverse effects (Vestal and Cusack, 1990).

Protein Binding

Effects of certain drugs on target organs may be altered if changes occur in protein binding. Following administration, a certain percent of drug in the serum is bound to protein, primarily albumin. The bound drug is in equilibrium with the unbound drug. Only the free drug is pharmacologically active. While bound, drug molecules cannot cross the blood-brain barrier, and metabolism and elimination of the drug cannot take place at the usual rates. Clinical effects of drugs can therefore be altered by plasma protein binding. The proportion of albumin among total plasma proteins decreases with age and with some chronic diseases (Wood-ford-Williams, et al., 1964; Greenblatt, 1979). Reduced protein binding of highly bound drugs can lead to a more intense clinical effect as is the case with the anti-coagulant warfarin (Coumadin, Du Pont Pharmaceuticals, Wilmington, DE) or as with the anticonvulsant phenytoin (Dilantin, Parke-Davis, Morris Plains, NJ) to faster elimination (Hayes et al., 1975).

It has been observed that acidic drugs generally have a high affinity for albumin, whereas many basic drugs show affinity for α_1-acid glycoprotein. The concentration of the latter protein increases with age (Abernethy and Kerzner, 1984). The clinical significance of this observation is not known at present. Studies have shown changes in protein binding of acidic drugs, such as naproxen (Naprosyn, Syntex, Palo Alto, CA) in the elderly. The concentration of Naprosyn not bound to plasma protein is twice as high in older patients (Upton et al., 1984). Although the exact relationship between the free drug level and the clinical effect of Naprosyn and most other drugs is not well established, the data do imply that a possible reduction in drug dosage or measurement of plasma free-drug concentration may be beneficial in patients of advanced age (Montamat et al., 1989).

Metabolism

The liver is the major site for biotransformation of drugs. The metabolism of drugs by the liver depends on the activity of microsomal enzymes responsible for drug transformations as well as on the rate of delivery of drugs to the liver. The latter is dependent on hepatic blood flow. It has been estimated that hepatic blood flow decreases by 40% from age 25 to 65 years (Ho and Triggs, 1984). In the case of drugs with rapid rates of metabolism, the rate-limiting step appears to be blood flow, and certain drugs with high hepatic extraction ratios show decreased clearance in the elderly (Vestal and Cusack, 1990). In the case of drugs metabolized by the hepatic enzyme systems, biologic variations among subjects as well as other factors such as smoking, for example, appear of greater significance than age (Vestal et al., 1979).

Renal Excretion

The kidneys eliminate drugs from the body only if they are in the polar, water-soluble form. Among the processes that govern renal excretion are glomerular filtration and tubular diffusion. The effect of aging on renal excretion of drugs is at present the best understood pharmacokinetic parameter of geriatric drug therapy. Age-related changes in renal function include decreases in glomerular filtration and renal blood flow. The number of functioning nephrons also decreases with age (Richey and Bender, 1977; Mayersohn, 1986). The rate of clearance of creatinine is an indication of the rate of renal drug elimination. Although interindividual variations exist, creatinine clearance can decrease by about 35% between the ages of 20 and 90 years in patients without evidence of renal disease. Both glomerular filtration and tubular secretion rates correlate with the decline in creatinine clearance with age (Rowe et al., 1976). Since creatinine clearance can be difficult to measure, plasma levels of drugs with predominant renal elimination should be monitored, particularly with chronic therapy in the elderly. Such drugs include the aminoglycoside, digoxin, chlorpropamide (Diabinese, Pfizer, New York, NY), cimetidine (Tagamet, SmithKline Beecham, Philadelphia, PA), and lithium (Vestal and Dawson, 1985).

Environmental Factors

Dietary intake can be an important factor in drug metabolism (Campbell and Hayes, 1974). Protein and certain micronutritional deficiencies, such as lack of vitamin C, can impair the metabolism of drugs (Krehl, 1974). Cigarette smoking induces hepatic microsomal enzyme activity but the effect on drug metabolism is variable (Vestal et al., 1979).

In general, the effects of aging on pharmacokinetic parameters of drug action prolong drug elimination half-lives, result in unpredictable changes in volume of drug distribution, and reduce total drug clearance. Although no consistent changes in albumin binding occur, free drug concentration in the elderly may be higher because of lower serum albumin concentrations (Lamy, 1980). For establishing dosage schedules, pharmacokinetic principles, particularly renal and hepatic factors, should be combined with clinical response of the patient to the established drug regimens, particularly for those agents for which age-related changes in their clinical actions have been observed. Table 5.2 lists some drugs that have been associated with age-related changes in pharmacokinetic parameters.

Drug–Receptor Interactions

The effect of drugs on target sites has been studied less extensively than the pharmacokinetic parameters discussed previously (Table 5.3). Both heightened and reduced drug effects, which have not been related to altered pharmacokinetic variables, have been suggested to be caused by changes in tissue sensitivity, altered homeostasis, or complications associated with chronic disease states in the elderly (O'Malley et al., 1980).

Table 5.2 Drugs associated with age-related changes in pharmacokinetics

Barbiturates
Benzodiazepines
Digoxin
Indomethacin
Meperidine
Morphine
Penicillin
Phenylbutazone
Phenytoin
Propranolol

Source: Lamy, 1980.

Table 5.3 Physiologic factors and pathologic conditions affecting drug action in the geriatric population

Physiologic Change	Pathologic Condition
Absorption	
Reduced GI secretions	Achlorhydria
Reduced GI blood flow	Diarrhea
Reduced absorptive surface	Malabsorption syndromes
Reduced GI motility	Pancreatitis
	Gastrectomy
Distribution	
Decreased cardiac output	Congestive heart failure
Decreased total body water	Dehydration
Reduced lean body mass	Hepatic failure
Reduced serum albumin	Renal failure
Increase in acid glycoprotein	Malnutrition
Increased body fat	Drug-drug interactions
Metabolism	
Reduced liver mass	Congestive heart failure
Reduced hepatic blood flow	Hepatic disease
Reduced enzymatic activity	Malnutrition
	Thyroid disease
	Cancer
	Microbial infection
	Drug-drug interactions
Excretion	
Reduced renal blood flow	Renal insufficiency
Reduced glomerular filtration rate	Hypovolemia
Reduced renal tubular function	

Adapted from Vestal and Dawson, 1985; Montamat, et al., 1989.

Table 5.4   Guidelines for geriatric drug utilization

Obtain a complete drug history, including use of all over-the-counter medications.

Review patients drug use on all office visits.

In general, when prescribing medications or using drugs for diagnostic purposes with geriatric patients, administer the minimal effective dosage.

Become familiar with the effects of age on the pharmacologic action of the drugs that the patient is using.

Become familiar with possible interactions between disease states and drugs.

Be alert to possible drug-induced ocular and systemic side effects.

Adapted from: Montamat, et al., 1989.

Enhanced clinical responses at drug levels below the therapeutic range have been observed with analgesics, psychoactive agents, and anticoagulants. In contrast, beta-adrenergic blocking agents and the calcium-channel blockers show decreased receptor sensitivities (Shepherd et al., 1977; Reidenberg et al., 1978); Vestal, 1979; Abernethy et al., 1986).

The mechanisms involved in age-related changes in drug responses are not well understood. Possible mechanisms, in addition to altered pharmacokinetics, may include changes in receptor density or affinity, changes in biochemical responses such as altered second messenger (for example, cAMP activity or glycogenolysis). Mechanical effects, such as altered vascular tone, have also been proposed (Wingard et al., 1991).

Some guidelines for drug utilization are present in Table 5.4.

SOME MAJOR DRUG GROUPS

A number of drugs are used more frequently in the geriatric population. Some require dosage reduction and close monitoring (Table 5.5).

Cardiovascular Drugs

Cardiovascular disease accounts for the majority of hospital admissions and hypertension, especially systolic pressure, increases after age 50 years.

Diuretics

Diuretics are commonly used in the elderly to treat hypertension above the age-corrected norm and congestive heart failure (CHF). Although the basic principles of therapy are not different, cautions resulting from altered pharmacokinetics and sensitivity do apply in the elderly. Thiazide diuretics often show a

Table 5.5 Pharmacological differences observed with certain drugs in geriatric patients

Drug	Clinical Observations
Alcohol	Special caution when sedative and hypnotics are used simultaneously
Analgesics	
Aspirin	Monitor for dose-related adverse effects and GI problems; analysis of plasma levels may be useful with chronic high doses; single doses require no dosage alteration
Morphine, meperidine	May require lower dosages for pain relief; may exhibit increased potential for side effects
Nonsteroidal anti-inflammatory agents	Adverse effects may be greater in elderly with certain drugs in this group; acute renal failure may be more frequent
Anticholinergic agents	Elderly appear more sensitive to anticholinergic drugs and drugs in general that exhibit anticholinergic properties; monitor for confusion, urinary problems, constipation, other anticholinergic effects
Anticoagulants	Elderly, especially women, may need lower dosages as observed with warfarin
Anticonvulsants	Increased plasma levels of phenytoin; monitoring of drug levels recommended to prevent dose-related toxicities
Anti-infective agents	
Aminoglycosides	Potential for accumulation exists; monitor plasma levels, especially if renal or hearing impairment exists
Amoxicillin and ampicillin	Reduction of dosage only if severe renal impairment exists
Tetracyclines	Dosage alteration probably not necessary; consider doxycycline in severe renal impairment
Cardiac drugs	
Digoxin	Higher incidence of side effects in elderly; monitor for side effects such as GI, CNS, and ocular
Calcium channel blocking agents	Diltiazem may have slower onset of action in elderly
Beta-receptor blocking agents	Propranolol exhibits higher plasma levels; serious side effects tend to be more common in elderly; bioavailability of labetalol increases with age
Antihypertensive agents	Incidence of postural hypotension and CNS effects may be higher with certain agents

Table 5.5 continued

Drug	Clinical Observations
Psychoactive agents	
Antidepressants	Elderly may be more sensitive to side effects, especially anticholinergic toxicity
Lithium	Higher incidence of side effects, e.g., neurologic; monitoring of plasma levels highly recommended especially if on concurrent diuretic therapy
Phenothiazines	Elderly more sensitive to sedative, anticholinergic, autonomic side effects; ocular side effects possible with high-dose, long-term use
Antianxiety agents	May accumulate to produce excessive drowsiness, reduced energy levels, aggravation of depression as has been reported with diazepam and chlordiazepoxide; lorazepam or oxazepam may be preferable in elderly; flurazepam shows increased prevalence of dose-related residual drowsiness
H₂ Receptor-blocking agents	Confusion has been reported with cimetidine; observe for changes in sensorium with cimetidine, ranitidine; half-life of ranitidine prolonged
Vitamins	Possibility of vitamin deficiencies exists in the elderly

Adapted from Tobias, 1988.

decreased natriuretic effect, particularly in patients with renal impairment. The loop diuretics, such as furosemide (Lasix, Hoechst-Roussel, Somerville, NJ) may be more effective. Volume depletion may lead to decreased cardiac output and electrolyte imbalance. Orthostatic hypotension and risk of hypokalemia and hyperuricemia is greater. Serum calcium levels may be increased. Use of any diuretic in the geriatric patient should be monitored closely, particularly if the patient is on multiple drug therapy (Andreasen et al., 1984; Baldwin and Vacek, 1989; Buechler and Malloy, 1989; Katzung, 1989).

Cardiac Glycosides

Preparations of digitalis have been used for more than 100 years for the management of CHF and atrial arrhythmias. Dosage levels between therapeutic and toxic effects are narrow, and the half-life of elimination of digoxin is increased by approximately 40% in the elderly (Reuning and Geraets, 1986). Close monitoring is essential to avoid potential side effects, which can include gastrointestinal (GI), cardiac, neurologic, and visual adverse effects. Nausea, anorexia, fatigue, depression, and confusion can be early signs of toxic levels of the drug (Lely and Van Enter, 1972). Cardiac side effects can include bradycardia and aggravation of CHF. The vision care practitioner should pay particular attention to possible visual effects, especially alterations in color vision. Several classes of drugs can affect digoxin serum levels when taken concurrently. Diuretics and certain calcium channel blocking agents, such as verapamil, has been observed to enhance the effects of digoxin. Phenytoin and the antacids have been reported to lessen its effects.

Antiarrhythmics

Patients on these drugs need careful follow-up because of their complex pharmacologic properties. The clearance of quinidine and procainamide decreases with age, with hepatic disease and CHF. Disopyramide (Norpace, G.D. Searle, Chicago, IL), because of its anticholinergic effects, is used less often in the elderly. Other drugs in this class, including flecainide and encainide, should be monitored closely in patients with hepatic or renal dysfunction because elimination of these drugs is slowed (Lamy, 1980; Tobias, 1988). Amiodarone (Cordarone, Wyeth-Ayerst Laboratories, Philadelphia, PA) has a long half-life, and its effects do not correlate well with serum drug levels. Toxicity, both systemic and ocular, is common (Bartlett and Jaanus, 1989).

Beta Adrenergic Blocking Agents

Beta adrenergic blocking agents are presently widely used in cardiovascular diseases. Studies have shown that the elderly exhibit a decreased clinical response to beta-blocking agents, such as propranolol (Inderal, Wyeth-Ayerst Laboratories, Philadelphia, PA) and timolol (Blocadren, Merck Sharp & Dohme, West Point, PA) (Vestal et al., 1979). The decreased responsiveness of this class of drugs in the geriatric population is presumed to be the result of their reduced interaction with cell receptors (Klein et al., 1986). Side effects are also higher. Depression is more common in the elderly. Advanced heart block and bradycardia can result from use of these drugs. Cardioselective beta-blocking agents can exacerbate bronchioconstriction. Beta blockers also decrease hepatic blood flow and can significantly reduce metabolism of other drugs (Parmley, 1981).

Calcium Channel Blocking Agents

Calcium channel blockers are being used with increasing frequency to treat angina, supraventricular tachyarrhythmia, and hypertension. Geriatric patients with hypertension appear to respond well to these agents. Dosage and frequency of administration should be monitored carefully in patients with renal or hepatic insufficiency. Concurrent use of the calcium channel blocking agent, verapamil, and digoxin can elevate serum levels of digoxin; therefore, the dosage of digoxin should be reduced (Abernethy et al., 1986).

Angiotensin Converting Enzyme (ACE) Inhibitors

ACE inhibitors are also in frequent use at present for control of hypertension and CHF. In general, these agents are well tolerated and effective in the elderly, but dosage reduction based on renal function has been suggested, because risk of acute renal failure, hypotension, and hyperkalemia exist (Lees and Reid, 1987).

Nonsteroidal Anti-inflammatory Drugs (NSAIDs)

It has been estimated that about half of the population over age 65 have symptomatic arthritis (Buechler and Malloy, 1989). NSAIDs are frequently prescribed and are also self-administered for various rheumatic problems and musculoskeletal pain. Use of one of these agents, ibuprofen, has particularly increased since it became available over-the-counter. The use of NSAIDs in the elderly is associated with risk of serious side effects. Aspirin, although an effective analgesic and anti-inflammatory agent, can cause serious GI irritation and also bleeding. It generally has limited usefulness as an anti-inflammatory agent in chronic use. When chronic anti-inflammatory effects are needed, the newer, longer-acting NSAIDs, such as sulindac (Clinoril, Merck Sharp & Dohme, West Point, PA), diflunisal (Dolobid, Merck Sharp & Dohme), diclofenac (Voltaren, Geigy, Ardsley, NY), and piroxicam (Feldene, Pfizer, New York, NY) may be preferred because of better patient compliance (Amadio and Cummings, 1986; Lamy, 1986). These agents are thought to exert their pharmacologic effects by interference with prostaglandin synthesis. Although prostaglandins appear to play a major role in the inflammatory response, they also play a vital role in the protective mechanism of the gastric mucosa and the autoregulation of renal blood flow.

A significant incidence of GI disease and renal impairment has been observed in elderly patients when anti-inflammatory dosages of NSAIDs are used. Acute renal failure appears more common in the elderly, especially those with renal disease or hypovolemia.

Diuretics, particularly the loop diuretics and the ACE inhibitors can interact with the NSAIDs and increase the risk of hyperkalemia (Lamy, 1986).

In general, it is recommended that use of NSAIDs in the elderly be monitored carefully for dose and possible adverse effects, particularly in patients with chronic disease and those on other medications. It also has been recommended that the dose be reduced initially and increased slowly to the desired clinical effect. Misoprostol (Cytotec, G.D. Searle, Chicago, IL), an analog of the E series prostaglandins with antiulcer properties, has been found useful in patients at risk for GI complications (Graham, 1989).

Sedative–Hypnotics

The half-lives of the barbiturates and benzodiazepines increase with age, particularly during the decade from 60 to 70 years. Decline in renal and liver function, decreased volume of distribution, reduction in lean body mass, and drug-receptor sensitivity have been suggested as the causative factors. When used in the elderly patient, benzodiazepines with relatively shorter half-lives, such as alprazolam (Xanax, Upjohn, Kalamazoo, MI), lorazepam (Ativan, Wyeth-Ayerst Laboratories, Philadelphia, PA), and oxazepam (Serax, Wyeth-Ayerst Laboratories) have been recommended (Buechler and Malloy, 1989). Among the possible adverse effects of these drugs, daytime drowsiness and ataxia are indications of excessive benzodiazepine dosage (Katzung, 1989).

Antipsychotic and Antidepressant Agents

The antipsychotic agents have been used extensively in the elderly, particularly in those who demonstrate agitated and disruptive behavior. However, full control of the patient's behavior is not always possible, and dosage should not be increased because side effects become prominent (Katzung, 1989). Before prescribing these agents, practitioners should ascertain that the patient's condition is not already the result of drugs being administered for other disease entities. The incidence of extrapyramidal effects, particularly akathisia (for example, restlessness and difficulty in sitting still) should not be mistaken as insufficient drug administration (Buechler and Malloy, 1989). Haloperidol (Haldol, McNeil Pharmaceutical, Spring House, PA) can be very effective in the treatment of symptoms associated with agitation, combativeness, and paranoia, but serious adverse effects can occur in the elderly. Depression is often misdiagnosed and untreated in the elderly. The symptoms associated with psychiatric depression, such as apathy and social withdrawal may be mistaken as senile dementia (Katzung, 1989). Again, before beginning therapy with an antidepressant drug, the possible effects of other medications that the patient may be taking must be taken into consideration. When an antidepressant drug is chosen, its sedative, anticholinergic, and cardiac side effects must be considered. Using these criteria, desipramine (Norpramin, Marion Merrel Dow, Kansas City, MO) and trazodone (Desyrel, Mead Johnson Pharmaceutical, Evansville, IN) are often the drugs chosen for geriatric depression (Buechler and Malloy, 1989; Salzman, 1985). There is some clinical evidence which seems to indicate that the elderly are clinically as responsive as younger patients, but side effects are more common in this age group (Katzung, 1989).

H_2-Blocking Agents

H_2-blocking drugs have been very useful in controlling various peptic and duodenal disorders. Their use is generally safe, but headaches and mental confusion can occur. Drug interactions with these agents, however, are of concern, particularly with cimetidine (Tagamet, SmithKline Beecham Pharmaceuticals, Philadelphia, PA) and ranitidine (Zantac, Glaxo Pharmaceuticals, Research Triangle Park, NC) (Sawyer et al., 1981). Both of these agents inhibit liver enzyme systems to varying degrees and thus prolong the half-lives of drugs metabolized by this mechanism, such as phenytoin, theophylline, and warfarin.

H₁-Blocking Agents

The classic H₁-antihistamines are distributed to all tissues, and because they are lipophilic, they also cross the blood-brain barrier. They undergo liver metabolism and the metabolites are excreted in the urine. The CNS effects of these drugs can manifest as stimulation or depression, with depression more common in adults, particularly the elderly. Sedation is generally the most common side effect associated with administration of diphenhydramine (Benadryl, Parke Davis, Morris Plains, NJ) and chlorpheniramine (Chlor-Trimeton). The elderly are also more sensitive to the cognitive effects of these agents and care must be taken in their use to minimize the anticholinergic effects associated with the classic antihistamine (Wingard et al., 1991).

The second generation of H₁ receptor antagonists such as terfenadine (Seldane, Marion Merrell Dow, Kansas City, MO) and astemizole (Hismanal, Janssen Pharmaceutical, Piscataway, NJ) do not penetrate the blood-brain barrier, and CNS depression is not a prominent side effect. The depressant effects of diazepam (Valium, Roche Products, Manati, PR) and alcohol appear also not to be enhanced by these agents (Kemp et al., 1985; Moser et al., 1978). Terfenadine is also available with pseudoephedrine as an antihistamine-decongestant combination product. Caution is advised with its use in the elderly because the two agents are more likely to have adverse reactions to sympathomimetics, such as palpitations, headache, and insomnia.

Anticholinergic Drugs

Anticholinergic drug toxicity is of concern, particularly in the elderly because they appear more susceptible to impaired autonomic effects on such organ systems as the bowels, bladder, and CNS. The elderly patient may be especially sensitive to the cognitive effects caused by the anticholinergic drugs and drugs in general with atropine-like effects. Loss of memory and delirium are common features of anticholinergic toxicity in the elderly. Use of scopolamine as a transdermal preparation has been associated with sudden loss of memory, disorientation, and delirium (Rozzini et al., 1988). Table 5.6 lists drugs with anticholinergic properties.

Table 5.6   Drugs with anticholinergic properties

Antipsychotics
Antidepressants
Antiepileptics
Antispasmodics
Antihistamines
Hypnotics

Antimicrobial Drugs

Mortality rates from infection are generally higher in older patients because of various factors, including reduced host-defense mechanisms and reactions to antimicrobials (Yoshikawa, 1990). Broad-spectrum antibiotics generally are preferred in the elderly, and the basic principles of therapy are the same as for younger patients. The age-dependent factor that must be considered is possible decrease in renal function. This is an important consideration with use of such anti-infective agents as the aminoglycosides, Vancomycin, fluoroquinolones, and amantadine (Symmetrel, Du Pont Multi-Source Products, Garden City, NY). Tetracyclines, with the exception of doxycycline and minocycline, are excreted by glomerular filtration and tend to accumulate in the presence of renal failure (Mallet, 1991).

In most elderly patients without moderately severe renal dysfunction, anti-infectives such as the penicillins, cephalosporins, and trimethoprim-sulfamethoxazole combination may be prescribed in standard doses.

Nonprescription Drugs

It has been estimated that more than 12 billion dollars is spent annually in the United States on over-the-counter (OTC) drugs. The geriatric population is believed to be a major consumer of OTC drugs, and most of this use is without prior consultation with a health-care provider (Lamy, 1986). Since nonprescription drugs can contribute to adverse drug reactions and drug interactions, it is important that all health-care practitioners monitor patients for OTC drug use (Stanaszek and Baker, 1983) (Table 5.7).

Among the OTC agents in frequent use are the analgesics, antacids, cough and cold remedies, laxatives, and vitamins.

Analgesics

The most frequently used OTC analgesics are acetominophen, aspirin, and, more recently due to its OTC availability, ibuprofen. All three drugs are effective in providing analgesia for mild-to-moderate pain. Tolerance does not seem to appear with chronic use.

Aspirin use in the elderly has been associated with adverse reactions. Symptoms of toxicity may appear at lower doses and may include irritability, deafness, and GI problems, including bleeding. Interaction with oral anticoagulants and uricosuric agents can occur. Chronic, high doses of aspirin can lead to kidney failure (Goldberger and Talner, 1975).

Acetaminophen has analgesic and antipyretic properties similar to aspirin and ibuprofen, but lacks anti-inflammatory effects. In pain associated with significant inflammation, the other two analgesics may be more effective.

Acetaminophen use in the recommended dosages generally is associated with less gastric irritation. It will not cause gastric bleeding or erosions, affect uric

Table 5.7   Over-the-counter drug interactions

OTC Drug	Prescription Drug	Possible Clinical Effect
Alcohol	CNS depressants	Enhanced depression
	Aspirin	Gastrointestinal bleeding
Antacids	Phenothiazines	Inhibition of phenothiazine absorption
	Tetracycline	Divalent cations, for example, calcium present in formulations impair absorption of tetracycline
Aspirin	Methotrexate	Enhanced clinical effects of methotrexate
	Anticoagulants	Enhanced anticoagulant effects
	Probenecid	Reduced uricosuric effect
Agents with anticholinergic effects, for example, antihistamines, cold and cough preparations	CNS depressants; anticholinergics	Enhanced anticholinergic effects
Phenylephrine; phenylpropanolamine	Monoamine oxidase inhibitors	Enhanced effects of these and other adrenergic agonists, for example, possible hypertensive crisis

Adapted from Lamy 1980; Stanaszek and Baker, 1983.

acid excretion, or potentiate the action of oral anticoagulants (Koch-Weser and Sellers, 1971).

Ibuprofen has analgesic, antipyretic, and anti-inflammatory effects. It is widely used for the relief of pain of various origins, including pain of rheumatic origin. Gastrointestinal irritation is a major adverse effect associated with its use.

Antacids

Antacids are frequently used for symptomatic relief of upset stomach, heartburn, and peptic ulcers. Antacids differ in palatability as well as in their ability to neutralize gastric acid. Sodium content of these products varies and should be considered in patients with CHF and decreased renal function. Effervescent formulations and those containing sodium bicarbonate are generally higher in sodium content (Lamy, 1980). Antacids can affect the absorption and elimination of drugs taken concurrently. By altering intestinal pH, absorption of acidic drugs can be increased and those of basic drugs decreased. By delaying gastric emptying, drug absorption from the intestine also may be altered. They also may affect urinary pH and thereby alter the excretion of acidic or basic drugs. It therefore is recommended that the use of these products be ascertained and their use monitored as closely as possible (Lamy, 1980).

Cough and Cold Preparations
Cough and cold preparations offer relief from symptoms associated with accumulation of secretions in the bronchial passages. These preparations can contain alcohol, dextromethorphan and other cough suppressants, antihistamines, bronchodilators, and decongestants. Alcohol can potentiate the effects of phenothiazines, sedatives, and certain of the antihistamines. The elderly also are more susceptible to the sedative effects of these agents. Elderly patients with asthma, glaucoma, and urinary tract problems generally are advised against the use of products containing antihistamines or other anticholinergic agents.

Bronchodilators and decongestants primarily contain adrenergic agonists. Use of these products can therefore lead to nervousness, dizziness, and insomnia. Because of their pressor effects, the use of these products is generally contraindicated in patients with high blood pressure, diabetes, and hyperthyroidism, and in the concurrent use of monoamino oxidase (MAO) class of antidepressants.

Laxatives
Laxative use among the elderly is also frequent. Disease, poor nutrition, diminished physical activity, and emotional factors can be possible causes of constipation. Chronic use of laxatives should be evaluated because it can lead to adverse effects such as disturbances in electrolyte and water balance (Lamy, 1980). It has been suggested that the safest laxatives for chronic use include the bulk formers and stool softeners.

Vitamins
Vitamin supplementation appears to be common in the elderly. While evidence for large-scale vitamin deficiencies are lacking, excessive intake appears common. Megadose intake of certain vitamins has been associated with renal and CNS effects. Niacin can alter liver function and raise blood levels of uric acid and glucose. Excessive intake of thiamine can result in cardiovascular and CNS effects (DiPalma and Ritchie, 1977). Vitamins A and D in particular can interfere with some laboratory tests (Lamy, 1980). Vitamin supplementation may be necessary in elderly patients with chronic drug use, certain disease states, and excessive stress.

REFERENCES

1. Abernethy, D.R. and L. Kerzner. "Age Effects on Alpha-1 Acid Glycoprotein Concentration and Imipramine Plasma Protein Binding." *J. Am. Geriatr. Soc.* 32 (1984): 705–708.
2. Abernethy, D.R., J.B. Schwartz, E.L. Todd, et al. "Verapamil Pharmacodynamics and Disposition in Young and Elderly Hypertensive Patients." *Ann. Intern. Med.* 105 (1986): 329–336.

3. Amadio, P. and D.M. Cummings. "Non-steroidal Antiinflammatory Agents: An Update." *Am. Fam. Physician* 34 (1986): 147–154.
4. Andreasen, F., V. Hansen, S.E. Husted, et al. "The Influence of Age on Renal and Extrarenal Effects of Furosemide." *Br. J. Clin. Pharmacol.* 18 (1984): 65–74.
5. Buecchler, J.R. and W. Malloy. "Drug Therapy in the Elderly." *Postgrad. Med.* 85 (1989): 87–99.
6. Baldwin, T. and J. Vacek. "Use of Cardiovascular Drugs in the Elderly." *Postgrad. Med.* 85, no. 5 (1989): 319–330.
7. Bartlett, J.D. and S.D. Jaanus. In: Bartlett, J. D. and S.D. Jaanus (eds.). *Clinical Ocular Pharmacology.* Boston: Butterworth, 1989, pp. 801–842.
8. Baum, C., D.L. Kennedy, M.B. Forbes, et al. "Drug Use in the United States in 1981." *J.A.M.A.* 251 (1981): 1293–1297.
9. Bhanthumnarin, K. and M.M. Schuster. "Aging and Gastro-intestinal Function." In: Finch, C.E. and L. Hayflick (eds.). *Handbook of Biology of Aging.* New York: Van Nostrand-Reinhold, 1977, pp. 709–723.
10. Buechler, J.R. and D. Malloy. "Drug Therapy in the Elderly." *Postgrad. Med.* 85 (1989): 87–99.
11. Campbell, T.C. and R.J. Hayes. "Role of Nutrition in the Drug-metabolizing Enzyme System." *Pharmacol. Rev.* 26 (1974): 171–197.
12. DiPalma, J.R. and D.M. Ritchie. "Vitamin Toxicity." *Annu. Rev. Pharmacol. Toxicol.* 17 (1977): 133–162.
13. Goldberger, L.E. and L.B. Talner. "Analgesic Abuse Syndrome: A Frequently Overlooked Cause of Reversible Renal Failure." *Urology* 5, no. 7 (1975): 728–735.
14. Goldberg, P.B. and J. Roberts. "Pharmacologic Basis for Developing Rational Drug Regimens for Elderly Patients." *Med. Clin. North Am.* 67 (1983): 315–331.
15. Graham, D.Y. "Prevention of Gastroduodenal Injury Induced by Chronic Nonsteroidal, Antiinflammatory Drug Therapy." *Gastroenterology* (1989): 675–681.
16. Greenblatt, D.J. "Reduced Serum Albumin Concentration in the Elderly: A Report from the Boston Collaborative Drug Surveillance Program." *J. Am. Geriatr. Soc.* 27 (1979): 20–22.
17. Greenblatt, D.J., M. Divoli, D.P. Abernethy, et al. "Physiologic Changes in Old Age: Relation to Altered Drug Disposition." *J. Am. Geriatr. Soc.* 30 (1982): S 6–10.
18. Hayes, M.S., M.S.S. Langinan, A.T.T. Short. "Changes in Drug Metabolism with Increasing Age." *Br. J. Clin. Pharmacol.* 2 (1975): 69–77.
19. Ho, P.C. and E.J. Triggs. "Drug Therapy in the Elderly." *Aust. N.Z. J. Med.* 14 (1984): 179–190.
20. Jernigan, J.A. "Update on Drugs and the Elderly." *Am. Fam. Physician* 29 (1984): 238–247.
21. Katzung, B. G. *Basic and Clinical Pharmacology.* Norwalk: Appleton Lange, 1989.
22. Kemp, J.P., C.E. Buckley, M.E. Gershwin, et al. "Multicenter, Double-blind, Placebo-controlled Trial of Trefenadine in Seasonal Allergic Rhinitis and Conjunctivitis." *Ann. Allergy* 54, no. 6 (1985): 502–509.
23. Klein, G., J.G. Gerber, J. Gal, et al. "Beta-adrenergic Receptors in the Elderly Are Not Less Sensitive to Timolol." *Clin. Pharmacol. Ther.* 40 (1986): 161–164.
24. Klein, L.E., P.S. German, D.M. Levine, et al. "Medication Problems Among Outpatients. A Study with Emphasis on the Elderly." *Arch. Intern. Med.* 144 (1984): 1185–1188.

25. Krehl, W.A. "The Influence of Nutritional Environment on Aging." *Geriatrics* 29 (1974): 65–76.
26. Koch-Weser, J., E. M. Sellers. "Drug Interactions with Coumarin Anticoagulants, Part 1." *New Engl. J. Med.* 285 (1971): 487–492.
27. Lamy, P.P. *Prescribing for the Elderly.* Massachusetts: Littleton PSG Publishing Company, 1980.
28. Lamy, P. "Renal Effect of Non-steroidal Antiinflammatory Drugs: Heightened Risk in the Elderly?" *J. Am. Geriatr. Soc.* 34 (1986): 361–367.
29. Lees, K.R. and S.L. Reid. "Age and the Pharmacokinetics and Pharmacodynamics of Chronic Enalapril Treatment." *Clin. Pharmacol. Ther.* 4 (1987): 597–602.
30. Lely, A.H. and C.H.F. Van Enter. "Non-cardiac Symptoms of Digitalis Intoxication." *Am. Heart J.* 83 (1972): 149–152.
31. Mallet, L. "Age-related Changes in Renal Function and Clinical Implication for Drug Therapy." *J. Geriatr. Drug Ther.* 5 (1991): 6–29.
32. Mayersohn, M. 1986. Special Pharmacokinetic Considerations in the Elderly. In: Evans, W.E. et al. *Applied Pharmacokinetics.* 2nd ed. Spokane, WA: *Applied Therapeutics.* 229–293.
33. Montamat, S.C., B.S. Cusack, R.E. Vestal. "Management of Drug Therapy in the Elderly." *New Engl. J. Med.* 321 (1979): 303–309.
34. Moser, L., K.S. Huther, J. Koch-Weser. "Effects of Trefenadine and Diphenydramine Alone or in Combination with Diazepam or Alcohol on Psychomotor Performance and Subjective Feelings." *Eur. J. Clin. Pharmacol.* 14 (1978): 417–423.
35. Novak, L.P. "Aging, Total Body Potassium, Fat-free Mass and Cell Mass in Males and Females Between Ages 18 and 85 Years." *J. Gerontol.* 27 (1972): 438–443.
36. O'Malley, K., T.G. Judge, J. Crooks. Geriatric Clinical Pharmacology and Therapeutics. In: Avery G.S. (ed.). *Drug Treatment.* New York: ADIS Press, 1980, 158–181.
37. Ouslander, J.G. "Drug Therapy in the Elderly." *Ann. Intern. Med.* 95 (1981): 711–722.
38. Parmley, W.W. "Beta Blockers in Coronary Artery Disease." *Cardiovasc. Rev. Rep.* (1981–1982): 655–662.
39. Reidenberg, M.M., M. Levy, H. Warner, et al. "Relationship between Diazepam Dose, Plasma Level, Age and Central Nervous System Depression." *Clin. Pharmacol. Ther.* 23 (1978): 371–374.
40. Reuning, R.H. and D.R. Geraets. Digoxin. In: Evans, W.E., Schentag, S.S., et al. (eds.). *Applied Pharmacokinetics: Principles of Therapeutic Drug Monitoring,* 2nd ed. Spokane: Applied Therapeutics, Inc., 1986, pp. 570–623.
41. Richey, D.P. and A.D. Bender. "Pharmacokinetic Consequences of Aging." *Annu. Rev. Pharmacol. Toxicol.* 17 (1977): 49–65.
42. Rowe, J.W., R. Andres, J.D. Tobin, et al. "The Effect of Age on Creatinine Clearance in Man: A Cross-sectional and Longitudinal Study." *J. Gerontol.* 31 (1976): 155–163.
43. Rozzini, R., M. Inzoli, M. Trabucchi, et al. "Delirium from Transdermal Scopolamine in Elderly Women." *J.A.M.A.* (1988): 260–478.
44. Salzman, C. "Geriatric Psychopharmacology." *Annu. Rev. Med.* 36 (1985): 217–235.
45. Sawyer, D., C.S. Conner, R. Scalley, et al. "Cimetidine: Adverse Reactions and Acute Toxicity." *Am. J. Hosp. Pharm.* 38 (1981): 188–197.
46. Schwartz, D., M. Wang, L. Zeitz, et al. "Medication Errors Made by Elderly, Chronically Ill Patients." *Am. J. Publ. Health* 52 (1962): 2018–2029.

47. Shepherd, A.M., D.S. Hewick, T.A. Moreland, et al. "Age as a Determinant of Sensitivity to Warfarin. *Br. J. Clin. Pharmacol.* 4 (1977): 315–320.
48. Stanaszek, W.F. and D. Baker. "Drug Monitoring in the Geriatric Patient." *Am. Pharm.* 23 (1983): 32–37.
49. Tobias, D. Geriatric Drug Use. In: Knoben, J.E., Anderson, P.O. (eds.). *Handbook of Clinical Drug Data.* Illinois: Drug Intelligence Publications, 1988; chapter 9.
50. Trounce, J.R. "Drug Metabolism in the Elderly." *Br. J. Clin. Pharmacol.* (1975): 289–294.
51. Upton, R.A., R.L. Williams, J. Velley, et al. "Naproxen Pharmacokinetics in the Elderly." *Br. J. Clin. Pharmacol.* 18 (1984): 207–214.
52. Vestal, R.E., A.H. Norris, J.D. Tobin, et al. "Antipyrine Metabolism in Man, Influence of Age, Alcohol, Caffeine and Smoking." *Clin. Pharmacol. Ther.* 26 (1979): 16–20.
53. Vestal, R.E., A.S.S. Wood, D.G. Shand. "Reduced Beta-Adrenoreceptor Sensitivity in the Elderly." *Clin. Pharmacol. Ther.* 26 (1979): 181–186.
54. Vestal, R.E. and G.W. Dawson. Pharmacology and Aging. In: Finch, C.E., Schneider, E.L. (eds.). *Handbook of the Biology of Aging,* 2nd ed. New York: Van Nostrand Reinhold, 1985, pp. 744–789.
55. Vestal, R.E. and B.J. Cusack. Pharmacology and Aging. In: Schneider, E.L., Rowe, S.W. (eds.). *Handbook of the Biology of Aging.* New York: Academic Press, 1990, pp. 349–383.
56. Wingard, L.B., T.M. Brody, J. Larner, et al. *Human Pharmacology.* St. Louis: Mosby Yearbook, 1991.
57. Woodford-Williams, E., A.S. Alvarez, D. Webster, et al. "Serum Protein Patterns in 'Normal' and Pathological Aging." *Gerontology* 10 (1964): 86–99.
58. Yoshikawa, T.T. "Antimicrobial Therapy for the Elderly. *J. Am. Geriatrics Soc.* 38 (1990): 1353–1372.

6

Normal Age Related Vision Changes

Meredith W. Morgan

This chapter will be limited to changes in visual function in the normal, healthy, aging eye free from obvious structural or pathologic anomalies. This restriction may raise some practical as well as philosophical problems, since few eyes that have survived 65 or more years of life are free from at least some slight sign of deterioration, degeneration, or past or present disease that can escape a scientific, sophisticated search. This chapter will use the concept of "normal" in much the same way as the average clinician states that an amblyopic eye is "normal" in that it has no immediately apparent structural or pathologic defect that could account for the reduced acuity. Such an eye is obviously not normal, since it has less than normal acuity. In an amblyopic eye, there is just no readily apparent cause for the reduced acuity. Conditions that apply to most aged eyes, such as miosis and the absence of accommodation, will be considered normal rather than abnormal or pathologic.

This approach is used for two main reasons: (1) pathologic and degenerative conditions affecting the aging eye are discussed in other chapters, and (2) departure from normal function is a clue that a more detailed and critical examination and search need to be made. This requires that the examiner know what normal function is. Unfortunately, most clinical optometric norms have been established by data from prepresbyopic subjects.

The major thrust of the discussion will be about the aspects of vision that are of chief concern to clinicians and ordinarily measured by them. Some attention, however, will be given to phenomena that today are primarily of interest to visual scientists, but that will someday also be of concern to optometrists. As a matter of fact, most of the significant changes in visual function of the aging eye, except for the loss of focusing ability and the increase in variability of measured functions, are not quantified by clinicians in the usual vision examination. As yet, nearly all ophthalmologists, as well as a majority of optometrists, assume that aging patients without significant motor imbalance and with good corrected visual acuity at distance and near must have satisfactory or normal visually controlled behavior and therefore need no therapy other than correction lenses. Some visual scientists, as well as some optometrists, are suggesting that there is a more sophisticated and comprehensive view of vision (Leibowitz, 1980).

The increase in variability or dispersion of measured function with increasing age applies to nearly all visual functions. This makes it extremely difficult to identify performance that is clearly subnormal. There are almost always some older persons who function as well as younger ones, but the number with "best performance" usually declines with age. For example, Weymouth (1960), using data supplied by Hirsch, reported that in the age bracket from 40 to 44 years, 93.5% of patients had a corrected visual acuity of 20/20 or better; in the age bracket from 70 to 74 years, however, only 41.9% had a corrected visual acuity of 20/20 or better, and 56.1% had a corrected visual acuity of 20/40 or better. Most of this decrease in the percentage of individuals with maximum acuity and the greater variability in best-corrected acuity is due to the effects of degeneration or disease conditions. Some of the decrease, however, cannot be accounted for on this basis. In the 70 to 74-year-old age group just referred to, 14.5% of the patients with corrected visual acuity of less than 20/25 had no clinically reportable degenerative or disease conditions — the eyes were clinically normal but visual acuity was not.

A good many of the apparent physiologic or psychological changes in visual function have a physical cause. Consequently, this chapter will first discuss changes in the structure of the eye that could result in a change in visual function and that are detected by clinicians in routine vision examinations. Most of the biometrical data that will be discussed is cross-sectional in nature; that is, the data were collected from different subjects, usually without regard to size or sex; at different times; and frequently by different examiners using different techniques. This means that differences in measurements between individuals attributed primarily to age can be only accepted tentatively. Most biometric data concerning the eye, such as length of the eyeball, depth of the anterior chamber, and radius of curvature of the cornea, are smaller for women than for men — smaller adult individuals have smaller eyes. For each decade during the past several decades, humans have become somewhat larger. Thus, changes that indicate that the eyes of older persons are smaller in any dimension may be due to the fact that older adult persons are, on average, smaller than younger adults.

CHANGES IN THE CORNEA WITH AGE

Corneal sensitivity to touch decreases with age. According to Millodot (1977), the threshold for touch almost doubles between the ages of 10 and 80, increasing rapidly after the age of 40. The cause for this decrease is not known. It is both an advantage and a disadvantage in fitting contact lenses — an advantage in that older patients adapt more readily to contact lenses, but a disadvantage in that corneal lesions may occur without creating significant subjective symptoms of pain. The practitioner, particularly with older patients, should not depend on the presence of symptoms to suggest that the integrity of the cornea need be examined carefully at regular intervals.

There have been reports of the increase in against-the-rule astigmatism in older people since before von Helmholtz. Most cross-section studies of refractive error and age comfirm this trend. Does this change in the meridian of greatest refractive power of the eye from the 90-degree meridian in youth to the 180-degree meridian in old age signify that the curvature of the cornea changes with age? In 1924, von Helmholtz believed that the natural form of the cornea was such that the meridian of greatest curvature was horizontal, but that the cornea was deformed in youth by the pressure of the lids so that the greatest curvature was vertical in youth. As the lid tension decreases and the ocular tissues harden with age, the cornea escapes back to its natural form.

The concept that the corneal curvature changes with age seems to be confirmed by the studies of Kratz and Walton (1949) and Phillips (1952). Kratz and Walton reported from a study of clinical records that the best estimate for the correction of astigmatism based on keratometric findings was achieved when the allowance for physiologic astigmatism in Javal's formula remained at 0.50 D for all ages. They argued that since the total astigmatism increases against-the-rule throughout life, the cause of the increase must be a change in corneal astigmatism. Their actual data, originally presented in graphic form, are summarized in Table 6.1. The data seem to support the concept that the number of patients having with-the-rule astigmatism decreases with age. Phillips' data from a clinical practice in Great Britain are shown in Table 6.2.

These data of Kratz and Walton and Phillips are unfortunately in relative terms showing the difference in power of the two principal meridians. It cannot be stated categorically that the vertical power, and hence the curvature, decreased or that horizontal power, and hence the curvature, increased.

In a longitudinal study of 46 patients over a period of 0.5 to 20 years, Exford (1965) reports that corneal power in both the horizontal and vertical meridians increased at a rate slightly less than 0.25 D per decade and that there was no observable trend that either meridian changed more rapidly than the other.

Mason (1940) reported on 475 eyes of people between the ages of 12 and 39 years and 475 eyes of people between the ages of 45 and 79 years. All eyes had at least a 0.25 D with-the-rule corneal astigmatism as measured using a keratome-

Table 6.1 Corneal astigmatism in Kratz and Walton study

Decade	Against-the-Rule Corneal Astigmatism (%)	With-the-Rule Corneal Astigmatism (%)	No Corneal Astigmatism (%)
2	18	80	2
5	11	78	11
8	30	20	50
9	75	25	0

Note: The number of patients at each decade is unknown.

Source: Based on Kratz, J.D., and W.G. Walton. "A Modification of Javal's Rule for the Correction of Astigmatism." *Am. J. Optom. Arch. Am. Acad. Optom.* 26 (1949): 302. *Am. J. Optom. Physiol. Opt.* Copyright 1949. American Academy of Optometry.

Table 6.2 Corneal astigmatism according to Phillips

Age (yr)	Against-the-Rule Astigmatism (%)	With-the-Rule Astigmatism (%)	No Astigmatism (%)	Number of Patients
10–20	6.8	75.5	12.7	164
20–30	8.2	72.3	19.5	268
30–40	17.7	64.1	18.2	204
40–50	25.6	46.9	27.5	320
50–60	31.7	40.5	27.8	356
60–70	33.9	37.7	28.4	239
70–80	35.0	37.2	27.8	140

Source: Based on Phillips, R.A. "Changes in Corneal Astigmatism." *Am. J. Optom. Arch. Am. Acad. Optom.* 29 (1952): 379. *Am. J. Optom. Physiol. Opt.* Copyright 1952. American Academy of Optometry.

ter. Of the younger group, 22% required against-the-rule corrections, whereas 41% of the older group required such corrections. Mason's data originally presented in graphic form are restated in Table 6.3.

The data of Mason indicate that some portion of the increase in against-the-rule astigmatism with age must be accounted for on some other basis than changes in corneal curvature, since even with matched corneal astigmatisms, more of the older group have against-the-rule astigmatism than do the younger group.

More recent data, however, indicate that indeed the power of the cornea does increase with age, particularly in the horizontal meridian. Baldwin and Mills found from a retrospective study of longitudinal data from private optometric practice that the horizontal meridian of the corneas of the same individuals became somewhat steeper over time. Their data are shown in Table 6.4.

Table 6.3 Comparison of corneal and ametropic astigmatism

With-the-Rule Corneal Astigmatism (D)	Ages 12–39 years		Ages 45–75 years	
	Against (%)	With (%)	Against (%)	With (%)
0.25	40	22	50	10
0.50	21	41	41	30
0.75	15	52	20	45
1.00	9	67	10	55
1.25	5	70	9	65
1.50	2	87	1	66
1.75	1	90	1	67
2.00	1	99	1	88

Note: The percentage of those with 0.00 D cylindrical correction for astigmatism has been omitted.
Source: Based on Mason, F.L. *Principles of Optometry.* San Francisco: Carlisle, 1940, pp. 400–401.

Table 6.4 The longitudinal change in the corneal and refractive astigmatism over approximately a 13-year period

Factor	Average Age: 52 Years		Average Age: 65 Years	
	Vertical	Horizontal	Vertical	Horizontal
Refraction	+ 1.09 D	+ 0.85	+ 1.91 D	+ 1.15 D
Change: 13 yr			+ 0.82 D	+ 0.30 D
Cornea	43.86	43.48 D	43.93 D	43.86 D
Change: power			+ 0.07 D	+ 0.33 D
Change: radius			− 0.01 mm	− 0.07 mm
Refractive Astigmatism	− 0.24 DC ax 90		− 0.75 DC ax 90	
Corneal Astigmatism	− 0.38 DC ax 180		− 0.07 DC ax 180	

Data taken from Baldwin, W., and D. Mills, 1981.

Anstice (1971) reported somewhat similar data as shown in Table 6.5.

Reporting only on the radius of a single meridian, Fledelius (1988) reported that the cornea steepens. Unfortunately, he did not give both meridians, but he did report separately on males and females. His data are given in Table 6.6.

Thus, with age it appears that the horizontal meridian of the cornea becomes steeper while the vertical changes very little. Consequently, there is an increase in the against-the-rule astigmatism.

CHANGES IN THE ANTERIOR CHAMBER WITH AGE

Weale (1962), quoting Johansen and Raeder, states that the depth of the anterior chamber decreases from an average of 3.6 mm in the age range of 15 to 20 years to an average of 3.0 mm by the age of 70 years because of growth of the lens. A decrease in the depth of the anterior chamber could make the angle of the anterior chamber at the root of the iris more acute, thus increasing the possibility of interference with aqueous outflow. Likewise, if all other factors remain constant, a decrease in the anterior chamber depth slightly increases the refractive

Table 6.5 Cross-sectional data of the differences in corneal and refractive astigmatism of patients between the ages of 25 and 39 and patients between the ages of 70 and 74

	Mean Astigmatism	
	Ages 25–39 Years	Ages 70–74 Years
Corneal	− 0.75 DC ax 180	− 0.15 DC ax 180
Refractive	− 0.30 DC ax 180	− 0.40 DC ax 90
Change, Corneal		− 0.55 DC ax 90
Change, Refractive		− 0.70 DC ax 90

Data taken from Anstice, J., 1971.

Table 6.6 Cross-section data of the mean corneal curvature of patients between the ages of 36 and 40 and patients about age 77

	Age 36–40 Years	Age near 77 Years
Radius of curvature, M	7.99 ± 0.29 mm	7.85 ± 0.27 mm
Radius of curvature, F	7.83 ± 0.20 mm	7.77 ± 0.27 mm
Change, curvature, M		−0.14 mm
Change, curvature, F		−0.06 mm

Data taken from Fledelius, H., 1988.

power of the eye, making the eye relatively more myopic. The chemical composition and refractive index of the aqueous appear to be independent of age.

CHANGES IN THE IRIS WITH AGE

One of the most significant changes in the older eye is senile miosis (Girren, et al., 1960; Weale 1963). In addition, the difference in diameter of the pupil in the light- and dark-adapted states becomes less and less. The cause of the miosis is not known, but it is thought to be caused by the atrophy of the dilator muscle fibers, an increased rigidity of the iris blood vessels, or both. In any event, the pupil becomes smaller at all levels of illumination, with only a slight increase in the latency of pupillary responses (Feinberg and Podolak, 1965).

This miosis reduces retinal illuminance and the diameter of retinal blur circles when the eye is out of focus. Consequently, at high levels of illumination, uncorrected visual acuity may appear to improve rather than decrease with age. Likewise, the range of clear vision at near through any addition appears to increase with age, giving the appearance of accommodative change.

This miosis makes it difficult to examine the fundus or other structures of the eye through the undilated pupil. Subjective refraction becomes more difficult because changes in lens power do not change the diameter of retinal blur circles as much as a similar change in eyes with larger pupils. This means that the optometrist must be prepared to use a 0.50 or 0.62 D instead of the usual 0.37 D crossed cylinder in the determination of the magnitude and the axis of any astigmatism. In other words, the older patient may be less sensitive to lens changes than the younger because of optical reasons rather than because of a decrease in observational abilities due to supposed senility.

CHANGES IN THE LENS WITH AGE

The lens of the eye continues to grow throughout life. Weale (1962), quoting Johansen and Raeder, states that the axial thickness of the lens increases by about 28% by age 70 years over that which existed at age 15 to 20 years. This means that if the lens is assumed to be 3.6 mm thick at age 15 to 20 years (the Gullstrand standard), then by age 70 it will be approximately 4.6 mm thick. The nuclear thickness remains constant while the cortical thicknesses increase. On the average, the anterior cortex increases by 0.6 mm and the posterior by 0.4 mm.

The transverse or equatorial diameter of the lens appears to increase at a somewhat slower rate than the axial thickness. (Weale, 1962; Mellerio, 1971; Brown, 1974) In the past, most authorities had assumed that if the lens becomes larger overall from the continuous laying down of new fibers just under the capsule posteriorly and just under the epithelium anteriorly, then it must also become flatter. To quote Duke-Elder (1961), "In this way the lens becomes continuously flatter with age. . . ."

Measurements of the curvature of the lens surfaces using slit-lamp techniques (Lowe and Clark, 1973; Brown, 1974) indicate that the radius of the central portion of the anterior lens surface decreases by about 0.1 mm per year between the ages of 40 and 70 years and that the radius of the central portion of the posterior surface remains almost constant (Figure 6.1).

Such an increase in curvature of the anterior lens surface is compatible with the observation that the axial thickness increases faster than the equatorial. It should be noted, however, that these comparisons of the physical parameters of the crystalline lens are based on cross-sectional data without regard to the physical size of the subjects.

The lens substance is not crystal clear, but is yellow; thus, as the lens thickens, it absorbs more and more light selectively (Coren and Gergus, 1972; Mellerio, 1971; Said and Weale, 1959; Weale 1973). This increase in absorption is mainly caused by the increased thickness rather than to any increase in pigment density per unit thickness. As the lens grows, it accumulates two fluorogens, one of which is activated by light of wavelength 345 nm and emits light of wavelength 420 nm (Lerman and Borkman, 1976; Satchi, 1973). In addition, the mass of some protein molecules of high molecular weight increases toward the nucleus of the lens. In some cases, the index of refraction of these high-mass molecules is greater than the index of their environment, and they can, under some conditions, act as scatter points for light (Spector, 1983).

The miosis and the growth of the lens does alter visual performance. According to Weale (1961, 1962, 1963) and Cullinin (1978), the amount of light reaching the retina in a normal 60-year-old is only about one-third that reaching the retina of a 20-year-old. This means that an older person must use significantly more light to achieve the same level of retinal illuminance as that achieved by a younger person. Mesopia and scotopia occur at higher levels of ambient luminance. In addition, the useful light reaching the retina may be attenuated by fluorescence and scatter. Both fluorescence and scatter tend to reduce contrast. The visual performance of an older person usually will be impaired at twilight.

The yellow pigment of the lens absorbs the short wavelengths more than the long. Thus, older people have a decreased sensitivity at the violet end of the spectrum. White objects may appear yellow, and the distinction between blues and greens is decreased. For example, the distinction between a light green wall and a blue green carpet will become less marked with age. Also the color differences between dark grey and dark brown will be less. Since there is great variation between older individuals of the same age, it is not possible to state that any given 70-year-old will have significant difficulty with color perception. This means that color vision of those over 55 years of age or so should be checked at regular intervals.

Contrary to the assumption of many clinicians, there does not seem to be much evidence that the index of refraction of the lens substance changes with age in the normal eye as defined in the introduction of this chapter (Parsons, 1906; Pierscionek, 1988).

The common clinical concept that the lens substance becomes significantly harder and less pliable with age is supported by the fact that the amplitude of accommodation decreases with age and ultimately becomes essentially 0 by the sixth decade of life. There is, however, little direct research data to support this concept. Fisher (1987) has stated that the reason the lens becomes more difficult to deform with increasing age is not because of lenticular sclerosis but rather because the capsule loses its elastic force, and the lens fibers become more compacted.

Likewise, there is little or no evidence of atrophy or sclerosis of the ciliary muscle (Weale 1962, 1963). In fact, the evidence seems to indicate hypertrophy of the ciliary muscle. Depending somewhat on the supporting pressure exerted by the vitreous, the mechanical aspects of the suspension of the crystalline lens in

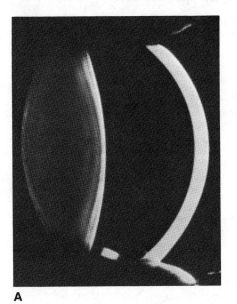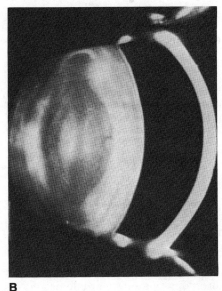

A   **B**

Figure 6.1 Biomicrospic photographs of the eye of a 10-year-old boy (A) and an 82-year-old man (B) to the same scale. These photographs clearly indicate the increase in lens thickness, the decrease in the depth of the anterior chamber, and the apparent increase in the curvature of the lens with increasing age. (From Brown, N., Exp Eye Res, 1974, 19:178)

relationship to the ciliary muscle must change as the lens increases in size with age. However, a change great enough to reduce the amplitude of accommodation to practically 0 should increase the static power of the eye as well as reaction time.

CHANGES IN THE VITREOUS WITH AGE

Millodot (1976) has found that the magnitude of the chromatic aberration of the eye decreases with age in both the phakic and aphakic eye. Millodot and Leary (1978) have found that the discrepancy between the magnitude of the ametropia determined by skiametry and subjective methods changes from plus to minus with increasing age of patients. Both of these observations can be explained if it is assumed that the index of refraction of the vitreous increases with age. This would also help explain the loss of reflectance of the fundus observed with an ophthalmoscope and the increase in hyperopia that occurs in the "normal" aging eye. Goodside (1956) has presented evidence that supports this hypothesis.

If the index of the vitreous increased enough to introduce a concave surface into the refractive system of the eye, in order to account for the decrease in chromatic aberration, the refractive power of the eye would become markedly reduced, and the increase in hypermetropia would be much greater than that reported for the aging eye. This decrease in power could be compensated for if there were a corresponding increase in the refractive power of the cornea and lens as the data seem to indicate. These changes must be investigated more fully before it can be stated that Millodot's hypothesis is correct or not.

In addition to a possible change in the refractive index, the vitreous appears to be subject to liquefaction and syneresis with age, which results in an increase in the speed and amplitude of the movements of vitreous floaters and a decreased support for the posterior lens surface. Ordinarily, muscae volitantes have no effect on vision except to give older people something to watch in an otherwise empty field or when bored. Sometimes, however, they can be very distracting during reading.

RETINAL AND NEURAL CONNECTION CHANGES WITH AGE

The changes in the retina and the neural connections that can accompany the normal aging process are largely inferential rather than directly observable in the normal eye. Consequently, this section will discuss the changes in visual function rather than observed changes in the retina or neural connections.

Clinicians usually assess the integrity of the retina and the visual system by direct observation (ophthalmoscopy and biomicroscopy); by the determination of corrected visual acuity; by the size and shape of the visual fields using various methods, including the Amsler grid; and by contrast sensitivity. On occasion, stereo-acuity may be determined, and even less frequently, performance on one of the color vision screening and glare sensitivity tests, may be determined.

In the absence of pathology, there is little decline in static corrected visual acuity with age up to about age 70 that cannot be accounted for by miosis and the increased density of the lens (Pitts, 1982). In general, however, the number of individuals achieving 20/10 to 20/25 visual acuity declines with age. According to the Framingham study (Kahn et al., 1977), 95.4% of individuals in the age group from 52 to 64 years have corrected acuity between 20/10 and 20/25. In the age group from 65 to 74 years, this percentage declines to 91.9, and in the age group from 75 to 85, it becomes 69.1. The major causes of this decline for the 75 to 85 age group are cataract (46%), macular degeneration (28%), glaucoma (7.2%), and general retinal pathology (7%). However, an apparent cause for the failure to achieve at least 20/25 acuity cannot be determined for about 10% of the patients between 75 and 85 years of age. As age increases, the number of patients apparently free from ocular disease, who achieve normal corrected acuity decreases.

The size of the visual field as measured under standard conditions decreases with age. That is, the $1/1,000$ isopter for the average normal 60-year-old will be inside that of an average normal 20-year-old (Burg, 1968; Dannheim and Drance, 1971), even when the pupil is controlled (Carter, 1982; Drance et al., 1967). This does not necessarily mean that neural function is diminished, since the density of the lens will reduce retinal illuminance even when pupil size is controlled. The retinal illuminance will be reduced even more by light scatter within the eye. Consequently, a slightly reduced field cannot be taken as positive evidence that there is reduced neural function. With multiple target presentations and short exposure times as frequently used in automated perimetry, there seems to be a more significant loss of field with age than with standard perimetry. (See section on spatial interaction.)

The presence of scotomas or areas of reduced sensitivity, as well as sudden changes in the visual field, are more important than a slightly reduced field. The clinician must make comparisons between recent fields. This means that the visual field should be determined and recorded at regular intervals in the aging patient.

Although individuals with excellent stereopsis do not necessarily have a good ability to judge distance, they do have good binocular motor and sensory integration. Thus, the determination of stereo-acuity can aid the optometrist in judging whether or not a patient's visual neural system is functioning properly. Likewise, the integrity of the monocular visual neural system can be judged from a determination of vernier acuity. Vernier acuity can be determined more easily in eyes with a poor optical system (with corneal or lenticular opacities) than can visual acuity, and hence it should prove useful in cataractous eyes.

Hofstetter and Bertsch (1976) have reported that stereo-acuity does not decline with age (up to age 42 at least) in individuals with good visual acuity. Pitts (1982) suspects that stereopsis would decrease with age after 50 years in a randomly selected sample of the population. Unfortunately, the author is not aware of a published study of the effect of aging on vernier acuity.

The changes in the ability to discriminate colors already have been discussed. Briefly, there is a shortening of the spectrum on the violet end, a loss of ability to discriminate blues from blue-greens, and a yellowing of white objects so that the older individuals may have difficulty discriminating between white and unsaturated yellow, between pastel violets and yellow-greens, and between dark browns and grays. These changes occur in the absence of disease and degeneration. Since subtle changes in color vision may be the first sign of disease, it is important that the color vision of aging patients be determined at regular intervals and that comparisons be made between the eyes of the same individual as well as with some normal standard.

The fact that mesopia and scotopia occur at lower levels of ambient illuminance in older individuals and not in younger people means that the difficulty with color discrimination that occurs after sunset occurs earlier in the evening for older persons.

It may well be that all the usual tests of sensory neural integrity show small but definite decrements in the absence of disease or degeneration.

In clinical testing such as the determination of visual acuity (spatial resolution), illumination, contrast and time are optimum rather than near threshold. Also, extraneous stimuli such as competing peripheral objects in the visual field are kept to a minimum. Usually the only significant competing objects in the field of view are optotypes adjacent to the one being resolved. In the real world, however, discrimination, identification, and resolution must be frequently made under low levels of illumination and poor contrast and with competing stimuli located nearby or peripherally to the object of regard and with some stimuli being presented on a variable time scale. Different stimuli have a masking effect on each other when adjacent in both space and time. Frequently, this masking effect becomes exaggerated or increased when there is a deterioration of some type in the visual system. Perhaps the best-known example of the effect is the significant improvement in the visual acuity of amblyopic eyes when optotypes are presented one at a time in a restricted field rather than a line or whole chart at a time.

The marked reduction in retinal illuminance with increasing age resulting from miosis, lens absorption, and light scatter already has been discussed briefly, but little has been said concerning contrast, spatial and temporal interaction.

CHANGES IN DARK ADAPTATION WITH AGE

Most investigators report that the absolute level of adaptation reached by the elderly is less than that reached by younger individuals. Whether there is a difference in the rate of adaptation, however, is unclear (Birren and Shock, 1950; Domey, et al., 1960). This change in the level of adaptation is probably caused by miosis and lens growth (Weale, 1962). Mesopia and scotopia occur at higher levels of ambient luminance in the elderly than in the young (Carter, 1982).

CHANGES IN RECOVERY FROM GLARE WITH AGE

Paulson and Sjostrand (1980) and Reading (1968), among others, have reported that elderly patients are more sensitive to glare than are younger patients. This is indicated by an increase in reaction and redetection time in the presence of a glare source.

Severn, et al. (1967a, 1967b) among others, have advocated a "photostress" test measuring the time required for functional recovery to a specified visual acuity after exposure to a measured flash of light.

CONTRAST SENSITIVITY CHANGES WITH AGE

Even in the absence of a glare source, Sekuler (1980) and Sekuler and Hutmann (1980) have reported that older individuals are only one-third as sensitive to low spatial frequencies (below 4 cycles/degree) as younger people. This loss of contrast sensitivity at low frequencies has not been borne out by a more carefully controlled investigation by Sekuler, et al. (1983). If care is used to be certain that the subjects have the proper optical correction and are free from disease and degenerative conditions, it becomes apparent that older people exhibit sensitivity losses predominantly at intermediate and high frequencies. This also reduces peak sensitivity and shifts it to lower frequencies. Most, *but not all,* of this loss is caused by the decreased retinal illuminance found in older subjects.

In addition, these same investigators report that older subjects experience difficulty in detecting and differentiating between relatively large complex targets, such as faces, at low contrast.

The investigation of the variations of the relationship between spatial frequency and contrast sensitivity and its meaning in visual perception is important and can be used to detect visual changes before there is a loss of visual acuity. It brings to mind the pioneering work of Luckiesh and Moss (1983) and Guth (1957, 1981). They developed a number of methods of determining the relationship between luminance, contrast, and target size (Luckiesh and Moss 1983).

ATTENTION FACTORS

Older individuals appear to have a decreased resistance to distraction and a decreased ability to selectively attend to one source of information in the presence of competing messages. They exhibit a decreased flexibility in observing all aspects of reversible figures (Hartman and Sekuler 1980; Kline and Birren 1975).

TEMPORAL INTERACTION

Kline and Orme-Rogers (1978) have presented evidence that indicates that the ability to separate visual events that happen serially declines with age. Events that appear as separate to younger individuals may be reported as smeared together by older observers. It is well known that there is a loss of flicker fusion sensitivity with age. This decrease in sensitivity persists even when the usual decrease in retinal illuminance is taken into account (Kuyk & Wisson, 1991). Both forward and backward masking effects increase with increasing age, and there appears to be "some major slowing in selective attention with pattern recognition processes" (Walsh, 1982).

SPATIAL INTERACTION

The interaction of different objects in the field of vision on the perception of each one separately or all as a whole complete picture is complex. The interaction may be as simple as that found by the interaction of adjacent optotypes (contour interaction) on each other, as found in the determination of visual acuity, or as complex as locating and recognizing a house number in a cluttered visual space while driving down a street.

There is very little decline in the ability of elderly subjects to localize suprathreshold peripheral objects in an uncluttered field, but performance declines somewhat when a central visual task is added. If, in addition to the central visual task, the peripheral field is cluttered, the decline in performance becomes significant. With age, there is a decrease in the size of the "useful" or "functional" field of view (Sekuler and Ball, 1986; Ball et al., 1988; Ball et al., 1990). This decline in peripheral localization ability occurs in the absence of any significant changes in the clinically determined visual field and appears to be related to attending to both a central task and, at the same time, attempting to localize another target in a complex field. The only significant correlation of this loss of functional field reported by Ball et al. is with answers by patients to questions concerning visual search and speed of processing such as, "Do you have to take more time now than you did in the past and be more careful doing things that depend on your vision such as driving, walking down stairs, etc.?"

Sekuler and Ball (1986) have found that peripheral localization in a cluttered field on the testing device can be improved with training. It is not known, however, whether this training actually results in improved performance in the real situation, but training undoubtedly makes the older observer more aware of the problem and may result in real improved performance.

DYNAMIC VISUAL ACUITY CHANGES WITH AGE

It is well known that visual acuity for moving targets is less than for stationary targets, and that the more rapidly a target moves, the greater is the decrease in dynamic visual acuity. Both Burg (1966) and Reading (1972) have reported that this decline in acuity with target velocity increases with increasing age. The cause for this decline is not known, but Goodson and Morrison (1979) have shown that dynamic acuity can be improved by training. The decline may be related to the decrease in the rate of smooth following movements, and the improvement with training may be caused by the improvement in these movements following visual training.

One of the consequences of aging is the failure of the organism to completely replace functional cells that have been injured, for example, by disease and trauma. This appears to be especially true of the nervous system. It has been reported (Dolman et al., 1980; Balazsi et al., 1984), for example, that the number of nerve fibers in the optic nerve decreases with age. This same decrease also takes place in the visual cortex where it has been reported that nearly half of the neurons drop out by age 70 years (Devaney and Johnson, 1986).

In view of the loss of neural function, it is more surprising that the aged human visual system performs as well as it does rather than to be surprised that there is some loss of acuity, adaptation, color vision, spatial and temporal resolution, or useful field, beyond that explained by physical changes in the iris and lens.

REFRACTIVE ERROR

As has already been reported, the horizontal meridian of the cornea becomes steeper with age and, as a consequence, it is not surprising that against-the-rule astigmatism also increases. The amount of changes reported by Hirsch (1959), Anstice (1971), and Baldwin and Mills (1981) is between 0.02 D and 0.04 D per year (longitudinal data) after age 40.

Along with this change in astigmatism, there is an increase in relative hyperopia and in the absence of visible lenticular opacities. According to Hirsch (1960), the rate of increase is between 0.03 D and 0.04 D per year after age 47. The cause for this increase in hyperopia is obscure. As Table 6.7 indicates, most of the apparent changes in the physical characteristics of the eye, determined from cross-sectional data, would lead one to expect a relative increase in myopia.

If one assumes the indices of refraction of the Gullstrand Simplified Eye (aqueous = vitreous = 1.336 and lens = 1.416), the 40-year-old eye should be a little more than 5.50 D hyperopic, and the 70-year-old eye should be almost exactly 3.00 D hyperopic — a 2.50-D increase in relative myopia.

The only really significant hyperopic-inducing change is the decrease in axial length. Sorsby, according to Grosvenor (1987), has reported much greater changes than that reported by Fledelius, but the Sorsby "older" grouping was from age 40 years upward, and the data were not included in Table 6.7.

Changes in the index of refraction, particularly a decrease in the index of the nucleus of the lens or an increase in the index of the vitreous, also could account for the real increase in hyperopia. Another possibility is that cross-sectional data

Table 6.7 Recent biometric data of the physical parameters of the eye. The refractive error was calculated using assumed indices of refraction

Parameter	Source	Age 40 Years	Age 60 Years
Cornea, r	Fledelius (1988)	7.91 mm	7.81 mm
Lens, r_1	Brown (1974)	13.4 mm	10.0 mm
Lens, r_2	Brown (1974)	−7.8 mm	−7.5 mm
Anterior chamber	Weale (1982)	3.2 mm	2.8 mm
Lens thickness	Hockwin (1987)	4.3 mm	5.0 mm
Axial length	Fledelius (1988)	23.5 mm	23.45 mm
Refraction	Calculated	+5.57 D	+3.05 D

of physical parameters over time are not reliable when making comparisons or determining growth. Present-day adults born in 1920 are, on average, smaller in most dimensions than present-day adults born in 1950. Consequently, smaller dimensions or sharper curvatures are suspect; on the other hand, larger dimensions or longer curvatures may be understated.

The cause of the increase in hyperopia must be determined by future research, taking advantage of the ever-increasing population who have had intraocular lenses (IOLs) for ten or more years. If the increase in hyperopia continues in these patients, the crystalline lens cannot be the chief contributor to the refractive change.

MOTOR SYSTEMS CHANGES WITH AGE

Accurate, steady fixation by either eye and by both eyes together is essential for normal binocular vision. Dannheim and Drance (1971) reported that under scotopic conditions, aging patients had difficulty with fixation. In contrast, the evidence derived from the maintenance of relatively good static visual acuity and good stereo-acuity, as well as the clinical evidence that aging patients usually have normal binocular vision, indicates that under photopic conditions, aging individuals maintain good, steady fixation. This has been confirmed by Kosnik et al. (1986).

Version Eye Movements

Sharpe and Sylvester (1978) compared the monocular pursuit eye movements of 15 patients between the ages of 19 and 32 years with those of 10 patients between the ages of 65 and 77 years. Even at relatively slow target movements, the older patients showed a decreased gain (increased lag) and consequently an increased number of saccades in order to maintain fixation.

Leigh (1983) claims that with advancing age, the range of voluntary eye movements becomes limited. If the individual follows a moving target, the restrictions are less marked. Vertical version movements seem to be restricted more than movements in other directions (Chamberlain, 1971).

In the author's clinical experience, however, most normal, vigorous aging patients do not exhibit marked restrictions of version movements, whether voluntary or following. In those instances in which the movements have appeared somewhat restricted, clinically acceptable version movements were restored by simple home vision training. In instances in which the voluntary and following movements were markedly restricted, the patient either had or was discovered to have neurologic disturbances.

Vergences

Tonic Vergence: Distance Heterophoria

Tonic vergence appears to increase somewhat with increasing years, as evidenced by increasing esophoria for distance fixation. The increase is about 0.03Δ per year after age 30 years. Hirsch et al. (1948) found the mean heterophoria to be just over a 0.5Δ exophoria at age 30, and nearly 0.4Δ esophoria by age 50. This variation has no clinical significance and is less than the error of measurement used in clinical testing.

Fusional (Disparity) Vergence

According to Sheedy and Saladin (1975), positive fusional vergence decreases with age, but negative fusional vergence does not. The decrease in positive fusional vergence is far greater than the increase in the near exophoria and thus appears to be a real loss in amplitude. In the author's clinical experience, however, positive fusional vergence in the elderly responds well to training; thus, the decrease in positive fusional vergence with age does not necessarily represent a permanent or serious loss.

Total Vergence

The total vergence as determined from the far point to the near point of convergence does not appear to change significantly with age (Duane, 1926; Mellick, 1949), but some reduction is to be expected.

Accommodative Convergence and Proximal Convergence

It is generally accepted that the loss of accommodation with age is the result of changes in the lens substance, ciliary body, or both. As already mentioned, Weale (1962, 1963) states that there is hypertrophy rather than atrophy of the ciliary muscle with age. Shirachi et al. (1978) believe that the loss of accommodation is due to the continued growth and hence the decreasing curvature of the lens itself and with a corresponding decrease in mechanical advantage of the ciliary muscle.

The loss of accommodation appears to be caused by changes in the lens or ciliary body rather than to changes in the underlying neural mechanisms. There may be some loss of blur appreciation, optically induced as opposed to retinal appreciation, because of miosis and perhaps some neural loss; however, these are minimal at the age at which accommodative ability first matches the depth of focus of the static eye. The fact that convergence is less effective in producing accommodation as age increases (Morgan, 1954; Fincham, 1955; Kent, 1958) may be explained by a reduction in the output of the effector mechanism, the lens and capsule. Thus, it appears that at the critical age at which accommodation reaches a minimum, approximately 55 years, aging affects neither the sensory output from the retina nor the motor neural input to the ciliary muscle.

In reality, a discussion of accommodation and accomodative-convergence is not germane to a discussion of the visual functions of the aging eye since presbyopia, in reality, is an affliction of middle age and not old age. By the time a person has become elderly, that individual has become fully adapted to a static eye with an accommodative amplitude equivalent to the depth of focus. Clinically, the near correction must be made more convex in some patients even after accommodation becomes minimal, but with the elderly, this increase in the addition is not to replace lost accommodation but rather to replace decreased contrast and resolution by increasing magnification.

Most elderly patients on fixating a near object through their reading correction present a near phoria, indicating more convergence than that of their tonic position. Most of this convergence is stimulated by the proximity of the target, but some of it may be caused by accomodative-convergence, even though the lens is not changed by the motor impulses to accommodate.

There is some direct evidence supplied by impedance cyclography (Saladin and Stark, 1975; Swegmark 1969) that neural impulses reach the ciliary muscle of presbyopic patients who have little or no accommodative response. In other words, presbyopic patients attempt to accommodate even when there is no direct feedback in the form of clearer retinal images. It is not known whether the origin of these impulses is reflex in nature because of blurring, nearness, or convergence, or whether it is voluntary.

There is also indirect evidence that the accommodative mechanism is probably activated in presbyopic individuals even though there is little or no gain in clearness of the retinal image. Sheedy and Saladin (1975) found that the mean near phoria of a group of young patients was 2.8Δ exophoria, whereas that for a group of presbyopes using a +2.50 D addition was 8.7Δ exophoria, or only approximately 6Δ greater than that for younger patients. If this increase in near exophoria were caused entirely by the loss of accommodation, the difference should be nearly 10 to 12.8Δ exophoria, because the average AC/A ratio is about 4Δ/1.00 D. Sheedy and Saladin also reported that the near fixation disparity for the younger patients increased from 0.17 minutes of arc of exo disparity to 6.62 minutes of arc through a +2.50 D addition. The older patients exhibited only 1.48' of exo fixation disparity through the same addition. In other words, presbyopic patients exhibit greater proximal convergence in both the disassociated and associated conditions than do nonpresbyopic patients under similar conditions. This increased proximal convergence could be conditioned gradually as accommodative convergence is lost with age, or it could be due, at least in part, to convergence stimuli derived from attempted accommodation.

VARIABILITY

The variability in visual performance between individuals appears to increase with age for virtually all tasks (Ratwinick, 1978). This alone tends to make it more difficult for a clinician to assess whether a below-normal performance on some visual task should be attributed to some optical or neural defect of an aging visual system or to just a normal decrease. As has been mentioned several times, such things as a decrease in dark adaptation, a shift in color perception at the violet end of the spectrum, and a report of increased sensitivity to glare may be attributed to miosis and growth of the lens rather than to a neural defect. However, these changes, although not indicative of degenerative conditions or disease, are nevertheless real and do represent actual decreases in function that may not be apparent from a routine visual examination. Consequently, elderly patients, in the absence of pathology, will have some decreased visual function that is reported by them but may be undetected by the clinician in routine examination.

Usual clinical procedures to not reveal such conditions as a reduction of temporal resolution or a shrinkage of the functional field; however, these losses usually result in subjective symptoms and complaints that, although real, may be vague and poorly described by the elderly patient and consequently overlooked by the optometrist, ophthalmologist, or internist. The elderly person may know that something is wrong, and it is not helpful to be informed by an optometrist or physician that everything is normal and nothing requires attention. For this reason alone, a good, simple, clinical measurement of spatial and temporal interaction and a method for the clinical determination of the size of the functional field is needed. In the meantime, however, more attention needs to be paid to the case history and to the elderly patient's report of visual problems.

All of these changes in visual function become much more critical under reduced visual conditions such as driving at night or in fog, where a further decrease in intermediate- and high-frequency information would be especially troublesome; when the rapid interpretation of successive visual stimuli are important, such as in reading road signs or detecting the shape of the sign in a unfamiliar location; or when reading poor-contrast printing or crowded printing under less-than-optimum levels of illumination.

Many of these conditions that result in decreased or more difficult visual performance cannot be avoided or corrected, but they can be explained to the elderly patient. Most elderly astute patients already know before they seek optometric care that they perceive more "slowly" and with less certainty than they did when younger. They seek vision care to eliminate or improve their visual performance or to seek assurance that nothing critical is wrong. The optometrist should be certain that patients understand the cause for their symptoms, and they should be advised about ways and means of improving their visual performance by using more light, substituting incandescent for fluorescent light, reducing driving speeds, avoiding looking directly into the headlights of oncoming cars at night, and closing one eye in the presence of momentary glare. With age, the best optical correction becomes increasingly important, as does the utilization of home visual training, where appropriate, to keep ocular movements free and full. Perhaps most important is an understanding and sympathetic optometrist who will someday be an aging viewer of the world and its wonders.

REFERENCES

1. Anstice J. "Astigmatism — Its Components and Their Changes with Age." *Am. J. Optom, Arch. Am. Acad. Optom.* 48 (1971): 1001–1006.
2. Ball, K., B. Beard, R. Roenker, R. Miller, D. Griggs. "Age and Visual Search: Expanding the Useful Field of View." *J. Optom. Soc. Am.* A5 (1988): 2210–2219.
3. Ball, K., C. Owsley, B. Beard. "Clinical Visual Perimetry Underestimates Peripheral Field Problems in Older Adults." *Clin. Vis. Sci.* 5 (1990): 113–125.
4. Balazsi, A., J. Rootman, S. Drasnce, M. Schulzer, G. Douglas. "The Effect of Age on the Nerve Fiber Population of the Human Optic Nerve." 97 (1984): 760–766.
5. Baldwin, W., and D. Mills. "A Longitudinal Study of Corneal Astigmatism and Total Astigmatism." *Am. J. Optom. Physiol. Opt.* 58 (1981): 206–211.
6. Birren, J.E., and N.W. Shock. "Age Changes in the Rate and Level of Dark Adaptation." *J. App. Psychol.* 26 (1950): 407–411.
7. Brown, N. "The Change in Lens Curvature with Age." *Exp. Eye. Res.* 19 (1974): 175–183.
8. Burg, A. "Visual Acuity as Measured by Dynamic and Static Tests: A Comprehensive Evaluation." *J. Appl. Psychol.* 50 (1966): 460–466.
9. Burg, A. "Lateral Visual Fields as Related to Age and Sex." *J. Appl. Psychol.* 52 (1968): 10–15.
10. Carter, J.H. "Predictable Visual Responses to Increasing Age." *J. Am. Optom. Assn.* 53 (1982): 31–36.
11. Chamberlain, W. "Restriction in Upward Gaze with Advancing Age." *Am. J. Ophthalmol.* 71 (1971): 341–346.
12. Coren S., and J.S. Gergus. "Density of Human Lens Pigmentation: In Vivo Measures over an Extended Age Range." *Vis. Res.* 12 (1972): 343–346.
13. Cullinin, T. "Low Vision in Elderly People: Light for Low Vision." Proceedings from a Symposium. London: University College, April 1978.
14. Dannheim, F., and S.M. Drance. "Studies of Spatial Summation of Central Retinal Areas in Normal People of All Ages." *Can. J. Optom.* 6 (1971): 311–319.
15. Devaney, K., and H. Johnson. "Neuron Loss in the Aging Visual Cortex of Man." *J. Gerontol.* 15 (1980): 836–841.
16. Dolman, C., A. McCormack, S. Drance. "Aging of the Optic Nerve." *Arch. Ophtholmol.* 98 (1980): 2053–2058.

17. Domey, R.G., R.A. McFarland, and E. Chadwick. "Threshold and Rate of Dark Adaptation as Functions of Age and Time." *Human Factors* 2 (1960): 109–119.
18. Drance, S.M., V. Berry, and A. Hughes. "Studies on the Effects of Age on the Central and Peripheral Isopter of the Visual Field in Normal Subjects." *Am. J. Ophthalmol.* 63 (1967): 1667–1672.
19. Duane, A. "The Norms of Convergence." In *Contributions to Ophthalmic Science,* W. Crisp and W.C. Finnoff (eds.). George Banta, 1926, pp. 24–46.
20. Duke-Elder, S. *Systems of Ophthalmology.* vol. IV. St. Louis, C.V. Mosby, 1961, p. 322.
21. Exford, J. "A Longitudinal Study of Refractive Trends after Age Forty." *Am. J. Optom. Arch. Am. Acad. Optom.* 42 (1965): 685–692.
22. Feinberg, R., and E. Podolak. "Latency of Pupillary Reflex to Light Stimulation and Its Relationship to Aging." In *Behavior, Aging and the Nervous Systems,* A.T. Welford and J.E. Birmen (eds.). Springfield, IL: Charles Thomas, 1965.
23. Fincham, E.F. "The Proportion of Ciliary Muscular Force Required for Accommodation." *J. Physiol.* (London) 128 (1955): 99–122.
24. Fisher, R.J. "The Mechanics of Accommodation in Relation to Presbyopia." In: Stark, L. and G. Obrecht (eds.). *Presbyopia.* New York: Professional Press-Fairchild Publications, 1987.
25. Fledelius, H. "Refraction and Eye Size in the Elderly." *Arch. Ophthalmol.* 66 (1988): 241–248.
26. Birren, J.E., R.C. Casperson, and J. Botwineck. "Age Changes in Pupil Size." *J. Gerontol.* 5 (1960): 267–271.
27. Goodside, V. "The Anterior Limiting Membrane and the Retinal Light Reflexes." *Am. J. Optom.* 41 (1956): 288–292.
28. Goodson, J.E., and T.R. Morrison. "Effects of Surround Stimuli upon Dynamic Visual Acuity." Paper presented at Tri-Service Aeromedical Research Coordinating Panel, Pensacola, Fla., December, 1979.
29. Grosvenor, T. "Reduction in Axial Length with Age: An Emmetropizing Mechanism for the Adult Eye?" *Am. J. Optom. Physiol. Opt.* 64 (1987): 657–663.
30. Guth, S.K. "Effects of Age on Visibility." *Am. J. Optom. Arch. Am. Acad. Optom.* 34 (1957): 463–477.
31. Guth, S.K. "Prentice Memorial Lecture: The Science of Seeing–A Search for Criteria." *Am. J. Optom. Physiol. Opt.* 58 (1981): 870–885.
32. Hartman, L.P., and R. Sekuler. "Spatial Vision and Aging: 2. Criterion Effects." *J. Gerontol.* 35 (1980): 700–706.
33. von Helmholtz, H. In *Physiological Optics,* vol. 1, James P.C. Southall (ed.). Optical Society of America, 1924.
34. Hirsch, M.J. "Changes in Astigmatism after the Age of Forty." *Am. J. Optom. Arch. Am. Acad. Optom.* 36 (1959): 395–405.
35. Hirsch, M. Refractive Changes with Age. In: Hirsch, M. and R. Wick (eds.). *Vision and Aging.* Philadelphia; Chilton, 1960.
36. Hirsch, M.J., M. Alpern, and H.L. Schultz. "The Variation of Phoria with Age." *Am. J. Optom. Arch. Am. Acad. Optom.* 24 (1948): 535–541.
37. Hockwin, O. "Biometry of the Anterior Eye Segment." In: Stark, L. and G. Obrecht, (eds.). *Presbyopia,* New York: Professional Press–Fairchild Publications, 1987.
38. Hofstetter, H.W., and J.D. Bertsch. "Does Stereopsis Change with Age?" *Am J. Optom. Physiol. Opt.* 53 (1976): 644–667.
39. Kahn, H.A., et al. "The Framingham Eye Study: 1. Outline on Major Prevalence Findings." *Am. J. Epidemiol.* 106 (1977): 17–41.
40. Kent, P. "Convergent Accommodation." *Am. J. Optom. Arch. Am. Acad. Optom.* 35 (1958): 393–406.

41. Kline, D., and J.E. Birren. "Age Differences in Backword Dichoptic Masking." *Exp. Aging Res.* 1 (1975): 17–25.
42. Kosnik, W., J. Fikre, and R. Sekuler. "Visual Fixation Stability in Older Adults." *Invest. Opthalmol. Vis. Sci.* 27 (1986): 1720–1723.
43. Kratz, J.D., and W.G. Walton. "A Modification of Javal's Rule for the Correction of Astigmatism." *Am. J. Optom. Arch. Am. Acad. Optom.* 26 (1949): 295–306.
44. Kuyk, T., and M. Wisson. "Aging Related Foveal Flicker Sensitivity Losses in Normal Observers." *Optom. Vis. Sci.* 68 (1991): 786–789.
45. Leibowitz, H., et al. "The Role of Fine Detail in Visually Controlled Behavior." *Invest. Opthalmol. Vis. Sci.* 19 (1980): 846–848.
46. Leigh, R.J. "The Impoverishment of Ocular Motility in the Elderly." In R. Sekuler, D. Kline, and K. Dismukes (eds.). *Aging and Human Visual Function.* New York: Liss, 1983, pp. 173–180.
47. Lerman, S., and R. Borkman. "Spectroscopic Evaluation and Classification of Normal, Aging and Cataractous Lens." *Ophthalmic Rev.* 8 (1976): 335–353.
48. Lowe, R., and B. Clark. "Radius of Curvature of the Anterior Lens Surface." *Br. J. Ophthalmol.* 57 (1973): 471–474.
49. Luckiesh, M., and F.K. Moss. *Seeing.* Baltimore: Williams and WIlkins, 1983.
50. Mason, F.L. *Principles of Optometry.* San Francisco: Carlisle, 1940.
51. Mellerio, J. "Light Absorption and Scatter in the Human Lens." *Vis. Res.* 11 (1971): 129–141.
52. Mellick, A. "Convergence: An Investigation into the Normal Standards of Age Group." *Br. J. Ophthalmol.* 33 (1949): 755–763.
53. Millodot, M. "The Influence of Age on the Chromatic Aberration of the Eye: 5." *Grafes Archiv fur Klinische und Experimentelle Ophthalmologie* 198 (1976): 235–243.
54. Millodot, M. "The Influence of Age on the Sensitivity of the Cornea." *Invest. Ophthalmol. Vis. Sci.* 16 (1977): 240–272.
55. Millodot, M., and D. Leary. "The Discrepancy between Retinoscopic and Subjective Measurements: Effects of Age." *Am. J. Optom. Physiol. Opt.* 55 (1978): 309–316.
56. Morgan, M.W. "The Ciliary Body in Accommodation and Accommodative Convergence." *Am. J. Optom. Arch. Am. Acad. Optom.* 31 (1954): 219–229.
57. Morgan, M. "Vision Through my Aging Eyes." *J. Am. Optom. Assoc.* 59 (1988): 278–280.
58. Parsons, J.H. *The Pathology of the Eye,* Vol. 3. London: Hodder and Staughton, 1906, p. 929.
59. Paulson, L.E., and J. Sjostrand. "Contrast Sensitivity in the Presence of a Glare Light." *Invest. Ophthalmol. Vis. Sci.* 19 (1980): 401–406.
60. Phillips, R.A. "Changes in Corneal Astigmatism." *Am. J. Optom. Arch. Am. Acad. Optom.* 29 (1952): 379–380.
61. Pierscionek, B., D. Chan, J. Emis, G. Smith, R. Augustyne. "Nondestructive Method of Constructing Three-dimensional Gradient Index Models for the Crystalline Lens." *Theory and Experiment* 65 (1988): 481–491.
62. Pitts, D.G. "The Effects of Aging on Selected Visual Functions: Dark Adaptation, Visual Acuity, and Stereopsis, and Brightness Contrast." In: R. Sekuler, D. Kline, and K. Dismukes (eds.). *Aging and Human Visual Function.* New York: Liss, 1982, pp. 131–159.
63. Pitts, D.G. "Visual Acuity as a Function of Age." *J. Am. Optom. Assoc.* 53 (1982): 117–124.
64. Ratwinick, J. *Aging and Behavior: A Comprehensive Investigation of Reserach Findings.* New York: Sprenger, 1978.

65. Reading, V.M. "Disability Glare and Age. *Vis. Res.* 8 (1968): 207–214.
66. Reading, V.M. "Visual Resolution as Measured by Dynamic and Static Tests." *Pflugers Archiv fur die Gesamte Physiologie* 338 (1972): 17–26.
67. Said, F.S., and R.A. Weale. "Variation with Age of the Spectral Transmissivity of the Living Human Crystalline Lens." *Gerontologica* 3 (1959): 1213–1231.
68. Saladin, J.J., and L. Stark. "Presbyopia: New Evidence from Impedance Cyclography Supporting the Hess-Gullstrand Theory." *Vis. Res.* 15 (1975): 537–541.
69. Satchi, K. "Fluorescence in Human Lens." *Exp. Eye Res.* 16 (1973): 167–172.
70. Sekuler, R. "Human Aging and Spatial Vision." *Science* 209 (1980): 1255.
71. Sekuler, R., and K. Ball. "Visual Localization, Age and Practice." *J. Optom. Soc. Am.* A3 (1986): 864–867.
72. Sekuler, R., and L. Hutman. "Spatial Vision and Aging: 1. Contrast Sensitivity." *J. Gerontol.* 35 (1980): 692–699.
73. Sekuler, R., C. Owsley, and L. Hutman. "Assessing Spatial Vision of Older People." *Am. J. Optom. Physiol. Opt.* 59 (1983): 961–968.
74. Severn, S.L., R. L. Tour, and R.H. Kershaw. "Macular Function and the Photostress Test: 1." *Arch. Ophthalmol.* 77 (1967a): 2–7.
75. Severn, S.L., R.L. Tour, and R.H. Kershaw. "Macular Function and the Photostress Test: 2." *Arch. Ophthalmol.* 77 (1967b): 163–167.
76. Sharpe, J.A., and T.O. Sylvester. "Effect of Aging on Horizontal Smooth Pursuit." *Invest. Ophthalmol. Vis. Sci.* 17 (1978): 465–468.
77. Sheedy, J.E., and J.J. Saladin. "Exophoria at Near in Presbyopia." *Am. J. Optom. Physiol. Opt.* 52 (1975): 474–481.
78. Shirachi, D., J. Lui, M. Lee, J. Jang, J. Wong, and L. Stark. "Accommodation Dynamics: 1. Range of Nonlinearity." *Am. J. Optom. Physiol. Opt.* 55 (1978): 631–641.
79. Spector, A. "Aging of the Lens and Cartaract Formation." In: R. Sekuler, D Kline, and K. Dismukes (eds.). *Aging and Human Visual Function.* New York: Liss, 1983, pp. 27–43.
80. Swegmark, G. "Studies with Impedance Cyclography on Human Ocular Accommodation at Different Ages." *Acta Ophthalmol.* 47 (1969): 1186–1206.
81. Walsh, D. The Development of Visual Information Processes in Adulthood and Old Age. In: Sekuler, R. et al. (eds.). *Aging and Human Visual Function.* New York: Alan Liss, 1982. p. 222.
82. Weale, R.A. "Retinal Illumination and Age." *Trans. Illuminating Engineering Soc.* 26 (1961): 95–100.
83. Weale, R.A. "Presbyopia." *Brit. J. Ophthalmol.* 46 (1962): 660–668.
84. Weale, R.A. *The Aging Eye.* London: Lewis, 1963.
85. Weale, R.A. "The Effects of the Aging Lens on Vision." *Ciba Foundation Symposium* 19 (1973): 5–20.
86. Weale, R.A. *Biography of the Eye.* London: H.K. Lewis and Co., 1982.
87. Weymouth, F. "Effect of Age on Visual Acuity." In: M.J. Hirsch and R.E. Wick (eds.). *Vision of the Aging Patient.* Philadelphia: Chilton, 1960, pp. 37–62.

7

The Optometric Examination of the Elderly Patient

Ian L. Bailey

The elderly are a special group within optometry's patient population. Many of their visual characteristics and their varied needs make them different from the younger segments of the clinical population. This chapter will focus on the special considerations commonly required in the provision of vision care for the older patient. It is inevitable that a chapter such as this will be laden with generalizations, since it emphasizes features that may be relatively common in the elderly even though they are by no means universal within, or unique to, this group.

Visual needs often are changed by retirement or by changes in life-style imposed by physical or sensory limitations acquired through aging. Aging brings inevitable changes to the visual system, such as loss of accommodation, reduced transmittance of the ocular media, and pupillary miosis. The visual system also tends to be affected by ocular pathologies, the most notable of which are age-related maculopathy, cataracts, glaucoma, and retinopathies. Changes in visual needs and normal and pathologic changes in the visual system create a wide diversity of special clinical problems. The clinician becomes obliged to apply special emphases and techniques, and special optical treatment or other rehabilitative attention often is essential.

It is the diversity of vision needs and characteristics that most distinguishes the elderly from the rest of the patient population. Therefore, when dealing with elderly patients, practitioners must use more imagination and flexibility in structuring the examination and treatment to suit these diverse individual needs.

CASE HISTORY

The goal of all case history taking is to obtain an understanding of the patient's problems and needs. The case history shapes the sequence and emphasis of examination and assessment procedures, the design of treatment programs, and the presentation of recommendations and advice. The rapport developed in the case history interview can be a most crucial factor in determining the success of any treatment that may follow. The optometrist must develop and display a genuine strong concern for the patient's expressed problems and needs and periodically remind the patient that it is the patient's needs that are motivating the investigative procedures and treatment considerations.

The patient's demands should be given some overt attention, but the optometrist should remain conscious of the possibility of an unspoken hidden agenda that might be harbored by either the patient or the optometrist. It can be useful for the clinician to mentally take stock and ask three questions: (1) What does this patient want? (2) What, in my opinion, does this patient need? And, (3) What is the real reason for the patient's being here today? These three questions sometimes will give rise to the same answer; especially in the elderly, however, differences in answers can be most important in decision making and presentation.

The case history should begin with the patient being asked to identify the main visual problem or problems. The optometrist should encourage a full elaboration of the present complaint by asking questions motivated by a genuine curiosity and a desire to fully understand the patient's problem. After the major presenting complaint has been explored adequately, the patient should be asked if there are other problems, and each of these should be pursued in turn. Some elderly patients, especially those who are lonely or have some doubts about their self-worth, may relish being the focus of attention, and the interview might become quite diverted. The clinician should be sensitive and tolerant toward such digressions.

When the patient exhausts the self-generated list of problems, some important topics should be raised, if they have not been covered already. These areas can be divided into four categories:

1. *Distance vision.* Patients should be asked about the adequacy of their distance vision for particular tasks, among which are recognizing faces, watching television or movies, driving, and reading street signs. Reactions to different illumination conditions may be included here.

2. *Near vision.* Reading is typically the most important near vision task. The optometrist should establish whether the patient can satisfactorily read books and magazines, private and business correspondence, and labels and price tags. Patients should be asked about the use of magnifiers and any special lighting conditions that are important to reading. Other near vision tasks such as handicrafts, maintenance chores, self-grooming tasks, and food preparation also usually warrant attention.

3. *Ocular and general health history.* Current and previous ocular health and general health conditions or treatment should be investigated. The clinician should determine whether the patient is currently taking any medication, and if so, consider any possible side effects. The patient's experience with glasses or other optical aids should be investigated, and any problems or shortcomings of previous optical treatment should be identified. When there has been some loss of vision, the

pattern of development of the loss should be established. The clinician should ask patients about their perception of the cause and prognosis of their ocular condition, and the treatment that has been given.
4. *Life-style.* With aging, particularly aging accompanied by loss of vision, there may be some major changes in the activities of daily life. The living environment may change; interests, aspirations, and habits may be altered; the capacity of independent travel and independent home management may be curtailed; and dependence on relatives, friends, or rehabilitation personnel may develop. The practitioner should be alert to such changes because they can significantly influence the needs of the patient.

Aging patients often have special fears and prejudices that require consideration. Most people have some fear of vision loss accompanying their advancing years. This fear becomes heightened when contemporaries suffer vision loss or begin to require attention or treatment for cataracts, maculopathy, or glaucoma. It is not uncommon for older patients to strongly fear impending blindness or serious vision loss, but they rarely admit this fear. The optometrist, therefore, should be careful to "read between the lines" during the history and identify such fears.

Incurring a partial or total vision loss inevitably is an emotionally traumatic experience for the individual concerned. Following the initial shock, a sequence of emotional reactions can involve depression, anxiety, disbelief, grief, denial, and anger. In time, however, the individual's emotional state stabilizes. Optometrists dealing with patients who have a recently acquired loss of vision should be aware of the probability of changing emotional attitudes. The finalization of prescribing decisions often must be delayed until the patient comes to reasonable terms with the visual limitations.

Patients who already have some loss of vision commonly fear that total blindness or substantially worse vision is inevitable. The practitioner should encourage the patient to discuss these fears. Often associated with the fear of blindness is a concern that some abuse of the eyes in the past will soon produce dreaded injurious consequences. Excessive reading, excessive fine work, poor illumination, wearing glasses, failure to wear glasses, wearing the wrong glasses, sitting too close to the television, using fluorescent lamps, or watching color television all can be believed to ruin vision, and such beliefs are most well developed in the elderly. Patients with these concerns should be given appropriate advice and reassurance. Patients who have already suffered some vision loss are particularly likely to be influenced by erroneous but commonly held beliefs that may lead them to expect a dismal visual future. Furthermore, a low-vision patient may proudly claim great virtue and restraint because he or she does not sit too close to the television, does not read any more than is essential, and does not use strong light, when, in fact, the avoided behaviors pose no threat to remaining vision and could provide the means for a broader and more enjoyable range of activities. Thus, optometrists should take special care to counsel their elderly patients about their future eye care needs and the prognosis for changes in their vision to insure that they really understand the status of their own vision.

When an individual retires, interests and priorities often change. Especially if there is some age-related disability, elderly people often curtail their social, vocational, and recreational activities. Withdrawal from social and other pleasurable activities can be passive and unconscious. It is important for the optometrist to understand the patient's range of daily visual activities. When there has been some vision loss, the extent to which the vision loss is restricting current activities or aspirations should be determined. A most useful approach is to ask patients to describe their typical daily activities. Ask what they do from the time they get out of bed in the morning until they go to bed at night. Such questioning often reveals the range of visual demands and, when there is restricted vision, often indicates the extent to which people are modifying their lives because of vision difficulties. The frustration and regret associated with a vision loss is often revealed by the question, "What things could you do when you had good vision that you cannot do now?"

In bringing the introductory interview to a close, the careful optometrist will summarize the priorities for the examination process that is to follow: "So, if I understand things correctly, the most important thing for us to concentrate on is your reading, especially for those bank statements. And we should thoroughly check the health of your eyes. Is this right?"

It can be reassuring to remind the patient that mutually agreed upon goals have been established and that these goals motivate all the examination procedures. Advising the patient of the purpose of various tests and relating them to the patient's symptoms emphasizes the clinician's concern and develops a stronger spirit of participation in the patient.

OCULAR HEALTH EXAMINATION

A thorough inspection of the external and internal aspects of the eyes using appropriate instrumentation is especially important in elderly patients. Statistically, they are much more likely to have significant ocular pathologic conditions or ocular signs of general health disorders.

The inspection of the interior of the eye can become more difficult than usual because of small pupils and lack of media clarity. Unless contraindicated, the pupils should be dilated to facilitate the examination. However, it is best to postpone the instillation of the mydriatic and the full ocular inspection until after the visual abilities have been tested. When ophthalmoscopy remains difficult, easier observation is possible using small-diameter illumination beams, observing from as close as possible, and perhaps reducing the illumination level. The examination of the eyelid, conjunctiva, cornea, anterior chamber, and iris requires special attention in elderly patients because of the relatively high prevalence of aging changes affecting these tissues.

Tonometry should be performed routinely on older patients because of the higher incidence of raised intraocular pressure or glaucoma.

During the examination of the eyes, the optometrist should explain what is being done. Older patients are almost invariably aware of cataracts and glaucoma, and they should be reminded that these and other ocular diseases are being given close consideration. They should be fully and clearly advised of the state of their own ocular health. This not only is part of the clinician's basic responsibility, but also reinforces the message that regular eye examinations are most important to older individuals. The details of discussions about ocular disease will vary according to the patient, the examiner, and their previous interactions. Even though the examiner can grow tired of giving essentially the same routine explanations to patient after patient, this responsibility should not be neglected or conveniently curtailed.

REFRACTION
Objective Refraction

Retinoscopy can be more difficult on older patients because of small pupils and media irregularities and opacities. However, it remains an important technique, and the examiner should make every effort to obtain a retinoscopic estimate of refractive error. When retinoscopy becomes unusually difficult, however, the clinician should be prepared to vary technique. Moving to closer-than-usual observation distances or moving off axis may provide an "easier" retinoscopic reflex; Mehr and Freid (1975) described this as *radical retinoscopy*. If a useful retinoscopic reflection cannot be obtained with the standard procedures, the clinician should, first of all, move closer and thus reduce the working distance, perhaps to as close as 5 cm in search of a satisfactory reflex. This can be most useful if there is unsuspected high myopia. If moving closer still provides no satisfactory reflection, it remains that hyperopia could be responsible. Placing a high positively powered lens (for example, + 14.00 D) at the patient's eye, beginning with a standard working distance, and if necessary, reducing the distance, may be useful in finding a difficult retinal reflection in patients with high hyperopia. Of course, when the retinoscopic working distance is changed, an appropriate allowance must be made in estimating the power of the refractive correction. Furthermore, moving off axis may produce some inaccuracy in both the spherical and astigmatic components; thus, this procedure is used only when axial viewing does not provide an adequate reflex.

When there are substantial lenticular irregularities due to cortical or posterior sub-capsular cataract, it may be impossible to obtain consistent or accurate results, because the apparent movement of the reflected light seems to be fragmented (moving in different directions or at different speeds). In these circumstances, a spot retinoscope may prove to be more useful than a streak retinoscope.

Objective optometers depend on light being reflected from the retina. Again, the small pupils and media opacities commonly found in older patients often cause less reliable results. Sometimes no result at all can be obtained.

Keratometry to estimate total astigmatism becomes more important when retinoscopy or objective optometer measurement fails. A record of corneal curvature is useful in quantifying any future changes.

Patients with low vision are often unable to make accurate judgments in subjective refraction procedures. Thus, it may be necessary to rely more than usual on objective refraction results.

Subjective Refraction

Subjective refraction often requires more time with older patients. Their sensitivity to blur may be reduced because of small pupils or because of media or retinal changes that affect visual discrimination. It becomes difficult for them to judge changes of image clarity in response to small refractive changes. Slower presentation of alternatives and sometimes repeated presentations can become necessary. However, older patients, lacking accommodation, do have a stable refractive state, which enhances the reliability of refractive error measurement.

When visual acuity is expected to be normal or near normal, a phoropter and the usual range of refractive techniques may be used. The bichrome (or duochrome) test, which is sometimes unreliable in younger patients, can be a more reliable test in older individuals. Again, small pupils make it difficult for the patient to discriminate the relative clarity of the red and green targets. Lenticular changes may cause the brightness of the green background to be reduced more than the red. It should be emphasized that clarity of the letters rather than the brightness of the red or green background is the criterion.

When the observation distance is 4 m or closer, an appropriate dioptric allowance (obtained by reducing the refractive correction by +0.25 D for a 4-m distance) should be made if clearest distance vision is being sought. With older patients, the binocular balancing of the spherical refraction becomes easy because of the stability of the accommodative state. Standard binocular balancing techniques may be used.

Astigmatism may be determined using crossed-cylinder techniques; the clock dial or related techniques also may be used. In the presence of media irregularities, however, the crossed-cylinder method is preferred. Clock dial, sunburst, paraboline, Humphrey, and similar techniques involving judgment of the clarity of lines in particular orientations all can produce anomalous results when there are refractive irregularities in the media. Similarly, the stenopaic slit method for determining astigmatism is contraindicated for patients with lens or corneal irregularities.

Refraction of Patients with Low Vision

Patients with low vision often require different refraction techniques. The phoropter should not be used. Patients should be free to move their heads and eyes to any preferred positions; they should not be shielded artificially from the ambient illumination; their eye movements and eye position should be observable by the clinician; and they should be aware that improvements achieved are due to simple lenses rather than the magic box that the phoropter might represent.

Trial lenses supported either in trial frames or in lens clips attached to the patient's current glasses should be used. However, trial frames tend to be clumsy, and often require repeated readjustment and repositioning. Furthermore, the vertex distance they provide is often larger than the eventual spectacle-lens vertex distance. These factors all become more bothersome when the refractive error is large. In general, therefore, trial lens clips (Halberg, Bernell, Jannelli, or Bommarito clips) that attach to existing glasses are easier to use. With trial lens clips used over the patient's current glasses, the frame usually sits securely and the lenses have a more appropriate vertex distance and pantoscopic tilt. These together enable a more accurate determination of the required refractive correction.

Working over the current glasses, the optometrist typically has to use only relatively low-powered lenses. This is useful, because low-powered lenses are easier to insert and remove from trial lens mountings and are usually available in finer steps of power.

Astigmatism usually can be measured more accurately when trial lens clips are being used. For either retinoscopic or subjective determination of astigmatism, the clinician at first should completely ignore any astigmatic correction that may be in the old glasses. The astigmatic component of the over-refraction is determined as though it were completely independent. There is no need for the axis and power of the overcorrecting cylinder to bear any relationship to the cylinder present in the glasses over which the refraction is being performed.

When the over-refraction has been completed, the glasses—with lens clips and trial lenses still attached—are taken to a focimeter, and the back vertex power of the combination is measured. This gives the total power required to optimally correct the refractive error. For example, a patient may be wearing a correction of 0.00 DS $=\!\!\Rightarrow\!=-4.50$ DC $\times$ 35, and the over-refraction in the trial lens clips may be $+0.75$ DS $=\!\!\Rightarrow\!=-1.25$ DC $\times$ 160. The examiner could do laborious calculations to determine the resultant power, but it is far simpler to measure the back vertex power of the combination with the focimeter. The resultant power will be found to be 0.00 DS $=\!\!\Rightarrow\!=-4.25$ DC $\times$ 27. This method is particularly valuable when the lens power is large.

In any new glasses, the pantoscopic tilt of the lenses and the vertical positioning of the optical centers probably will be quite similar to those in the existing glasses. Any power errors that may have resulted from the aberrational effects created by tilt and position of the lens will be compensated for by the over-refraction, and a more appropriate refractive correction determination will be obtained.

Patients with low vision are often less sensitive to refractive changes. In general, the poorer the acuity, the poorer is the sensitivity to change. However, this is far from being a universal rule. Sometimes patients with visual acuities of 20/500 will be able to respond reliably to 0.50 D of change, and patients with 20/60 acuity may not be able to respond to 1.50 or 2.00 D of change. It is best for the clinician to begin the refraction with an open mind and wait for the patient's responses to reveal individual sensitivity to blur.

Refracting a low-vision patient begins with directing the patient's attention to visual acuity chart letters at (or close to) the patient's limit of resolution. Initially, the steps of dioptric power should be large enough to allow the patient to recognize changes in clarity easily.

Holding a plus lens in one hand and a minus lens of equal power in the other (say, $+6.00$ D and -6.00 D), the optometrist may ask the patient to make judgments involving 6.00 D of change ($+6.00$ D to plano or -6.00 D). When using hand-held lenses, it is often advisable to fabricate the plano presentation by holding lenses of equal and opposite power together rather than using no lens at all. Some patients have already decided whether or not they want a change of correction, and this can influence their response to "with" to "without" comparisons.

Once the patient can make confident responses to dioptric changes, the size of the changes should be reduced systematically in the process of pursuing the refractive error. When large steps of dioptric power are being used, the clinician may be guided by the strength of the patient's response. This may be revealed by the patient's choice of words, tone of voice, or quickness of response. For example, upon the introduction of a $+6.00$ D lens, the patient might respond, "That's blurry." Upon switching to the -6.00 D lens, the patient says firmly, "That's much worse." To a plano presentation ($+6.00$ D with -6.00 D), the patient responds, "That's better." Upon returning to the $+6.00$ lens, the patient says, "That's a little blurry again." From this sequence, the examiner has learned that plus is strongly preferred to minus and that there is a consistent but mild preference for 0.00 over $+6.00$ D. It appears the refractive error is positive—closer to 0.00 than $+6.00$, but not very close to 0.00 D, since there was such a strong difference between $+6.00$ D and -6.00 D. At this stage, a reasonable guess at the spherical refraction error would be in the range of $+1.50$ to $+2.25$ D. It also can be argued that the patient can discriminate dioptric changes of at least ± 3.00 D.

The spherical refraction process continues making use of bracketing, going from an excess of plus to an excess of minus. It is finalized when changing from plus to minus in the finest discriminable step elicits a response indicating that both presentations appear slightly but equally blurred.

On completing the spherical power determination, the optometrist can begin the astigmatic determination with some knowledge of the patient's responsiveness to refractive blur. This knowledge can guide the practitioner in choosing the power of the Jackson cross-cylinder that is to be used. In a general optometric office, ± 0.25 D and a ± 0.75 D hand-held cross-cylinder should be available. The lower-power cross-cylinder is useful for normal patients, and the ± 0.75 D cross-cylinder will be strong enough for the majority of low-vision patients with poorer discrimination. The test target observed during the Jackson cross-cylinder refraction is usually a selected letter or letters on the Snellen chart at or close to the limit of the patient's acuity. Remember that the flip cross-cylinder test works best when the spherical equivalence of the test lens combinations is kept constant.

After the astigmatism has been measured, it is prudent to check the spherical component. If any significant change is necessary, the power of the cylindrical correction should be rechecked.

VISUAL ACUITY MEASUREMENT

Visual acuity measurement requires a little more care in elderly patients than in younger ones. Older patients are more affected by test illumination and the distribution of light within the luminous environment. Thus, more care than usual should be taken to insure that the chart illumination is at a standard level (80 to 320 candelas per square meter) and that troublesome glare sources are eliminated from the field of view. Illumination conditions may need to be changed while visual acuity is being measured. Because older patients are more likely to acquire changes in their vision, for reference purposes, it is important that the best practical measure of visual acuity be made.

When visual acuity is reduced, nonstandard techniques become necessary. Projector charts, which are suitable for the measurement of normal visual acuity, should not be used for low-vision patients. Most do not provide the contrast or adjustability in range of luminance that is available with printed board or transilluminated charts. Also, projector charts lack flexibility to extend the range in order to measure poorer acuities. With printed charts it is easy to alter the observation distance over a wide range.

For all visual acuity measurement, it is wise to record acuity by giving partial credit for rows that were only partially read correctly (20/20 − 2, or 20/15 + 1, and so forth). Optometrists who do not always use the same chart should always make note of the chart that was used.

Visual Acuity Measurement in Low-Vision Patients

Chart design can influence the visual acuity score, and this can become most important when there is disturbed macular function. The number of letters per row and the relative spacing between letters and between rows can cause substantial variations in visual acuity scores. Many low-vision patients require a reduced observation distance, and the practitioner should be aware that, with some charts, changing observation distances can influence the acuity scores obtained.

First, scaling may change. Many charts have a size sequence of 200, 100, 80, 60, 50, 40, 30, 25, 20, and 15. At 20 feet, an acuity of 20/200 might be recorded, indicating that the patient read the 200-foot symbols but failed to read the 100-foot symbols. On changing to a 10-foot observation distance, it may at first be anticipated that the acuity score will be 10/100. Consistency with the 20-foot measurement only requires that the acuity be at least 10/100, but not as good as 10/50. Thus, the acuity score could be recorded as 10/100, 10/80, or 10/60 and still be consistent with the 20/200 finding. Only when the chart follows a logarithmic (or constant-proportion) size progression can this scaling problem be avoided.

Second, changing to a closer observation distance often alters the nature of the task at threshold. The number of letters per row may increase, and the relative spacing between optotypes may change. With macular dysfunction, contour interaction becomes much more important than usual, and increasing the number of letters per row or reducing spacing can significantly reduce the acuity that can be achieved. A patient who reads a single 20/200 letter with ease might not be able to read any of three closely spaced letters on a 100-foot row when the viewing distance has been changed to 10 feet.

Visual acuity scores will be more valid and more impervious to change with changing observation distance if the task is made essentially the same at each size level. This requires that almost equally legible symbols be used, that there be the same number of symbols in each row, that the spacing between symbols and between rows be proportional to symbol size, and that size follow a geometric (or logarithmic or common-multiplier) progression. Bailey-Lovie charts and their derivatives follow these principles (Bailey and Lovie, 1976; Ferris et al., 1982).

Bailey-Lovie charts were designed to avoid problems encountered in low-vision work. Their size range extends from 200- to 15-foot symbols. With the chart as close as two feet, acuities of 2/200 (equivalent to 20/2000) may be measured. The Feinbloom Visual Acuity Chart is a popular chart designed for low-vision work. The size progression is irregular, and there is wide variation in spacing and in the number of symbols at the different size levels. Nevertheless, the Feinbloom chart does have attractive features: the size range extends to 700-foot symbols, symbol size progresses in relatively small (albeit irregular) steps, and the page-turning mode of presentation can be psychologically encouraging to patients who have become accustomed to reading very few letters correctly when tested on more common charts. The Feinbloom chart also uses numbers rather than letters. Although these numbers may not be uniformly legible, they can be useful to patients who are not familiar or facile with the English alphabet.

Low-vision patients may have their visual acuity significantly altered by relatively minor changes in illumination. Thus, the recommended procedure is to make the first measurement of acuity at the standard or customary illumination level. Then, referring the patient to the smallest letters that can be read, ask if there is any change when illumination is increased or decreased. When externally illuminated panel charts are being used, the illuminance may be controlled by moving the luminaire closer to the chart or by turning off other room lighting and moving the luminaire away from the chart or shielding it in some convenient manner.

When there is macular dysfunction, it can be informative to note the manner in which the patient reads the chart. Many patients perform much better when reading letters at the start or the end of rows and perform poorly when attempting to read more central letters. This usually indicates problems from central scotomas and may lead the clinician to expect some limitation of the patient's potential to read efficiently. When there is evidence or suspicion of macular disturbance, it can be useful to direct the patient to fixate above, below, to the right of, or to the left of a row of letters that has been found to be difficult. Any reported changes in visibility can indicate whether eccentric viewing strategies may facilitate reading the chart.

ASSESSMENT OF NEAR VISION

Some aspects of the near vision assessment become much easier with elderly patients. Because older patients lack accommodation, their working distance becomes highly predictable from the power of the addition being used. The range of clear near vision depends on pupil diameter and the size of the test target detail. With newsprint or something similar as the target, the range of clear vision is often measured to be about 1.00 D. With charts having a size range that goes smaller than the patient's resolution limit, and providing that the patient always looks at the smallest print that can just be read, the range of clearest vision is often found to be reduced to about 0.25 D.

For patients with normal distance visual acuity, an equivalent near-vision performance usually will be achieved. Occasionally, near visual acuity may be significantly worse if there are central lenticular opacities that have a more harmful effect on vision when the pupil constricts in response to viewing near objects. More rarely, acuity can improve at near distances because peripheral opacities are rendered less important by pupillary constriction.

The quantity and quality of illumination should be optimized, and elderly patients generally should be given advice on how to arrange their lighting for prolonged near visual tasks. An adjustable lamp with an incandescent (60- or 100-watt) bulb provides an almost universally useful means of controlling the task illumination. The task illuminance can be increased by moving the lamp closer to the material, and the bulb or bright spots from the reflector of the lamp should not be directly visible to the patient.

The most appropriate near-vision addition can be determined in various ways, but it is the desired viewing distance that dominates the decision for the typical elderly patient. A variety of methods may be used to determine the power of the addition; the range of clear vision, biochrome, or cross-cylinder at near techniques all can work satisfactorily on older patients. After the clinician has determined the power of the required addition while using test charts at the desired working distance, performance should be tested using magazines, newspapers, bank statements, or whatever represents the patient's most common or most important near vision tasks.

Given a particular visual acuity, the size of resolvable detail is determined by the working distance. If patients request clearer vision than they obtain with their present glasses, even though the present glasses are in correct focus for the desired working distance, the clinician must increase the addition, thereby simultaneously reducing the working distance. More exotic optical devices also can be considered.

If a change in the power of the addition is to be considered, the clinician should be conscious of the magnitude of resolution improvement that can be expected. Almost all distance visual acuity charts use a size progression ratio of about 5:4 in the region of 20/20 (50, 40, 30, 25, 20, and 15). Changing viewing distance by a 5:4 ratio (50 cm to 40 cm, 40 cm to 32 cm, and so forth) should proportionally increase resolution capacity equivalent to one line of improvement. Since dioptric power is inversely proportional to viewing distance, the addition must be increased by a ratio of 5:4 to achieve improvements that may be thought of as "one line." Thus, 1.50, 2.00, 2.50, 3.25, 4.00, and 5.00 D is a series of lens powers in which each step represents about one line of acuity improvement. Note the close similarity between the numbers in this sequence and the size progression in the 20/20 region of the distance visual acuity chart. With this sequence as a reference, the clinician can deduce that a patient with a +2.50 D addition will get only a marginal improvement (one-third of a line) by having the addition increased to +2.75 D. A +3.25 D addition is required to provide a resolution improvement that could be described as "one full line."

Optometrists usually measure and record the near visual acuity. The near visual acuity record should specify both the observation distance and the size of the smallest print that may be read. It is preferable to specify print size in M units or points. M units express the distance in meters at which the lowercase letters subtend 5 minutes of arc. Points indicate print size according to the units used by printers and typesetters. It is common (albeit inappropriate) to express print size as a reduced Snellen equivalent, a fraction that expresses the equivalent distance visual acuity required to read that particular print when it is viewed from 40 cm. This method becomes clearly inappropriate when the viewing distance is other than 40 cm. It is confusing and inaccurate to record *20/20 at 30 cm,* since this expression, as it is most commonly used, is intended to indicate that the visual acuity is in fact less than equivalent to 20/20.

Print that is truly equivalent to 20/20 at 40 cm can be said to be 0.40 M units in size. Using the M unit notation, near visual acuity can be expressed as a true Snellen fraction. Print that is 0.40 M (20/20 at 40 cm) viewed at 40 cm would demand an acuity of 0.40/0.40 M; if the same print were just legible at 30 cm, the acuity would be 0.30/0.40 M. The M unit system is far more appropriate and more consistent with the methods traditionally used to measure distance visual acuity. Fortunately, the Jaeger system is becoming less commonly used, as its lack of standardization is becoming well known.

In patients with normal or near-normal vision, there is usually fairly close concordance between the near and distance visual acuities. The visual task for the near visual acuity measurement usually involves reading typeset print, which is more complex than reading the fairly widely spaced letters found on the distance visual acuity charts. Such differences in complexity do not have much influence on acuity scores in the normally sighted. In patients with disturbed macular function, however, task complexity can cause major inconsistencies in acuity scores. It is quite common for patients with macular degeneration to have a near or reading acuity score that is twofold or worse than the distance letter chart acuity.

Near visual acuity measurements with reading charts often serve as a basis for determining the magnification that a low-vision patient might require to satisfactorily perform a complex task at near. Distance visual acuity measurements taken with letter charts are much less reliable for this purpose.

Many satisfactory reading charts are available for testing normally sighted patients. Reading charts with larger size ranges and more systematic design features have been designed by Bailey and Lovie (1980), Keeler (1956), and Sloan (1959).

ASSESSMENT OF BINOCULAR VISION

As patients grow older, they are more likely to develop some ocular motor difficulties because of changes affecting the neuromuscular mechanisms and the structural tissues around the eyes. In examining binocular coordination, care should be taken to observe the version movements of the eyes as they move in the six cardinal eye-movement directions (right, left, up and right, down and right, up and left, and down and left). A relative lagging of one eye indicates an oculomotor dysfunction that warrants a more detailed evaluation of the noncomitancy.

The cover test should be carefully and routinely performed at distance and near for older patients. Older patients lack accommodation and have no stimulus to accommodative convergence; thus, they show more exophoria at near. Vertical deviations are also more common in the elderly. Phorias or tropias should be measured at both distance and near using loose prisms. When large near exophoria is found, the strength of the fusional vergence mechanism can be judged by the facility and speed with which the patient makes vergence eye movements to obtain fusion when a base-out prism (say, 10Δ diopters) is introduced before one eye. Poor fusion responses tend to indicate a need for prescribing prisms.

Although it is common practice to measure the near phoria with the test target close to eye level, it is more appropriate to have the target lower so that downgaze is required. This is more representative of the habitual reading eye posture, particularly if the patient holds or touches the near fixation target.

A variety of subjective tests are available for measuring heterophoria in younger patients, and these often provide different measures of the heterophoria. However, there is more consistency in the older patients because of their lack of accommodation, so the choice of method used to measure heterophoria becomes less important.

When there is a potentially significant heterophoria, the optometrist must decide if prism is to be prescribed, and if so, how much. There are many reasonable approaches to these decisions (see Chapter 10). Fixation disparity, rules involving fusional reserves, and rules based on phoria magnitude can all be useful in indicating how much prism should be prescribed. It can be prudent to check the advantage obtained from the prism by introducing the prism of the indicated power and orientation and asking the patient to report on the clarity or ease of vision while observing fine print. The prism is then removed and reintroduced after a pause, but with the base direction changed 180 degrees. If a patient with exophoria does not prefer base-in to base-out prisms, judged by changes in clarity or by relative difficulty in adapting to the change, the decision to prescribe prisms should be carefully reconsidered. With vertical prism, the prism power magnitudes are usually smaller, and it may be more convenient to make this kind of change by keeping the prism in the same orientation but transferring it to the other eye, changing from 2 BUR to 2 BUL and so on.

Anisometropia creates special problems, especially relating to vertical phorias. Younger anisometropes can tilt their heads forward or back as needed to achieve viewing through the optical centers of the lenses and thus avoid differential prismatic effects. Older patients wearing bifocals must move their eyes in downgaze to view through the bifocal segment when they read.

When patients are already wearing a bifocal correction for anisometropia, decision making is easier. Unless there has been a substantial change in refractive error, the patient's need for vertical prismatic correction can be tested at distance and at near using methods such as those already described using the patient's old glasses. Patients with anisometropia often exhibit significant vertical heterophoria at near, but they will lack symptoms and will not show any strong preference for having the correcting prism in place. Each case should be considered individually. When the anisometropia is newly acquired—perhaps because of a myopic shift in one eye—symptoms and adaptation difficulties are more likely. Some practitioners prefer to prescribe some overall vertical prism to minimize such vertical phoria problems at near. Others choose to prescribe bifocals with no special prism compensation but may warn the patient of possible symptoms and adaptation difficulties; this strategy avoids prescribing special prism until it has been demonstrated that the patient has failed to adapt.

The remedies for the bifocal problems in anisometropia are to use slab-off or other prism-controlled bifocals, executive bifocals where there is no prism present at the dividing line, Franklin split-lens bifocals, or asymetrical bifocal segments (for example, Ultex in one eye and flat-top in the other); or to revert to separate distance and reading glasses. Fresnel press-on prism can be cut so they are confined to the bifocal segment region. Although they are not often used as a permanent solution, they can be useful in investigating the potential value of a prismatic correction in the bifocal segments.

Several tests can determine whether a patient truly does have binocular vision in a particular situation. Good stereo-acuity, the ability to see both monocular targets on a fixation disparity test, and fusion with the Worth four-dot test are useful standard criteria. The simple bar-reading test is sometimes overlooked; holding a pen midway between the eyes and the page of print should not obscure any print if simultaneous binocular vision is present.

VISUAL FIELD MEASUREMENT

Visual field losses are more common in elderly patients than in younger ones. Field defects may come from chorioretinal pathology, glaucoma, optic atrophies, and intracranial disorders. When measuring visual fields, the clinician should be conscious of the purpose of conducting the test:

1. Is it to screen for otherwise unsuspected pathologic conditions?
2. Is it to seek evidence that will confirm the presence of an already suspected pathologic condition?
3. Is it to monitor the progress of a previously identified field defect?

4. Is it to evaluate the impact that the field loss already known to be present will have on the person's ability to function?

The test parameters (target size and luminance, as well as background luminance) and strategies for presentation will vary accordingly. See Anderson (1982) and Bedwell (1982) in the Suggested Readings list at the end of this Chapter for more information on visual fields testing.

For screening, test spots should be just comfortably detectable, and a systematic broad search should be made of the whole visual field. For confirming tentative diagnoses, the test targets should be just detectable — and only just detectable — in the region where the field defect is most likely to occur. The test target presentation should be confined largely to this region of the visual field, and the motion of dynamic targets should be such that the direction is at right angles to the probable border of the scotoma.

To monitor the progression of visual field defects, the stimulus condition must be as similar as possible to those used previously. Again, any target motion should be orthogonal to the known border of the scotoma.

For functional evaluation of the visual fields, binocular observation should be permitted. Relatively easy to see targets should be used.

Automatic or semiautomatic visual field screeners have become more popular over the last decade. These instruments present static targets in a controlled and repeatable manner. In general, they eliminate many of the problems associated with technique and bias that can so easily contaminate the results with the traditional, operator-controlled, dynamic target tests. The automated field screeners are available in tangent screen and bowl perimeter form. Several have been subjected to studies that establish norms and recommend the stimulus variables most suitable for different age groups. The popularity of automated screeners may grow further, but the tangent screen and bowl perimeter will remain very important to clinical practice.

Low-vision patients may have some special problems associated with visual field measurement. Central fixation, which is often a problem, can sometimes be overcome by providing a cross target centered on the fixation point. Elastic cord, masking tape, or even chalk may be used on the tangent screen to provide a cross through the central point. The patient is instructed to look toward the center of the cross, even though he or she may not see the actual intersection. Flashing the target can make it easier for the patient to maintain central fixation, because patients are less tempted to move their eyes to check on the presence of the target if it is flashing.

Functional visual field testing is important in low-vision patients. Whenever frank scotomas are found on the tangent screen or bowl perimeter, a much coarser test of functional detection ability should be made using larger and more visible targets. A hand or piece of writing paper may be used as a target against a black screen to establish whether the scotoma is truly absolute.

The Amsler grid can be a most useful test of central visual function, characterizing disturbances of central vision. Patients may report absences, fading, or distortion in parts of the grid pattern while they maintain fixation on its center. When patients report observable changes, the practitioner may gain insights into the nature of the visual disturbance and perhaps may be better able to predict or understand the patients' functional difficulties. Sometimes a patient will not recognize scotomas, as "filling in" seems to occur. Indeed, the normal physiologic blind spot usually cannot be observed on Amsler grid patterns. Useful information is obtained about the patient vision function when visual disturbances are reported on the Amsler grid test. When no visual disturbance is observed by the patient, however, no definite conclusion should be made about the presence or absence of scotomas.

COLOR VISION TESTING

The purpose of testing color vision is twofold. First, the identification of color vision anomalies can assist in the diagnosis or detection of pathologic changes in the visual system. Second, altered color vision can cause some difficulties with color discrimination tasks, and the possibility of such functional difficulties should be discussed with the patient.

Color vision usually changes as the patient ages because of yellowing of the crystalline lens and physiologic and pathologic changes in the macular region. Such defects tend to be tritanopic, the most obvious manifestations being a reduction of discrimination in the blue and blue-green regions of the spectrum.

The test of choice for the routine assessment of color vision in older patients is the Farnsworth Panel D-15 test, in which 15 colored chips are arranged so that they appear to be in order according to chromatic similarity. Patients having normal aging changes affecting their color vision typically make only a few small-magnitude errors of the tritanopic type. When there is retinal pathology, however, the number and magnitude of errors in arranging the D-15 targets become greater. In cases of substantial retinal pathology, the magnitude of errors in arranging the D-15 test targets becomes large, and the pattern of the errors is more random (see Chapter 6).

OTHER TESTS OF OCULAR OR VISUAL FUNCTION

A variety of clinical tests of visual functions can be useful in identifying the presence of ocular pathologic changes, for making diagnostic distinctions, or for explaining functional difficulties resulting from the pathology. Contrast sensitivity losses of small magnitude are common in the elderly, and more severe losses of contrast sensitivity accompany many of the ocular diseases that are associated with aging. There are three basic approaches for measuring contrast sensitivity. The traditional method is to present sinusoidal grating targets at selected spatial frequencies. Then contrast is varied to determine the minimum contrast at which the striped grating pattern can be detected for each of the spatial frequencies. The Contrast Sensitivity Function is a graph showing how contrast sensitivity varies with spatial frequency (see Chapter 13). The grating displays may be presented on oscilloscope or video screens or on printed chart displays (Ginsburg, 1984). The second method is to measure visual acuity with low-contrast letter charts that effectively determine the spatial frequency limit for resolution at selected contrast levels (Regan, 1988). The third method is to present a sequence of large targets, such as large letters or edge targets (Pelli et al., 1988; Bailey, 1987; Verbaken and Johnston, 1986), in which there is a progression of reducing contrast, and the lowest contrast at which the target can be recognized is the measure of contrast sensitivity.

Disability glare is more of a problem in older patients because all develop increased intraocular light scatter as a result if inevitable aging changes in the lens of the eye. Light scatter becomes more pronounced with the development of cataract or with disorders affecting the cornea or the vitreous. Tests of disability glare can be useful for monitoring the development of cataract or other medial opacities or for the prediction of functional difficulties that may be experienced under glare conditions. Recently, low-contrast letters charts with a surrounding field of glare have proven to be sensitive measures of disability glare (Regan, 1991; Bailey and Bullimore, 1991). A more analytical assessment of light scatter and glare can be made by a method introduced by Van den Berg (1986) in which scattered light from a flashing bright annulus of light can induce a flickering appearance in a steady, central, spot target. Introducing counterphase flicker of variable intensity into the central spot provides a means of nulling the flickering appearance induced by the light scattered from the annulus. This effectively quantifies the scattered light.

Retinal adaptational mechanisms may be impaired by some age-related eye diseases, and dark adaptation and glare recovery tests may identify such losses. Sophisticated instrumentation is available for testing dark adaptation and glare recovery, but some relative or functional assessments may be made by testing the patient's ability to see objects in very dim light or by measuring the time taken for maximum visual acuity to return following exposure to a strong light such as from a penlight held close to the eye. Differential diagnosis of pathologic conditions may be facilitated by the use of electro-retinograms, electro-oculograms, fluorescein angiography, measurement of responses to flicker, special tests of color vision function, and visually evoked cortical potentials (see Chapter 13).

PRESCRIBING SPECTACLES FOR THE NORMALLY SIGHTED

Most older patients require optical correction for both distance and near vision tasks. Driving, watching television and movies, spectating the public events, and referring to distant informational signs cause good distance vision to be important for most individuals. At near, tasks ranging from writing and reading personal and business correspondence; reading labels on foods and medicines; reading price tags; reading directories; and recreational or educational reading of books, newspapers, and magazines are all part of regular daily life for most people. It is clearly desirable for most people to have easy access to clear distance and near vision.

Bifocals, trifocals, or progressive addition lenses are worn by older patients. Small in number are the emmetropes who do not need distance glasses, myopes who do not need near vision glasses, and the people who choose to use only single vision glasses and change their spectacles whenever they change from distance to near viewing.

In considering trifocals, the starting point is usually the questions, What is the person's range of clear near vision with the most appropriate reading glasses? And, are there important intermediate distance tasks that will not be seen with adequate clarity if simple bifocals are used? Trifocals typically have an intermediate segment that is half the power of the stronger reading segment.

Progressive addition lenses have two benefits. One is that they are preferred by people who do not like the appearance of the dividing line of the standard bifocal or trifocal segments. The other benefit is that progressive addition lenses provide a channel of progressively increasing power between the distance viewing point and the near viewing point. In effect, this provides a continuous sequence of focus for all possible intermediate distances. Objects at intermediate distances will be seen clearly when the head and eyes are positioned so that the most appropriate portion of the lens is being used. The patient can experience some diminished clarity and some spatial distortion when viewing through the areas in the lower half of the lens that are outside the channel of progressive power change. Many patients are not bothered by this, whereas others find it annoying and distracting.

The size and position of bifocal or trifocal segments should be chosen to suit the patient's functional needs and particular wishes. The width of the field of clear near vision, prismatic jump, and chromatic effects can influence the recommendations made.

Older patients are more likely to have ametropias of high magnitude. In progressive myopia, the magnitude of refractive error can continue to increase throughout life. Fairly large myopic shifts can occur from changes in the crystalline lens. On the other end of the scale, many older patients become highly hyperopic if intraocular lens implants are not used following cataract extraction.

High refractive errors require special consideration. When performing the refraction, care should be taken to insure that the vertex distance and pantoscopic angle of the lenses being worn are similar to those expected to be present in any new glasses that might be worn in the future.

The position of the optical centers relative to the patient's pupil can become much more significant when lens powers exceed about 8.00 D. The basic principle guiding lens positioning is that the optic axis of the lens should point toward the center of rotation of the eye. Lens designers assume this when they select lens parameters to avoid aberrational effects. The center of rotation is typically about 27 mm behind the spectacle plane.

It follows that pantoscopic tilt of the spectacle plane is a key factor in determining the vertical placement of the optical centers. The greater the pantoscopic angle, the lower are the centers. A simple method for measuring pantoscopic tilt is to take a protractor with a plumb line (or a straightened paper clip) attached to its center. The base of this protractor can be held so that it is against or parallel to the spectacle plane. With the patient's head in its natural or habitual posture, the plumb line will indicate the most usual pantoscopic tilt. To compensate for the effects of pantoscopic tilt, the optical centers should be made lower than the center of the pupils by 1 mm for each 2 degrees of pantoscopic tilt. Ten degrees of pantoscopic tilt is quite common, and for this, the height of the optical centers should be 5 mm below the pupil center. This is about level with the corneal limbus. The correctness if the optical alignment can be verified by having the patient tilt his or her head back while fixating a bright light at an appropriate distance. The optometrist, with the eye close to the light, should observe the reflex from the cornea in line with those from the lens surfaces (see Chapter 11).

Aphakic spectacle corrections often require special lens design considerations. Bifocals, and rarely trifocals, become virtually essential. The prescribing practitioner is obliged to consider a number of lens design options. For example, should the lens material be plastic to minimize weight, glass because of its scratch resistance, or higher-index glass to minimize thickness? Aspheric lens surfaces are likely to be used, and the purpose may be to enhance appearance by reducing thickness and sagittal depth, or to provide imagery of better quality when viewing through more peripheral regions of the lens. Some aspheric lenses available today have been designed primarily to achieve a better cosmetic appearance. Others are designed to minimize aberrational effects. In general, this kind is a little less effective in minimizing thickness. The responsible optometrist stays abreast of developments in lens design and is prepared to consider the weight, appearance, durability, and aberrations of the lenses. Of course, many of the problems associated with spectacle lenses of higher power can be avoided or minimized by the use of contact lenses.

PRESCRIBING FOR LOW-VISION PATIENTS

Most elderly patients with low vision can benefit from optical aids to enhance their visual performance. The optimal aids for individual patients depend on the range and relative importance of the visual tasks they wish to perform, their vision characteristics, and their psychological attitudes toward their disability and to the use of optical aids. Patients who need low-vision aids usually need more than one special optical aid. In prescribing optical aids, magnification is usually the first optical parameter considered. The field of view, distribution of image quality, image brightness, adjustability of focus, appearance, portability, convenience, cost, working distance, and maintenance requirements are other factors that enter the decision-making process. It is convenient to consider optical low-vision aids under three headings: (1) magnifiers for distance vision (telescopes), (2) magnifiers for near vision, and (3) nonmagnifying aids to vision (see Chapter 12).

Magnification for Distance Vision: Telescopes

Telescopes are commonly used by low-vision patients to enhance the resolution of detail in signs, distant faces, television, movies, or other visual displays and scenery. Many elderly patients with low vision need to travel independently; if their vision is not adequate for driving, however, they may have to rely on public transportation. Dependence on public transportation, in turn, necessitates reading bus numbers, street signs, and traffic signals.

Prescribing a telescope (or telescopes) for a low-vision patient involves both determining the required magnification and selecting an appropriate telescope.

Achieving the Required Acuity

The determination of the required telescope magnification is straightforward. The clinician determines visual acuity with best spectacle correction and estimates the resolution performance required to meet the patient's specific needs. Most commonly, an acuity performance of 20/30 to 20/40 is set as a practical and useful goal, but higher resolution is sometimes sought. When acuity is poor, the goal may be reduced to about 20/60. If acceptable telescopes do not improve visual acuity to 20/80, the value of a telescope prescription becomes questionable.

Calculating the required magnification is simple; it is a matter of ratios. For example, a patient with a visual acuity of 20/200 who wishes to read bus numbers might require 6 × magnification to reach about a 20/30 level of performance.

Most low-vision patients do obtain the expected improvement in resolution. Exceptions may occur when using charts on which the task is made more difficult (more letters, closer spacing, or both for the smaller letters). In these cases the improvement may be less than simple theory predicts. The optometrist should verify that the patient does in fact obtain the expected visual acuity with the magnification originally predicted. Occasionally some modification of the magnification value will be necessary.

Certain techniques are important when testing patient performance with telescopes, especially with elderly patients. For best vision, the telescope must be focused properly. The greater the magnification, the more critical this becomes. If the patient has only a small refractive error, the clinician may focus the telescope for his or her own eye, observing from the correct viewing distance. Only small focus adjustments then should be required of the patient. When patients have higher refractive error, the clinician may use a trial lens to simulate the patient's refractive error and again adjust the telescope. Thus, for a 6.00 D myope, the clinician should look through a telescope while holding a +6.00 D lens between the telescope eyepiece and his or her own eye (or glasses, if worn) and, being careful to be at the correct observation distance, focus to obtain clearest vision. The telescope should then be close to correct adjustment for the patient. Remember that adjustments that increase the telescope length add plus power to correct hyperopic refractive errors or to focus for closer viewing distances. Shortening the telescope length adds minus power.

Many telescopes of 6 × or greater magnification do not provide enough focusing range to enable a focus for the commonly used 20- or 10-foot distances. Should there be an insufficient range of focus, the clinician can effectively simulate optical infinity by moving the chart to 4 m (12.5 ft) and then hold a +0.25 D trial lens against the objective of the telescope. A chart observation distance of 2 m with +0.50 D lens in front of the telescope achieves the same effect.

It is necessary to insure in-focus vision when determining whether or not the patient achieves the resolution goal sought. The clinician should always verify that the prescribed telescope does indeed focus at the distance required. The patient's actual working distance should be established in the field or alternatively simulated in the office or local environment. The patient's observation distance may be 30 ft (say, a lecture theater) or 8 ft (an overhead menu at a fast-food restaurant); whatever this observation distance is, however, it should be simulated, and the clinician should check that the telescope's focusing range is adequate.

When more than one viewing distance is required, it may be necessary to prescribe a removable lens cap of appropriate power to achieve the change in focus. Now there are several series of monocular telescopes with very wide focusing ranges and these have become widely used in the low-vision clinical community.

Another important optical parameter is the exit pupil of the telescope, which defines the size of the beam of rays that can emerge from the telescope. The exit pupil almost invariably can be calculated by dividing the diameter of the objective lens by the magnification of the telescope. Thus, an 8 × 20 telescope has an 8 × magnification and a 20-mm objective lens diameter; the exit pupil size is 20 ÷ 8, or 2.5 mm. An 8 × 40 telescope has a 40-mm objective, and thus has a 5-mm exit pupil. Telescopes of 4 × 20, 6 × 30, 8 × 40, and 10 × 50 all have 5-mm exit pupils.

The exit pupil can determine image brightness. If the exit beam is smaller than the eye pupil diameter, the image brightness is reduced as though the eye pupil had constricted to become the same size as the exit pupil of the telescope. An 8 × 20 telescope with a 2.5-mm exit pupil used by an eye with a 5-mm pupil will cause a fourfold decrease in retinal image illuminance. The effective diameter of the pupil is reduced by a factor of 2, so the effective area is reduced by a factor of 4. If the exit beam of the telescope is larger in diameter than the eye pupil, the image brightness should not be reduced except for the loss by reflectance and absorption. Lens coatings can reduce this kind of light loss.

This discussion of image brightness and telescopes applies to the observation of most objects. Different arguments and conclusions apply to the observation of stars, because the size of the retinal images of point sources is not affected by the magnification of the telescope.

Telescopes with smaller exit beams are generally more difficult to use, especially if the patient is inexperienced or has unsteady hands. It is more difficult to maintain a small exit beam in alignment with the eye pupil.

Older patients who have difficulty using telescopes to view the visual acuity chart are helped if the magnification is lower, the exit pupil is larger, or the field of view is larger. Sometimes, it is necessary to develop the patient's skills gradually by beginning with telescopes of lower magnification. Patients with alignment difficulties can be assisted by reducing the room lighting and increasing the illumination on the chart. Then, if the telescope is not aligned properly, the exit beam will be visible as it illuminates the iris, sclera, or eyelids. The patient can be guided so that the exit beam enters his or her pupil. Even when the telescope is aligned, it may be necessary for the clinician to continue to help maintain alignment and assist with the focus adjustment. In general, older patients need significantly more training and guidance to become proficient in using telescopes.

Selecting a Telescope

Once it has been verified that a patient can achieve the desired visual acuity with the use of a telescope of a particular magnification, the clinician must select the type of telescope that produces the required magnification and most conveniently satisfies the patient's needs. The prescribed telescope may be monocular or binocular. Binocular telescopes tend to be preferred when the visual acuity is similar for the two eyes. Some patients find binocular telescopes easier to hold because the two eyecups can touch the eyebrows and provide some support or tactile feedback to help the patient maintain proper alignment. However, binocular telescopes are bulky and heavy, which detracts from their portability and comfort.

Patients who use telescopes to assist in their independent travel abilities usually prefer telescopes that are light in weight, concealable, easily carried in pocket or purse, and easy to use. Wrist straps, neck cords, or small finger ring mountings may help keep the telescope easily accessible for use as needed. Difficulties in holding a higher powered telescope with adequate steadiness can sometimes be reduced or eliminated by the use of a tripod, monopod, or other supporting structure.

Telescopes mounted in a spectacle frame or similar mounting have their advantages. They can prove most useful when observation with the telescope is for protracted periods (for example, when watching sporting events, stage presentations, or movies). Ready-made sports glasses, which are a pair of adjustable telescopes mounted in a spectacle-style frame, can be relatively inexpensive. Hook-on monocular telescopes can be attached to existing distance spectacles, thereby simultaneously correcting the refractive error and providing magnification.

Patients often request a spectacle-mounted system for viewing television. Generally, it is better to have the patient move closer to the television. Because telescopes restrict the field of view, in many television-viewing situations telescopes will not allow the patient to see the whole screen at one time. Many older patients resist sitting close to the television, as they believe it is harmful to the eyes. Such misconceptions should be corrected.

Bioptic telescopes are spectacle-mounted telescope systems that are arranged to enable an easy transition from viewing through the telescope portion to viewing through the lens in which the telescope is mounted. These systems are more commonly prescribed for younger adults, but some older patients benefit from them. Bioptic telescopes can be used in driving, permitting the wearer quick access to telescope viewing for short-term observation of signs and traffic signals. Many state departments of motor vehicles permit driving with bioptic telescopes provided that the usual visual standard is met when the wearer observes through the telescope, and vision through the nontelescope section must be of a particular standard. Drivers wearing bioptic telescopes may have some general or individual restrictions on their driver's licenses. Older patients who use a bioptic telescope system for driving often want a bifocal addition for viewing the speedometer and other gauges and displays.

Spectacle-mounted bioptic telescope systems are available in magnifications up to $8 \times$, but $3 \times$ and $4 \times$ seem to be most useful. The small field and difficulties with steadiness and with aiming the telescope make the higher magnification bioptic telescopes harder to use.

Older patients, who are often self-conscious about their visual handicap, may be reluctant to even consider the use of a telescope. Most patients whose visual acuity is 20/60 or poorer should be given information about telescopes so they can understand their potential advantages. Encouraging patients to borrow a telescope for use at home for a week or so can produce some appreciation of the benefits and may change attitudes about telescopes.

Magnification for Near Vision

Optical magnification to provide low-vision patients with assistance for near vision tasks can be considered in six categories: (1) high-addition reading glasses, (2) hand-held magnifying glasses, (3) stand magnifiers, (4) head-mounted loupes, (5) near vision telescopes, and (6) videomagnifiers and projection magnifiers.

There are three basic steps in prescribing a magnifier to provide a level of resolution that will meet the patient's visual needs: (1) determining the magnification or power required; (2) deciding what kind of magnifier (hand-held, stand, and so forth) would be most appropriate; and (3) given the magnification demand and the kind of magnifier, determining which of the available models has the best combination of features to satisfy the patient's requirements.

Determining Magnification Requirements

Magnification for near vision can be a difficult topic to discuss, because there are many conflicting definitions of *magnification*. To illustrate the difficulty, a 5.00 D lens held at a full arm's length might produce an apparent magnification of $5 \times$, and the resolution could be $2 \times$ better than that obtained with a previous 2.50 D addition that gave clear vision at 40 cm, yet the manufacturer may have this magnifier labeled $2.25 \times$; to cap it all, the clinician may recall a simple formula ($M = F/4$) which suggests that the magnification should be $1.25 \times$. The word magnification implies a comparison and demands the question, Compared with what? Because there are several alternative answers to this question, there are several alternative definitions of magnification, and it is not always clear which definition is most appropriate (as the example illustrates).

Much of the potential confusion surrounding the use of the term magnification can be avoided by using the concept of Equivalent Viewing Distance (EVD) to quantify the magnifying effect that optical systems provide. The EVD is the distance at which the object subtends the same angle as that being subtended by the image seen with the magnifying device. For example, a $4 \times$ photographic enlargement of a sample of print that is viewed from a distance of 40 cm presents the observer with an image whose angular size is equivalent to that obtained if one were to view the original print sample from a distance of 10 cm, that is, the EVD is 10 cm. Similarly, a video-magnifier giving an image that is enlarged by 10 while being viewed from a distance of 50 cm provides an EVD of 5 cm.

Many optical magnifiers can be used to create an image at optical infinity, in which case the EVD is equal to the equivalent focal length of the magnifier. A $+20$-D lens being used to give an image at infinity will provide an EVD of 5 cm. Frequently, optical magnifiers give an enlarged image that is located at a finite distance. The EVD is then the eye-to-image distance divided by the enlargement ratio (or transverse magnification). For example, consider a fixed-focus stand magnifier that gives an image that is enlarged by a factor of 3 and is located 20 cm behind the lens of the magnifier. A patient using this magnifier so the separation between the eye and magnifier is 10 cm will achieve an EVD of $(10 + 20)/3 = 30/3 = 10$ cm. For a given patient, systems that provide the same EVD will yield the same resolution.

A presbyopic patient would be expected to obtain the same resolution with each of the following optical systems:

1. A $+12.5$ D spectacle addition; print at 8 cm.
2. A $+12.5$ D hand-held magnifier regardless of how far it is held from the eye while the patient uses distance vision glasses.
3. A $2.5 \times$ telescope with a $+5$-D cap to provide a 20-cm working distance.
4. A stand magnifier with a $+20$-D lens whose image is 20 cm (5 D) below the lens and the patient uses a $+2.50$-D addition. The separation between the object and the magnifier must be 4 cm (25 D), and the enlargement ratio will be $5 \times$. The expected eye-to-image distance is 40 cm; eye-lens separation is 20 cm.
5. A closed-circuit television magnifier giving an enlargement of $10 \times$ when the viewing distance is 80 cm ($+1.25$-D addition).

All five systems provide an EVD of 8 cm (or Equivalent Viewing Power of $+12.5$ D). All will afford a resolution equal to that which would be expected if the patient were to hold the object of interest 8 cm from the eye while maintaining a clear image by accommodation or using an addition. In any evaluation of near vision performance, the patient should wear the appropriate addition and hold the test material so that it is in sharpest focus.

Determining the Power Required

Although it is possible to use distance visual acuity in estimating how much dioptric power is required to enable a patient to read print of a certain size, this is not the surest approach. Letter charts used for distance vision and reading cards used for near vision present tasks of quite different complexity; there is no strong concordance between letter chart acuity and reading chart acuity, especially when there are macular disturbances. Presbyopic patients almost invariably have a reading correction, and the most convenient and appropriate way to begin the power determination is to measure the patients' reading acuity while they use their existing reading correction. For example, a patient might have eyeglasses that incorporate a +3.00 D addition. Holding the test card at 33 cm, this patient might be able to read 2.5-M print (which could, on some charts, be labeled *20 points* or *20/125.*).

The EVD required to reach a resolution goal then can be determined by simple ratios or proportions. For example, it might be decided that the patient should be able to read material of newsprint size (1-M, 8 points, or 20/50 in size). Whatever units are used, it can easily be seen that a 2.5 × improvement in resolution is required. This improvement in resolution can be achieved by changing the viewing distance from 33 cm by a factor of 2.5 ×, so that an EVD of 13 cm is indicated. For this presbyopic patient, the power of the addition needs to be increased from 3.00 to 7.50 D. The clinician should then verify that the patient does, in fact, achieve satisfactory reading of the 1-M print (8 points or 20/50) that had been set as the goal. This usually is done in spectacle format with a trial frame or trial lens clip.

When working over existing bifocals, the lens clip might not allow full access to the bifocal portion of the lens. In such a case, the lens clip can be raised so that only the distance portion of the lens is being used, and the full required addition can be introduced into the lens clip. Special care must be taken to insure that an appropriate working distance is being used, as some older patients strongly resist working at close distances.

Selecting the Magnifying Aid

Once the dioptric power that will give the desired reading resolution performance has been determined, the optometrist must decide which of the various aids should be used to provide the required EVD.

Spectacle lens corrections afford the widest fields of view, leave both hands free to support or manipulate task materials, are convenient to carry, and are relatively inconspicuous. Their disadvantage is the close working distance they may impose. If a spectacle prescription is to be issued, the lens form must be considered. Will it be single vision lenses, bifocals in a usual configuration, bifocals with high placement of the segments, special series lenses, or aspheric lenses? Binocularity issues should be addressed. If binocular vision is to be achieved (it is usually achievable if addition powers are +10.00 D or less), the prism or decentration must be considered. Fonda (1981) recommends as a rule of thumb that 2 mm of total decentration be given for each diopter of addition power. Thus, there should be 8 mm of total decentration for a 4.00-D addition, 16 mm for an 8.00-D addition, and so on. This method provides a small net amount of base-in prism.

Many patients with low vision must perform near-vision tasks monocularly, either because there is substantial inequality between the two eyes or because the required lens powers are too high. Even though the other eye might not be used during the main reading tasks, some attention should be given to whether it should be totally occluded or blocked with a frosted lens, or whether some lens should be worn in front of that eye. Perhaps a simple balance lens will be indicated, but often monovision possibilities should be considered. It may be useful to have a single vision lens before the poorer eye to give in-focus distance viewing or to provide an intermediate or near vision focus. A bifocal or trifocal lens before the poorer eye might best satisfy the patient's overall visual needs and convenience.

Hand-held magnifiers have as their main advantage the adjustability of working distance. In one extreme, the patient can hold the magnifying glass in the spectacle plane, in which case the reading material will need to be in the appropriate focal plane. At the other end of the scale, the magnifier may be held at a full arm's length; again, the test card will need to be in the proper focal plane. The further the lens is held from the eye, the smaller is the field of view. Provided patients are using their distance glasses, the resolution can be determined directly from the equivalent power of the hand-held magnifying lens. The EVD will be the focal length of the magnifier. Bifocal wearers should not view through their bifocal segments unless the magnifier is being held close (that is, closer than one of its focal lengths) to the spectacle lens. Holding the magnifier against the reading addition in spectacles effectively provides the sum of the two powers. The combination then will act as a strong spectacle lens.

Hand-held magnifiers provide portability and flexibility. They are ideally suited for looking at price tags, reading maps, and checking labels on containers in a store.

Stand magnifiers, which are most commonly used for reading tasks, are particularly helpful to elderly patients, since hand steadiness is not very important. If strong dioptric powers are required, and even if there are no hand steadiness problems, stand magnifiers provide a level of easy and reliable control not attainable with spectacles or hand-held magnifiers. For reading tasks of limited duration (for example, reading telephone books and television schedules, checking bills, and reading greeting cards), stand magnifiers can be of most value. Some even incorporate a light to illuminate the task. Stand magnifiers may be somewhat bulky and therefore less convenient to carry, and the working situation becomes much more rigidly defined.

The optometrist must understand a few basic optical principles in order to prescribe stand magnifiers intelligently. First, fixed-focus stand magnifiers produce images that are relatively close to the lens of the magnifier. Rarely is the image farther than 50 cm behind the magnifying lens, and most image locations are in the range of 3 cm to 40 cm behind the lens surface. Consequently, presbyopic patients must wear a reading correction to obtain a clear view of the image.

The image location and the power of the spectacle addition determine the separation required between the magnifier and the spectacles. If the image of the magnifier is 10 cm below its surface, and the patient is focused for 40 cm because of a +2.50-D reading addition, the required separation is 30 cm. Had the spectacle addition been 5.00 D, the required separation would have been 10 cm. The clinician should know the image location for the stand magnifier being used.

The second basic optical principle to be understood is that the image produced by the stand magnifier is larger than the original object. The net effect of the magnifier is to produce an image that is both larger and more remote than the original object. The power of the magnifier lens and the object-lens separation determine the size of the image. The enlargement ratio (which may be called the *transverse magnification*) is constant and should be known to the clinician, since it influences the final resolution.

Third, when the patient views the enlarged image formed by the magnifier, the resulting EVD can be determined by dividing the eye-to-image distance by the enlargement ratio. Alternatively, the equivalent viewing power may be determined by multiplying the accommodation demand by the enlargement ratio. If a stand magnifier forms an image that is 20 cm below the lens and the enlargement ratio is 3×, then a patient whose eye is 10 cm above the lens will have eye-to-image distance of 30 cm, so the EVD = 10 cm. The accommodation demand is 3.33 D, so that the EVP = 10 D. The EVD can be used in predicting the resolution that the patient will be able to achieve with the system.

The following demonstrates some of the important considerations that should be made when using stand magnifiers. Two widely used stand magnifiers made by Combined Optical Industries Ltd. are considered here:

Magnifier	COIL 5428	COIL 5123
Labelled Power	+20.00 D	+28.00 D
Equivalent Power	+17.50 D	+24.00 D
Image Position	15 cm	25 cm
Enlargement Ratio	3.6 ×	7.0 ×

Consider a patient who can just read 3-M print at 40 cm with a 2.50-D addition. With these glasses in place, this patient should position the spectacles 25 cm from the COIL 5428 so that this separation and the image distance total 40 cm. Similarly, the required separation from the COIL 5123 is 15 cm.

Here, the EVD achieved when using COIL 5428 is 40/3.6 = 11.1 cm (or, EVP = 2.5 × 3.6 = 9.00 D). The patient's resolution will improve by a factor of 3.6, so the smallest print legible should become 3/3.6 = 0.83 M. For the COIL 5123, the EVD = 40/7 = 5.7 cm (or, EVP = 2.5/7 = 17.50 D). With this magnifier, the resolution would be improved by a factor of 7.0, so that the predicted resolution limit would be 0.43 M.

If the addition were changed to 3.00 D, then required separations would change to 18 cm for the COIL 5428 and 8 cm for the COIL 5123. The EVD values achieved would be 9.2 and 4.8 cm (EVP = 10.9 and 21 D). The resolution limits would then become 0.69 M (from 3 M × [9.2/40]) and 0.36 M (from 3 M × [4.8/40]).

Unfortunately, manufacturers specify neither image location nor the enlargement ratio; even their nominal lens powers or magnification ratings often defy logic or understanding. However, there are simple in-office methods for measuring these key optical parameters (Bailey 1981a, 1981b, 1981c).

Head-mounted loupes are positive-powered lenses that are mounted so they sit in front of the spectacle plane. They are mainly used for viewing manipulative tasks. A wide variety of such devices is available. Some are single lenses that attach to the spectacle frame or spectacle lens, and the lens generally is mounted on a pivoting bracket that allows the lens to be conveniently removed or inserted into the line of vision. These provide monocular viewing, and lens powers usually range from 10.00 D up to about 30.00 D. Binocular loupes, which are available in powers up to about 10.00 D or 12.00 D, usually incorporate some prism or decentration to facilitate convergence. Some binocular loupe systems attach to spectacles, but most are mounted on a headband that positions the lens bracket 2 cm or so in front of the spectacle plane. Many can be flipped up and down as needed. Another potential advantage of head-mounted loupes is that the mounting of the lenses an inch away from the spectacles means the task may be moved 1 inch farther away from the face. For some manipulative tasks, this change in viewing distance will be useful.

Near vision telescopes (sometimes called *telemicroscopes*) are not so commonly prescribed for older patients, but their distinct advantages sometimes make them essential. Near-vision telescopes are called for when a certain level of dioptric power is required to achieve a given resolution goal, but the patient is compelled to have a long working distance and unrestricted or bimanual access to the task. Performing surgery and viewing computer terminals are two tasks for which near-vision telescopes are often prescribed, but they can be valuable for many other tasks. The advantage of near-vision telescopes is the increased working distance, but this must be balanced against the principal disadvantage, the reduced field of view. The depth of focus is also quite small, so the working distance must be accurately maintained.

Near-vision telescopes can be created most simply by adding a lens cap to the objective lens of a distance telescope. The EVD achieved by the system can be computed easily; it is simply the focal length of the lens cap divided by the telescope magnification. For example, a system made from placing a 4.00 D lens cap on the front of a 2.5 × telescope will create a focus for 25 cm. The EVD = 25/ 2.5 = 10 cm (EVP = 4.00 × 2.5). This will provide the same resolution as any other system that achieves an EVD of 10 cm. In this example, the working distance will be 25 cm, as this is set by the focal lens of the lens cap. Other near-vision telescope systems to achieve an EVD = 10 cm could be created by combining a 2.00-D lens cap and a 5 × telescope (working distance = 50 cm), a 3.00-D cap and a 3.3 × telescope (working distance = 33 cm), a 5.00-D cap and a 2.0 × telescope (working distance = 20 cm), or many other combinations. The critical optical parameters in the prescribing of near-vision telescopes are the working distance and the resolution the patient will achieve.

Videomagnifiers and projection magnifiers produce enlarged images on a screen. Closed-circuit television systems use electronics to achieve the enlargement, whereas projector systems enlarge with optics. Videomagnifiers offer some special additional advantages over optical systems. A wide range of magnification is usually available, and masks and border enhancement can be created electronically to improve visual performance. Because such high transverse magnification or enlargement ratios can be achieved, it is usually possible for patients to read the videomagnifier display from a comfortable viewing position.

The EVD achieved with a videomagnifier can be calculated by dividing the actual viewing distance by the enlargement ratio. For older patients, the viewing distance commonly corresponds to the power of their general purpose bifocals. A patient with a 2.50-D addition, for example, viewing an image that is 3 times larger than the original from 40 cm, will have a system with an EVD of 40/3 = 13.3 cm (EVD = 2.5 × 3 = 7.50 D). If it had previously been determined by testing with spectacle lenses that an EVD of 10 cm was required to achieve a particular resolution goal, and the patient was expected to view the screen from 40 cm, then the videomagnifier should be arranged to provide a 4 × enlargement.

Rarely do optical magnifiers used in low vision achieve EVD values greater than 2 cm (EVP = 50 D), but many videomagnifier systems can easily provide EVD values of 1.0 cm or less (for example, a 30-cm observation distance and a 30 × enlargement) without imposing extreme constraints that reduce comfort or potential efficiency. Because videomagnifiers can provide such high magnification while allowing comfortable viewing postures, reading comfort and endurance are the main benefits provided by these systems. Low-vision patients with a moderate to substantial loss of vision who need to read for long periods or need very high magnification should be considered possible candidates for videomagnifier systems.

For all near-vision magnification systems, care should be taken to adjust the illumination to suit the patients' needs. Most older, low-vision patients require more illumination than usual, but they are more susceptible to glare. Consequently, more than the usual attention should be paid to positioning the luminaire and the task material so that potentially troublesome glare is avoided.

A device that has proved useful for glare control is the typoscope, or reading mask. This is a black card with a rectangular aperture that is usually made large enough to accommodate three lines of one-column-width print. The typoscope can enhance reading acuity and comfort by reducing glare from white paper close to the immediate fixation point. This device also serves as a line guide and helps patients with field defects to maintain their place when reading.

Yellow filters also are found to be beneficial by some patients, who report that they make vision apparently clearer and more comfortable. Illumination control by varying the quantity and quality of the task and ambient lighting, as well as by the use of the typoscope and yellow filters, should all be included routinely in the assessment of the patient's near vision magnification.

Nonmagnifying Aids to Vision

Contact lenses can offer special advantages to some low-vision patients. They can substantially reduce the effect of corneal irregularities that are due to corneal or anterior eye scarring or other causes. When the corneal distortion is more pronounced, soft contact lenses are not as effective, since some of the corneal distortion may be translated to the front surface of the lens. Hard lenses can be more effective in nullifying the optical effect of distortion, but they are more likely to cause potentially troublesome pressure spots on the distorted cornea. The other major optical benefit of contact lenses is that they substantially reduce aberration and prismatic effects that can produce vision difficulties with the use of stronger spectacle lenses. Because the contact lenses move with the eye, the visual axis of the eye is always close to the optic axis of the correcting lens; this means that peripheral aberration problems are eliminated or at least greatly reduced. Differential prismatic effects that occur with spectacle corrections for anisometropia are much better controlled with contact lenses. Aphakic patients often experience perceptual and depth judgment difficulties when they are introduced to spectacle corrections, and they may be bothered by the field restriction and the jack-in-the-box effect created by the high plus spectacle lens. These effects are avoided or minimized by using contact lenses.

Filters also can be beneficial to many elderly patients. For reasons that are not fully understood, many patients with retinal disorders and some with cataracts report seeing better when yellow filters or some other "minus blue" filter is worn (see Chapter 6). Older patients, especially those with visual disorders, tend to be more sensitive to very bright light; thus, sunglass filters (sometimes very dense ones) are often required. The approach to prescribing tints is largely empirical. Decisions are based on reported symptoms and the patient's expressed perception of the effect of the filters.

Visual-field defects accompanying pathologic changes can produce functional difficulties for patients, especially in mobility tasks. Three kinds of optical devices can help patients with particular kinds of visual field defects: reversed telescopes, hemianopic mirrors, and partial prisms.

Reversed telescopes can be useful for patients who have developed a concentric loss of visual field such as occurs in advanced retinitis pigmentosa or glaucoma. Reversed telescopes obviously reduce visual acuity, but they can provide an enlarged visual field. Most patients who use reversed telescopes only do so for navigational purposes, and then only when the local environment contains repetitive or potentially confusing details. An example of such a situation is an intersection at which many roads or paths meet. Most reversed telescopes are hand held and are of a moderate range of magnification (2 to 6×).

Hemianopic mirrors can help some patients with homonymous hemianopia. A mirror is mounted on the nasal eyewire of the spectacles in front of the eye that is on the same side as the field loss. The mirror is angled so that it is about 10 degrees with respect to the primary line of sight; it is about 20 mm to 40 mm in width. For a patient with a right homonymous hemianopia, therefore, the mirror would be mounted on the nasal portion of the right eyewire and angled slightly toward the right eye. By reflection, this mirror will present part of the right-hand field of view to the right eye. This segment from the blind field seen through the mirror will appear to the right eye to be reversed and unstable, and it will be projected so that it seems to be superimposed on the left-hand field. The purpose of the mirror is to provide some awareness of events and hazards on the blind side. The patient must learn not to give close attention to detail seen in the mirror. When the patient becomes aware of an object or event deserving attention, the head should be turned so that the full inspection and any decision making is made with the benefit of direct vision. Only a small minority of hemianopic patients have mirrors prescribed, but optometrists nevertheless should consider them as a possibility for each hemianopic patient.

Partial prisms are the third kind of optical device prescribed to help patients with field problems. Their main use is in hemianopias, but they can also be useful when there has been a concentric loss of visual field. Partial prisms are usually in the form of Fresnel membrane prisms of high deviation (20 to 30Δ) that are placed on the lens so that they are totally within the blind field when the patient looks straight ahead. The base direction of the prism is always away from the primary line of sight. When the patient makes an eye movement toward a blind part of the field, the prism will be encountered after a certain degree of deviation.

The prism optically shifts things in from the periphery. This means that smaller eye movements will be required to view more peripheral objects on the blind side. Expressed another way, an eye movement of a given magnitude allows the patient to see further to the periphery when viewing through the prism. The prism creates a blind spot, and the patient may be distracted by apparent jumping or disappearance of objects when eye movements traverse the edge of the prism. The prisms are placed so they will remain unnoticed within the patient's blind field most of the time when relatively normal, small-magnitude eye movements are being made. When the patient wants to inspect more peripheral regions, large eye movements are called for; these are supplemented by the effect of the prism.

A fairly typical configuration of the partial prisms for a right hemianope would be a 30Δ base-out prism mounted on the right lens so that it covers the full vertical height of the lens beginning at a point about 6 mm to the right of the primary viewing point. On the left lens there would be a much smaller area of prism (30Δ base in), and again the vertical edge of the prism would be about 6 mm from the primary viewing point. Because Fresnel membrane prisms can be removed and replaced easily, it is not difficult or expensive to experiment with this kind of correction.

Training in the Use of Optical Aids

Adaptation, practice, and training are often necessary if patients are to receive maximum benefit from their low-vision aids. Many aids demand that new skills be learned. Older patients are generally less able to adapt, and they require more training. For example, structured, guided practice in techniques for sighting and focusing with telescopes can be vital to success. Furthermore, it is often useful to give initial training with telescopes that have lower magnification and larger exit pupils, since these are easier to use.

A variety of skills may need to be developed for reading; these include positioning the head, the eyes, the aid, and the material to achieve clear focus and then making the required relative movements to enable the most fluent reading. Sometimes only brief instruction is needed, whereas other situations may require extensive training and supervision.

Many low-vision patients have central scotomas, and their visual performance and efficiency may improve if they can learn eccentric viewing strategies. Similarly, many patients may need training in more efficient scanning and search techniques.

It is a good policy to insure that a patient is able to use any optical aid with reasonable proficiency before it is issued. Training the patient in the most efficient use of an aid or the eyes can be the key to success for many patients.

ADVICE AND RECOMMENDATIONS

When all the clinical data have been collected, the optometrist should pause and take stock. Has all the relevant information been uncovered? Again, the following question would be asked: What does the patient really want? What do I want the patient to have? Really, why did the patient come to see me?

The clinician should decide on the treatment options and then consciously consider the strategy for presenting recommendations and advice. For example, should others be present when the advice is given, and to what extent should they be involved? What issues need to be given strongest emphasis, and what should be sidestepped or downplayed? How strongly should the treatment recommendations be advocated? What does the patient really need to know? What will the patient like to hear, and what will not be accepted easily?

The advice and recommendations the optometrist submits to elderly patients need not be confined to optical and visual matters. As a health-care practitioner, the optometrist has a responsibility to the patient's general health, and any need for rehabilitative attention that may contribute to the patient's overall well-being should be discussed. The optometrist can be a critical link in the health-care chain, taking the initiative in directing patients toward appropriate and broadly based care for their health and well-being.

Optometrists should remain well informed about the availability of health care and other support and social services available in the local community. In particular, the optometrist should maintain contacts with the medical community and rehabilitation counselors or social workers, as well as be familiar with the activities and services of organizations serving the visually handicapped or senior citizens.

REFERENCES

1. Bailey, I. L. "Locating the Image in Stand Magnifiers." *Optometric Monthly* 71, no. 6 (1981a): 22–24.
2. Bailey, I. L. "The Use of Fixed-Focus Stand Magnifiers." *Optometric Monthly* 71, no. 8 (1981b): 37–39.
3. Bailey, I. L. "Verifying Near Vision Magnifiers." *Optometric Monthly* 72 (1981c): 34–38.
4. Bailey, I. L. "Mobility and Visual Performance Under Dim Illumination." In: *Night Vision-Current Research and Future Directions.* Symposium Proceedings, Committee on Vision of the National Research Council and the National Academy of Science, Washington D.C.: National Academy Press, 1987, pp. 220–230.
5. Bailey, I. L. and M. A. Bullimore. "A New Test of Disability Glare." *Optom. Vis. Sci.* 68 (1991): 911–917.
6. Bailey, I. L., and J. E. Lovie. "New Design Principles for Visual Acuity Letter Charts." *Am. J. Optom. Physiol. Opt.* 53 (1976): 740–745.
7. Bailey, I. L., and J. E. Lovie. "The Design and Use of a New Near-Vision Chart." *Am. J. Opto. Physiol. Opt.* 57 (1980): 378–387.
8. Ferris, L., A. Kassoff, G. H. Bresnick, and I. L. Bailey. "New Visual Acuity Charts for Research Purposes." *Am. J. Ophthalmol.* 94 (1982): 91–96.
9. Fonda, G. E. *Management of Low Vision.* New York: Thieme-Stratton, 1981.
10. Ginsburg, A. P. "A New Contrast Sensitivity Vision Test Chart." *Am. J. Optom. Physiol. Opt.* 6 (1984): 403–407.
11. Keeler, C. H. "On Visual Aids for the Partially Sighted." *Trans. Ophthalmol. Soc. UK* 76 (1956): 605–614.
12. Mehr, E. B., and A. N. Freid. *Low Vision Care.* Chicago: Professional Press, 1975.
13. Pelli, D. G., J. G. Robson, and A. J. Wilkins. "The Design of a New Letter Chart for Measuring Contrast Sensitivity." *Clin. Vis. Sci.* 2 ((1988): 187–199.
14. Regan, D. "Low-Contrast Charts and Sine Wave Grating Tests in Ophthalmological and Neurological Disorders." *Clin. Vis. Sci.* 2 (1988): 235–250.
15. Regan, D. "Specific Tests, Specific Blindnesses: Keys, Locks and Parallel Processing, The 1990 Prentice Award Lecture." *Optom. Vis. Sci.* 68 (1991): 489–512.
16. Sloan, L. L. "New Test Charts for the Measurement of Visual Acuity at Far and Near Distances." *Am. J. Ophthalmol.* 48 (1959): 807–813.
17. Van den Berg, T. J. T. P. "Importance of Intra-ocular Light Scatter for Visual Disability." *Doc. Ophthalmologica.* 61 (1986): 327–333.
18. Verbaken, J., and A. W. Johnston. "Population Norms for Edge Contrast Sensitivity." *Am. J. Optom. Physiol. Opt.* 63 (1986): 724–732.

SUGGESTED READINGS

1. Anderson, D. R. *Testing the Field of Vision.* St. Louis: CV Mosby, 1982.
2. Bailey, I. L. "The Aged Blind." *Austr. J. Optom.* 58 (1975): 31–39.

3. Bailey, I. L. "Telescopes: Their Use in Low Vision." *Optometric Monthly* 69 (1978): 634–638.
4. Bedwell, C. H. *Visual Fields*. London: Butterworth, 1982.
5. Borish, I. W., S. A. Hitzeman, and K. E. Brookman. "Double Masked Study of Progressive Addition Lenses." *J. Am. Optom. Assoc.* 51 (1980): 933–943.
6. Faye, E. E. *The Low Vision Patient*. New York: Grune and Stratton, 1970.
7. Faye, E. E. *Clinical Low Vision*, 2nd ed. Boston: Little, Brown, 1984.
8. Hirsch, M. J., and R. E. Wick. *Vision of the Aging Patient*. Philadelphia: Chilton, 1960.
9. Jose, R. T. *Understanding Low Vision*. New York: American Foundation for the Blind, 1983.
10. Kitchin, J. E., and I. L. Bailey. "Task Complexity and Visual Acuity in Senile Macular Degeneration." *Aust. J. Optom.* 63 (1981): 235–242.
11. Lederer, J. "The Effects of Age on Visual Functioning." *Aust. J. Sci.* 32 (1969): 79–86.
12. Lovie-Kitchin, J. E., E. J. Farmer, and K. J. Bowman. *Senile Macular Degeneration*. Brisbane, Australia: Queensland Institute of Technology, 1982.
13. Morgan, M. W. *The Optics of Ophthalmic Lenses*. Chicago: Professional Press, 1978.
14. Rosenbloom, A. A. "Low Vision." In: G. Peyman, D. Sanders, and M. F. Goldberg (eds.) *Principles and Practice of Ophthalmology*. Philadelphia: W. B. Saunders, 1980, pp. 241–277.
15. Rosenbloom, A. A. "Care of Elderly People with Low Vision." *Visual Impairment and Blindness*. June 1982, pp. 209–212.
16. Sekuler, R., D. Kline, and K. Dismukes. *Aging and Human Visual Function*. New York: Allan R. Liss, 1982.
17. Sloan, L. L. *Reading Aids for the Partially Sighted*. Baltimore: Williams and Wilkins, 1977.
18. Weale, R. A. *The Aging Eye*. London: Lewis, 1963.
19. Weale, R. A. *A Biography of the Eye: Development, Growth, Age*. London: Lewis, 1982.

8

Designing Spectacles for the Elderly Patient

Meredith W. Morgan
Albert L. Pierce

PRESCRIBING LENSES FOR THE ELDERLY PATIENT

The most frequent change in the lens prescription of the average, healthy, elderly patient is the addition of between +0.50 DS and +1.00 DS either to the previous major lens correction, the segment, or divided between the two. Also, there usually is a slight increase in against-the-rule astigmatism. (See Chapter 6.) If the change is an increase in myopia, it has been the writer's experience that this is associated most frequently with either the development of cataracts or with uncontrolled blood glucose. Consequently, if there is a myopic change, special attention should be paid to these possibilities before prescribing. Also, if the change is more than plus or minus 0.75 DS, the patient probably will notice a change in near working distances required by the new prescription. This change should be explained carefully to the patient before the new prescription is ordered and before the patient discovers this for himself or herself. Undoubtedly the new prescription will enhance resolution at critical working distances, but because the patient has no accommodation, it also will decrease resolution at some other distances.

Older patients usually can be considered "expert" bifocal or trifocal spectacle wearers in that most of them have been successfully wearing multifocal lenses for many years. Consequently, they have a well-established concept about what to expect from a new pair of glasses both in terms of comfort and performance. If, for any reason, the new pair is not going to perform up to their expectations, the optometrist should carefully explain to them, in terms that they can understand, just why this will occur. A few patients may have never made the adjustment to constant use of multifocal lenses and may resort to part time use, when necessary, of near work lenses that may be single vision or multifocal. The reasons for this rejection of constant wear spectacles should be determined before a new correction is prescribed.

In general, the rules for prescribing spectacles for elderly patients are exactly the same as the rules for prescribing for younger, presbyopic patients. There are, however, some special considerations, both physical and optical, that may be complicating factors.

The physical problems that can arise from a new prescription involve appearance (style), comfort, and stability. These may be aggravated by loose, fragile skin in the areas supporting the weight of the spectacles. Generally, these problems can be minimized by keeping the weight of the glasses to a minimum and by increasing the bearing area of the frame. This may be difficult because of style, a matter of personal taste influenced by current trends and advertising, matters over which the optometrist has little control.

The optical considerations involve both the resolution ability of the patient's visual system as well as characteristics of the spectacles themselves. These two primary considerations are not independent but are frequently dependent. To some extent, it is true that the better the patient's visual system the easier it is for the patient to detect optical shortcomings in the correction. While this may be true, a more important consideration arises when the patient's visual system is operating near the border between what is frankly low vision and that which can be considered normal vision. The optical correction itself under these circumstances must be the very best that it can be in order to maintain the patient's visual performance as near "normal" as possible. In all situations, the performance of the lenses because of careless refraction, aberrations, inaccurate interpupillary distances, incorrect pantoscopic and faceform tilt, should not detract from optimum possible performance. At all times, the optometrist should be "prescribing for visibility" (Davis, 1990).

Special Lens Considerations

The choice of lens material to be used will be governed by a number of factors relating to the lens power and the type of frame selected. For example, in rimless frames, holes must be drilled for mounting, and fabricating regulations require plastic lenses. Polycarbonate is the first choice. It has a higher index of refraction (1.586) than CR-39 (1.4885), which results in a slightly thinner lens. Polycarbonate also is far superior to regular CR-39 in safety. The lens is virtually unbreakable, even when ground to a knife-edge thinness. Polycarbonate absorbs almost 100% of the ultraviolet (UV) radiation after coating (it screens 97% of the UV radiation up to 400 nm). Finally, mounting polycarbonate lenses to the frame allows the holes to be threaded; thus, the lenses are held tightly to the frame without the usual loosening effect.

While the use of high index plastics is highly desirable for the above-stated reasons, they do have one serious drawback, and that is they have lower nu values and hence greater dispersion. This can result in a lateral chromatic aberration that at best reduces image contrast, resulting in a reduction of acuity or, at worse, in visible color fringes along high-contrast edges of the visual scene. The blurring of lateral chromatic dispersion is a function of the magnitude of the aberration which, in turn, is a function of the prismatic power and the nu value of the lens material. This can become a significant problem in corrections greater than ± 4.00 DS (Morgan, 1978; Hampton et al., 1991).

Since the prismatic power of a lens increases as the distance from center of the lens increases, this lateral chromatic dispersion is greater through the edge of lenses than it is in the central portion. Unfortunately, individuals who wear multifocal lenses are forced to use portions of the major lens away from its center when looking through the segments. This means that the quality of the image through a round top segment may be better in convex lenses than it is through flat top segments. (The base-down prism created by the add neutralizes the base-up effect of the major lens.) The reverse of course is true for concave lenses. Maximum resolution is obtained where the prismatic displacement is zero through the portion of the lens being used.

All lenses prescribed for elderly patients should offer UV protection, cutting off radiation below approximately 400 nm. This is especially true of pseudophakes who have lost the retinal protection offered by the yellow-tinted crystalline lens. If the patient complains of glare, or if it is noticed during the examination that there is considerable back scatter from the patient's eye when using the ophthalmoscope or retinoscope, tints that absorb into the blue region of the spectrum should be tried. Forward scatter is usually the cause of disability glare, but its magnitude cannot be determined by the magnitude of the back scatter noticed by the examiner. Sometimes the particles creating the scatter are of such size that short wavelength light is scattered more than is light of long wavelength. In this case, a tint that absorbs blue will reduce scatter and hence reduce veiling glare. Such tints may help protect the crystalline lens and the retina from photic damage. There have been several attempts to quantify disability glare such as the BAT test of Holladay and the disability glare test of Bailey and Bullimore (Zigman, 1986; Holladay et al., 1987; Pitts, 1990; Bailey and Bullimore, 1991).

GENERAL LENS DESIGN CONSIDERATIONS FOR THE OLDER PATIENT

For the average older patient, the primary consideration in choosing a lens design and type is how well the patient was performing with the previous correction. Except for the dramatic change in vision that occurs with the onset of aphakia or the change in visual requirements that may occur at retirement, changes in both vision and visual requirements are usually very gradual in the healthy, aging patient. Even at retirement, the change may not be great, since among the active elderly, avocations already may be more important and demanding than vocations at the time of retirement.

Before changing the lens type or design from that previously worn, the optometrist must answer the following question: Are there any compelling reasons to change the type and design of the lenses that the patient is now wearing? As has already been mentioned, most elderly patients are experienced spectacle wearers, and unless there has been some significant change in the lens prescription or in the patient's visual requirements, the same type and design of lenses should be prescribed, providing performance was adequate. The optometrist must carefully question and listen to the expert, the elderly patient. Some of the factors that need to be considered, in addition to the change in correction, are performance distances, desired visual field sizes, freedom of head and eye movements, acuity of vision required and desired, visual performance through the edges of the old lenses, weight of the new correction, and appearance. The primary considerations are the adequacy of the old lens design and type and the changes desired or needed.

Performance Distances

Patients must be questioned about working distances used and the need for visual performance at these distances. If a patient must perform well at various distances, multifocal lenses or progressive addition lenses should be considered (Borish, et al., 1980; Schultz, 1983). One of the few advantages that results from the miosis of aging is that the depth of field increases, which in a sense replaces lost accommodation.

Desired Visual Field Sizes

Patients also must be questioned about the usefulness of the size of field, particularly through the segments of their old lenses. If the field is too small, it may be made larger by increasing the segment size, reducing the vertex distance of the lenses, or increasing the working distance (reducing the power of the addition). Whether any of these solutions is possible must be determined for each patient. Fortunately, another advantage of aging miosis is an increase in the size of the field of view for segments of the same size and power.

The size of the field of view decreases, however, as the total power through the segment becomes more convex. For this reason, when the power of the distance correction is greater than $+5.00$ D, great caution must be exercised in prescribing trifocals. The intermediate field may be too small to be useful, and, in addition, it displaces the near segment lower in the lens, where optical performance is poorer. Certainly trifocals are virtually useless in aphakic corrections of $+10.00$ D or more.

Freedom of Head and Eye Movements

To view objects through specific regions of a lens, the head, the eyes, and the object of regard must be in a specific location in relation to one another. If the patient does not have good vertical movement of the head and eyes for any reason, placement of the segment becomes even more critical than it usually is. Lack of free head and eye movement may limit the effectiveness of trifocals, because the intermediate segment occupies space and forces the near segment to be placed lower in the lens. This also may limit the usefulness of progressive addition lenses, because the distance between the area of clear distance vision and clear near vision is fixed; the region of clear near vision may be too low in the lens for it to be usable by the patient for extended periods, as when reading. The limitation of head movement may be caused by a short neck or a lack of facility in adjusting the head, eyes, and object into the proper relationship. The optometrist should observe each patient in action to determine the extent and ease of head movement possible.

Acuity of Vision Required and Desired

The optometrist must determine the acuity required and desired by the patient for visual tasks. Sometimes these are not the same, since some individuals always want to see the "gnats eye," whereas others are happy if they can just recognize what they are looking at. Still others, because of their vocation or avocation, must be able to resolve critical detail and may be willing to adapt to a short viewing distance to achieve the necessary resolution (low-vision patients do this all the time).

Several aberrations, such as marginal astigmatism and chromatic dispersion, tend to destroy the ability of a lens to create sharp images. Both these aberrations increase as the visual angle increases toward the edge of the lens — particularly as the power of the lens increases, as the index of refraction increases, or as the v value of the lens material decreases. Thus, if it is important to achieve really excellent resolution at near through a segment, the segment must be placed high in the lens, the proper base curve for minimum astigmatism should be chosen, and high-index lens materials should be avoided. Remember that as optical imagery by the lens is improved, the range of acceptable vision is increased.

Visual Performance Through the Edges of the Old Lenses

If the correction exceeds ± 4.00 or ± 5.00 D, the optometrist should determine if the patient has noticed distortion or blurring through the edges of the old lenses. The patient can be instructed to look at the edge of a doorway monocularly while turning his or her head from left to right and back again. The patient then is asked to note whether the edge remains straight or becomes curved as the line of sight passes into the periphery of the lens. Likewise, the patient may be questioned about sharpness of vision. Some care should be exercised in subjective perception testing to avoid suggesting to older patients that they should see the doorway curved, the floor tilted, and so forth. In other words, the questions asked should not suggest the answers. Usually, the well-adapted spectacle wearer will not notice distortion but may notice a decrease in clarity. Some patients, however, do not adapt to distortion subjectively and avoid it by not using the edges of their lenses. If this is the case, the optometrist should consider the use of lenses of deeper base curve (Katz, 1983; Morgan, 1978).

Distortion may become especially annoying when high-index glass is used. To limit the marginal astigmatism and distortion to that present in crown glass lenses of the same power, high-index lenses must be made on steeper base curves; however, this tends to defeat the purpose for which the high-index glass was used in the first place. Jones (1980) has calculated that a +6.00 D lens of crown glass with a back surface power of −4.00 D has the same marginal astigmatism for a 30-degree eye rotation as a +6.00 D lens with a −6.50 D base curve made of glass of 1.700 index.

Weight of the Lenses

If patients complain that their old spectacles weigh too much and the optometrist wishes to avoid using the procedures to be described, lenses made of CR-39 or polycarbonate should be considered. These should be geometrically centered in a frame of the smallest acceptable eye size, and the lenses made as thin as possible. For lenses between +5.00 D and −5.00 D, high-index glass will not produce a lighter-weight lens, even though the lens is thinner. In powers outside this range, however, high-index lenses will be both thinner and lighter.

Weight is primarily a function of lens thickness and eye size (equivalent diameter). Jones (1980) has calculated that for a −6.00 D lens with an equivalent diameter of 50 mm, a 10% increase in weight would result from any one of the following: (1) 10% increase in specific gravity (density), (2) a 1.00 D increase in power, (3) as little as 0.25-mm increase in thickness, or (4) somewhat less than 1-mm increase in equivalent diameter.

Appearance

In general, aging patients have the same complaints about the appearance of their spectacles as do young patients, but they may be somewhat more philosophical and reticent about expressing their complaints. Furthermore, many aging patients are willing to forget glamour for the sake of comfort. Nevertheless, the chief complaints about appearance are lack of style (usually too small), visible segments, edge thickness and internal reflections, too much lens bulge, and enlarged eyes with aphakic corrections.

Style, of course, is a matter of taste and advertising. It should be pointed out to the patient that comfort and good visual performance sometimes are not compatible with high style; choices must be made. One of the best choices is two pairs of spectacles: an everyday, at-home, comfortable, high-performance pair, and a high-style, tolerable-performance pair for social occasions.

Segments can be made virtually invisible by prescribing round-top, fused-segment bifocals made in light pink tinted glass with the surfaces coated. The other solution to this problem is to prescribe one of the progressive addition lenses.

Edge thickness in concave lenses can be reduced by making the lens smaller, thinner, or of higher-index glass. Frequently, only the latter is practical.

Lens bulge — that is, how much the lenses protrude in front of the plane of the frame — is a function of the lens power, equivalent diameter, base curve, index of refraction, and thickness. Presumably, nothing can be done about lens power, and little can be done about reducing thickness below that required. However, the other factors can be controlled to some extent. Altering the base curve and the index of refraction may change the optical performance of the lens, as already described. However, the patient may not complain about, or even notice, a slight decrease in visual performance in the absence of a comparison standard. Also, some of the decreases in performance are very slight and can be appreciated only after very precise and careful determinations. One of the wonders of the world is the adaptability of the human sensory mechanisms.

Internal reflections and the visibility of the lenses can be reduced by anti-reflection coatings. This will not reduce the edge thickness or the bulge, but it will make both less noticeable.

Little can be done about the magnification of the patient's eyes as seen through the lenses, except to keep the vertex distance and the lens thickness to a minimum. Magnification is less noticeable when the power of the lens decreases gradually toward the periphery, as it does in some so-called full-field high-plus lenses.

Complaints about weight, bulge, and magnification are greater as the correction becomes more convex. This is especially true of aphakic lenses made on so-called corrected base curves. In addition, these lenses create a ring scotoma around the edge of the lens because of the ever-increasing prismatic displacement of objects viewed further and further out toward the edge of the lenses, which suddenly drops to zero displacement as the line of sight passes to edge of the lens. This creates the so called "Jack-in-the-box" phenomenon in which objects jump in and out of the fields of view as the wearer moves the eyes behind the lenses. All of these problems can be minimized if the front curvature of the lens gradually flattens after the central 30 mm or so. This creates a peripheral zone of gradually decreasing power, gradually decreasing prismatic displacement, and gradually decreasing magnification. Also, the lenses can now be made thinner and lighter with less bulge. Patients' eyes viewed through such lenses do not appear to be magnified as much as through regular aphakic lenses because the magnification increases gradually from the edge of the lens to the center, and since the power of the lens at the edge is less, the magnitude of edge scotoma is reduced. All these gains are achieved by some loss in edge resolution, but generally the trade-off makes the lenses more acceptable to the patient.

High-index lenses deserve special mention. As the mean index of refraction goes up, the v value decreases and dispersion increases. Patients may see colored fringes around some objects viewed through the edges of their lenses, or they may report a blurring of vision. As the index goes up, reflection from the surface increases, so the lenses become less transparent and more visible. Antireflecting coating is effective in eliminating this problem, and all high-index lenses should be coated as a matter of routine. The specific gravity of high-index glass is greater than that of plastic or crown glass. As a rule, only when the lens power is greater than 5.00 D will the decreased thickness result in a lighter lens.

Specific tradenames of lenses and glass have been avoided, because these change with time. The reader is urged to maintain a file of trade publications, such as "Frame Product Guide," published annually in Newport Beach, CA, and journal articles to stay abreast of current developments (Bennett, 1983).

FRAMES AND MOUNTINGS

The relationship between the older patient and the optometrist can be made into a frustrating and unhappy one for both by improperly fitting spectacles, which either hurt the patient's nose, ears, or both, or which slide down the nose. The most accurate lens prescription and the most scientifically designed lenses are useless if the spectacle frame cannot be tolerated or if it fails to hold the lenses in the proper position. It therefore behooves the optometrist to be certain that the patient secures a well-designed, well-made, and well-fitting frame that is stable and holds its adjustment.

The unique problems associated with the aged patient were well defined more than three decades ago by Archer and Eakin (1960). Many of their suggested methods of treatment still are considered appropriate in dealing with the spectacle problems of today's older generation. The balance of this chapter will discuss methods for offering better care to the ever-increasing number of older patients.

The basic design of the traditional frame has changed very little during the past 50 years. Ever-changing fashion trends, of course, have profoundly influenced certain styling changes, and many of the extreme designs have negatively affected the comfort and fitting qualities of certain styles. Within variations, however, the basic geometric fitting principles have remained virtually unchanged. Today's contemporary frame styles still depend on the patient's nose for the prime support base; almost two-thirds of the entire spectacle weight is concentrated there. Most of the weight in the majority of cases is transferred directly to the sides of the nose through the contact pads of the bridge. The temples also play an important stabilizing role in maintaining control and positioning of the front section of the spectacles. The nose, however, remains the single most important area when fitting spectacles to the older patient.

AGE-RELATED PROBLEMS

In the professional care and treatment of the older patient, practitioners must remember they are seldom dealing with an amateur when it comes to wearing spectacles. Most elderly patients have worn a spectacle correction for many years. During a lifetime they have accumulated their full share of spectacle-related difficulties. Thus, they usually consider frame adjustment problems and occasional fitting difficulties as minor annoyances that are worth the benefits received. Through experience, these patients usually have developed a high degree of patience, tolerance, and understanding. Thus, to be plagued with additional spectacle problems during the later years of life is both ironic and sad.

Some older people develop an age-related physical impairment that interferes with the normal placement and wearing conditions of spectacles. The bony structure of the nose, which is the main support base for the spectacles, does not change with age, but the skin and connective tissue surrounding the nasal area do change. The skin often becomes parchment-like and extremely thin, and fragile and loose. The gradual change in the skin's texture and its loss of resilience result in a weakened footing for the weight-bearing surfaces of the spectacles. The skin no longer can support the continual downward gravitational pull of the spectacles, so it folds and becomes irritated and painful.

The aged patient, either because of mental impairment or a reluctance to complain, may ignore an irritation until it has advanced to a serious stage. In any event, the plan is to reduce the weight-bearing load of the spectacles. Abstinence from wearing all forms of spectacles would be a natural solution, but this is usually impossible because the patient may not be able to go without spectacles during the recovery period. Reduced pressure at the weakened area of the nose will insure air circulation and promote healing of the abused skin tissue. The following represents a general approach to solving this problem:

1. Use temporary or permanent accessories of various kinds that can be applied quickly to the frame. Some available devices are shown in Figure 8.1.
2. Modify the bridge contour, particularly in fixed-bridge frames.
3. Custom design and construct a frame that meets the specific requirements of a particular patient.

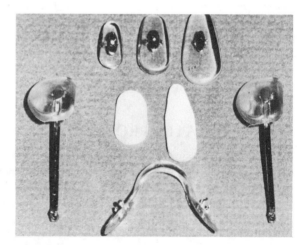

Figure 8.1. Attachments to change the weight-bearing surface of frames: (Top) pads of different sizes; (Center) stick-on cushions; (Right and Left Sides) Usden Crutch, and (Bottom) Flexit-Fit bridge.

Adjustable Bridge Control Techniques

The vast majority of frames worn by the older population are equipped with some type of adjustable nose piece. Frequently, this causes problems when the nasal skin's natural resilience has deteriorated as a result of the aging process.

Foam stick-on nose pad cushions may ease the discomfort caused by a previously worn ill-fitting frame. However, they should never be used as a permanent means of correction, as the real reason for a fitting problem may be masked by the cushion pad itself.

Pad size, shape, and texture are very important. The patient's frame may have small, hard, plastic pads, which should always be replaced. The most suitable nose pad for the aged individual is a soft, flexible, polyvinyl pad. Its size depends on factors relating to the spectacle weight and the type of nose to be fitted. As a general rule, the fitter should use a pad size that will distribute the bearing load over as great an area as possible.

The Usden Crutch technique is recommended for extreme or advanced cases where the skin and tissue have become seriously damaged. If the skin shows signs of marked irritation or redness, complete rest from the irritating spectacles may be necessary to prevent further complications. Relief is possible through the use of the Usden Crutch, a device that easily attaches to the patient's spectacles. The simple attachment consists of two 1 1/2-inch-long extension bars that are fastened to the underside of each temple hinge assembly. On the end of each bar is a large polyvinyl pad. By adjusting each of the bars, the pads can be positioned so as to rest on the cheek. This results in a slight vertical elevation of the entire front so that the regular nose pads will be clear of skin contact (Figure 8.2). The patient should be referred to a physician if the condition appears to be serious or if the inflammation does not show definite signs of improvement after a few days of Usden Crutch wear.

Flexit-Fit (Hilco Corp. Plainsville, MA) bridges offer one of the best opportunities for increasing the weight-bearing surface of the spectacle load to an absolute maximum (Figure 8.3). The individual nose pads are replaced by a one-piece, polyvinyl strap that forms a U-shaped bridge. When properly attached to the pad arms, the strap can be adjusted to allow major contact over the crest region rather than at the sides of the nose. Removing the weight from the sides and redirecting it to the more firm foundation of the nasal crest will lessen the strain on the worn and weakened side tissue.

Temple grips (Huggies) also act as temporary aids in fighting the effects of irritating spectacles. Temple grips slipped over the ends will prevent slippage and also add to overall comfort. Pad cushions and temple grips, however, never should be considered a "cure" for frame ailments. They never should act as a substitute for a well-fitted and properly adjusted frame.

Solid or Fixed Bridge Control Technique

Aside from Usden Crutch, no longer commercially available, the most effective treatment for solid bridge fitting problems involves a molding treatment.

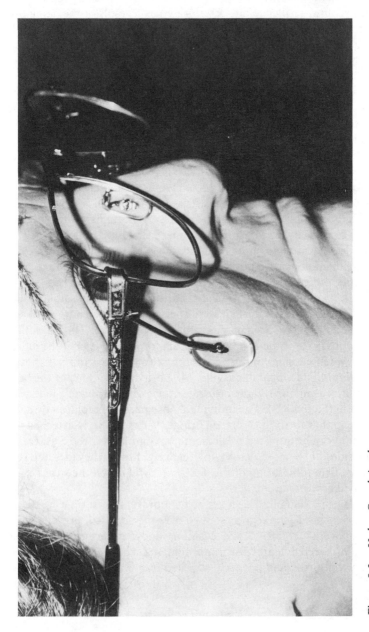

Figure 8.2. Usden Crutch in place.

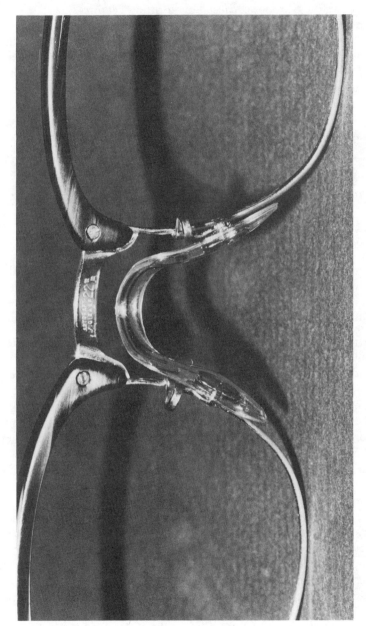

Figure 8.3. Flexit-Fit Bridge in place.

Add-on foam cushions are seldom effective. Perhaps the best approach is one that uses a compound developed by the dental profession, Coe-Soft, a soft relining plastic that eases the discomfort caused by ill-fitting dentures.

When applied to the bridge area of a frame, Coe-Soft forms a soft, nonslip lining between the hard surfaces of the frame and the delicate tissue of the nose. Nontoxic and nonirritating, Coe-Soft offers one of the best and least expensive methods of controlling irritation resulting from this type of nose-fitting problem. The material bonds itself readily to all acetate or acrylic frame materials.

It is equally effective for adjustable pads when inner changeable polyvinyl pads are not available. Applied to the surface of hard plastic nose pads, it forms an outer layer of soft flexible plastic that molds itself to the exact contour of the nose.

Saddle Conversion for Adjustable-Pad Bridges

The saddle conversion technique used for adjustable-pad bridges takes advantage of the adjustable features of the bridge to form a new network for the saddle fit. This procedure may appear to be complicated, but after a few practice sessions with an old frame, all fears and hesitation will be dispelled quickly. The entire operation is an in-office procedure and requires no unusual equipment.

The steps in the procedure follow:

1. After the nose pads have been removed, each of the adjustable arms must be straightened and then rebent into a horizontal position. The ends of each pad arm should meet or overlap in the center of the bridge. This will form the rough network or inner reinforcing core for the construction of the plastic portion of the saddle bridge. The frame then should be placed on the patient's face. Adjustments to the metal core over the crest of the nose will regulate the frontal positioning of the spectacles. Exactness of the bridge fit is not important at this stage. Establishing the correct eyewire distance on the vertical positioning of the spectacle front are the two most important adjustments to be completed. (See Figure 8.4).
2. Jet Acrylic, a dental plastic used in the restoration of teeth and denture materials, should be mixed and applied to the metal network of the newly formed bridge bar. A sufficient quantity of the plastic should be applied while the mixture has a soft, puttylike consistency. The saddle design can be shaped with the use of a small spatula. Continual applications of the mixing liquid will keep the material soft and pliable. After shaping the bridge, and while the material is still pliable, the frame should be placed carefully on the patient's face. The back side of the newly formed saddle should be lightly pressed against the face to mold the soft plastic to the shape of the nose. (A thin film of mineral

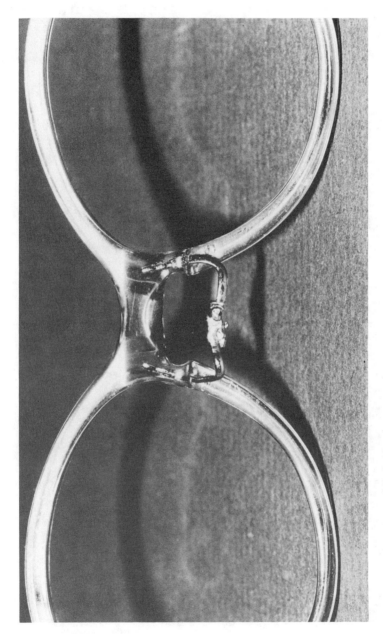

Figure 8.4. Forming saddle bridge form guard arms.

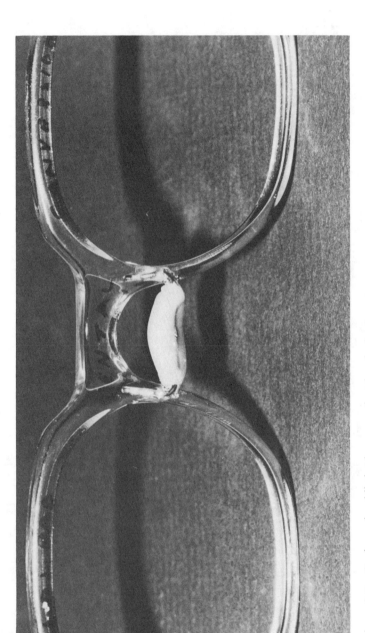

Figure 8.5.   Re-formed saddle bridge covered with soft plastic.

oil applied to the nasal region prior to this step will prevent the skin from sticking to the soft plastic.) Within 10 minutes, the material will begin to harden. The frame then should be removed from the face and placed in a container of warm water. After approximately 30 minutes, the hardening process will be completed.
3. The final phase involves filing, sanding, and polishing to complete the saddle piece. Figure 8.5 shows the finished product.

CRITERIA FOR GERIATRIC SPECTACLE DESIGN

Failure will still occur despite the best efforts. Assuming that none of the treatment plans discussed so far have offered a workable solution to the problem, what is the next procedure? An entirely new spectacle design needs to be created. Although circumstances and conditions may alter certain design features, the following are suggested guidelines for solving this problem.

The frame should be strong, but lightweight. It should be no larger than absolutely necessary to accommodate the facial size. For centering purposes, the frame PD should be equal to the distance interpupillary separation. The bridge should be adjustable, with the DBL as small as possible. The temples should preferably be of a cable type, with covers over the mastoid ends. Finally, the frame style and color must be pleasing to the patient.

REFERENCES

1. Archer, J.E., and R.S. Eakin. The Fitting and Adjusting of Spectacles for the Older Patient. In: Hirsch, M. and Wick R. (eds.) *Vision of the Aging Patient.* Philadelphia. Chilton. 1960, pp. 202–213.
2. Bailey, I., and M. Bullimore. "A New Test for the Evaluation of Disability Glare." *Optom. Vis. Sci.* 68 (1991): 911–917.
3. Bennett, I. "The Changing World of Lenses." *Optometric Management* (Sept. 1983): 29–50.
4. Borish, I., S. Hitzeman, and K. Brookman. "Double Blind Study of Progressive Addition Lenses." *J. Am. Optom. Assoc.* 51 (1980): 933–943.
5. Davis, J. Prescribing for Visibility. In: Sheedy J. (ed.). *Environmental Optics.* Philadelphia: J.B. Lippincott, 1990, pp. 131–155.
6. Hampton, L., N. Roth, I. Meyer-Arendt, D. Shuman. "Visual Acuity Degradation Resulting From Polycarbonates." *J. Am. Optom. Assoc.* 62: 760–765, 1991.
7. Holladay, J., T. Peger, J. Trujillo, and R. Ruis. "Brightness Acuity and Outdoor Visual Acuity in Cataract Patients." *J. Cataract Refract. Surg.* 13: 67–69, 1987.
8. Jones, W.F. "High Index Glass: The Manufacturer's View." *Manufacturing Optics International.* (Nov. 1980): 33–36.
9. Katz, M. "Distortion by Ophthalmic Lenses Calculated at the Farpoint Sphere." *Am. J. Optom & Physiol. Opt.* 60: 944–959, 1983.
10. Morgan, M. *The Optics of Ophthalmic Lenses.* Chicago: Professional Press, 1978, pp. 309–327.

11. Pitts, D. Ultraviolet Protection. In: Sheedy J. (ed.). *Environmental Optics.* Philadelphia: J.B. Lippincott, 1990, pp. 95–115.
12. Schultz, D. "Factors Influencing Patient Acceptance of Varilux-2 Lenses." *J. Am. Optom. Assoc.* 54 (1983): 513–529.
13. Zigman, S. Recent Research in Near UV Radiation and the Eye. In: Urbach F. and Gange R. (eds.). *The Biological Effects of UVA Radiation.* New York: Praeger, 1986.

9

Contact Lenses and the Elderly Patient

Edward S. Bennett
Melvin J. Remba
Barry A. Weissman

Contact lenses have assumed an important, if not vital, role in the visual rehabilitation of patients of all ages encompassing a wide variety of ocular conditions. Until recently, the focus of the contact lens practitioner has been primarily fitting and management of the healthy, young, myopic and hyperopic patients. These individuals are typically easier to fit because they have a more stable tear film, uncomplicated refraction, enhanced dexterity in handling the lenses and, in many cases, greater motivation. However, it is unfair and unwise to rule out any patient because of age. The visual benefits, resulting patient satisfaction, and enhancement of the quality of life, often can be greatest with the older patient population. As a result of these considerations, it is apparent that an increase in prescribing and fitting the older patient with contact lenses is a definite trend among eyecare professionals. The reasons for this change in attitude for both patients and clinicians are the following (Phillips, 1986; Benjamin and Borish, 1991):

1. The "baby boomers," individuals who were fitted with contact lenses during the late 1960s and 1970s and remained enthusiastic lens users, are now reaching presbyopic age; therefore, the interest in presbyopic contact lens correction is increasing.
2. Contact lens manufacturers are devoting a great amount of resources to multifocal contact lens clinical research and development. As a result, improved bifocal lens correcting concepts and designs, in both rigid and soft materials, are being introduced on a regular basis.
3. Clinical expertise and new technology have increased the number of conditions that can be treated or aided by contact lenses.
4. One of the biggest barriers — the psychological acceptance of contact lenses by middle-aged and older people — is being broken down; older people want contact lenses!

5. The population over retirement age is increasing; the average life span in the industrial countries is increasing as well.

The purpose of this chapter is to discuss ocular conditions common to the older patient population and the role of contact lenses in the visual correction of these conditions. Conventional contact lenses will not be emphasized because they are not within the scope of this chapter. The specific areas to be addressed will be (1) presbyopia and (2) therapeutic applications. Contact lens application in aphakia, less used now than in previous years because of the wide use of IOLs, are discussed in Chapter 11. Patient selection, lens design alternatives, fitting considerations, problem-solving, and psychological aspects of contact lens use by the elderly will be discussed.

PATIENT SELECTION

Patient selection is always an important component of eventual success in contact lenses; this is especially true with the elderly patient. Prior to fitting, it is extremely important for the practitioner to perform the necessary history, questioning, and testing procedures to assess the patient's suitability and potential for successful contact lens wear and to rule out any contraindications. If these pre-fitting procedures are not performed, or performed inadequately, contact lens-induced complications and patient dissatisfaction with lens wear can result. The following criteria can serve as a checklist for the initial selection of the older patient (Mannis and Zadnik, 1986):

Factors for Success:

- Definite need of visual correction
- Strong motivation to use contact lenses
- Insight into the rationale for contact lens wear and care
- Good personal hygiene
- Manual dexterity
- Adequate ocular adnexal function

Factors for Failure:

- Poor sociologic support system
- Poor understanding of necessary hygiene
- Poor manual dexterity
- Abnormalities or chronic disease of the external eye
- Unrealistic expectations

Obviously, some of these factors pertain more to those individuals wearing daily wear, (that is, presbyopic) lenses, whereas some pertain more to the extended wear/bandage/therapeutic contact lens wearer.

Patient motivation is an extremely important factor for success because perseverance is an essential part of the visual adaptation necessary with any presbyopic fitting system. Not only do first-time wearers need to be patient during the

2- to 4-week adaptation process, something they have not had to be concerned with for the 50, 60, or more years they have lived, but they also have to learn how to handle and care for the lenses, and, in some cases, they have to adapt to multiple imagery that is inherent in most bifocal lens designs. Whereas the younger patient usually is motivated by cosmetic factors, the older patient may have other motivating factors, including visual and medical considerations. A monocular aphake with good phakic vision in the opposite eye, for example, is likely to be highly motivated to wear the lens successfully in order to gain binocularity. Many elderly patients will exhibit anxiety about their possible inability to handle the lens(es); therefore, encouragement and reinforcement by the practitioner and staff members is vital. The practitioner has to balance the visual or medical requirements of patients against their motivation, temperament, physical disability, degree of activity, and handling difficulties. Usually, patients already wearing contact lenses make the transition to a presbyopic contact lens correction much easier than first-time presbyopic candidates.

The importance of comprehensive patient education cannot be underestimated. Many older patients have little idea of what a contact lens is, and what options are available to them. The practitioner must take great care in explaining to the patient exactly what is involved in lens care, handling, cost, and follow-up office visits. If the patient is very elderly, it is beneficial to have a spouse, son, or daughter present both at the initial discussion and, at minimum, the first few visits to insure that advice and instruction are understood completely and can be reinforced. In addition, for older or infirm patients, assistance from family members may be required for insertion and removal of a daily-wear lens or removal and disinfection of an extended-wear lens. A person who lives alone or is in any form of self-care facility may not be a good candidate for contact lens wear, especially if poor manual dexterity is present.

ANATOMIC AND PHYSIOLOGIC CHANGES

General anatomic and physiologic changes in the older eye are discussed in Chapter 6. Nevertheless, there are several important changes that must be considered as they pertain specifically to the prospective contact lens wearing elderly patient (Phillips, 1986; Benjamin and Borish, 1991).

Eyelids

With age, a reduction occurs in muscle tone, amount of orbital fat, and elasticity of the skin of the eyelids. The lower lids of elderly individuals may not retain sufficient elastic "memory" to resume their customary place against the surface of the globe. This can be disadvantageous in the case of alternating bifocal contact lenses in which it is important for the prism ballasted and truncated inferior edge to rest against the lower lid margin, and not to sag into the lower fornix. The upper eyelid also loses elasticity as a patient ages. Blepharochalasis is often present, and tonic retraction of the upper lid by Muller's muscle is diminished so that ptosis is likely. As the superior eyelid has an important role in contact lens centration and movement — especially rigid lenses — it is valuable to evaluate lid tension prior to fitting. If rigid (non-prism ballasted) lenses are indicated, the use of both a lenticular construction with rounded edges and optimal peripheral thickness profile are important to facilitate removal. Loss of lid elasticity, common with many older patients, often requires alternative methods of lens insertion and removal (to be discussed).

It is also important to rule out appositional abnormalities that would interfere with lens wear (that is, ectropion, entropion, and lagophthalmos), although the latter two conditions could benefit from soft lens wear to "blanket" the cornea from eyelash-induced foreign body irritation (Mannis and Zadnik, 1986). Trichiasis should be ruled out and, if present, epilation should be performed prior to fitting. Evidence of chronic blepharitis (that is, irregular lid margins, seborrheic discharge, collarettes, ulcerations, or chalazia) should discourage (but not contraindicate) contact lens wear.

Tear Film

Tear flow tends to gradually reduce with age. Aging tends to decrease the number and function of secretory cells responsible for lubricating the corneal surface. Goblet cells of the conjunctiva and the mass of the lacrimal glands decrease with age, resulting in a progressive reduction of tear production (Weale, 1982). This decrease may be as much as a factor of four, resulting in the so-called "dry eye." Reduced tear flow often can result as a complication of rheumatoid arthritis in the form of Sjogren's syndrome. In addition, overnight ocular exposure resulting from incomplete lid closure also compromises the lacrimal lubrication system by evaporation effects (Benjamin and Borish, 1991). Therefore, these patients, especially if an extended-wear schedule is prescribed, should be advised against sleeping under a ceiling fan and avoid any forms of air drafts during the day, which typically act to evaporate tear fluid.

Careful evaluation of the tear film quality and quantity is essential and aids in selecting the best lens type. As reduced tear flow results in an increase in the amount of lens surface deposition, leading to blurred vision, discomfort and possible papillary hypertrophy, the selection of a wettable lens material, and a wearing schedule compatible with tear-film function is important. Frequent use of ocular lubricants is often necessary. If a soft lens is selected, a planned replacement or disposable lens program is indicated. Unless absolutely necessary, extended wear is contraindicated in cases of dry eye or lacrimal dysfunction.

Conjunctiva

Slit-lamp examination of the conjunctiva will determine whether it is thickened and insensitive because of previous infection or trauma. The presence of pingueculae and other elevations of the conjunctiva can physically elevate the lids away from complete contact with the cornea, creating "lid gap." This accelerates corneal desiccation in the case of rigid lens wear, and pingueculae are known to be irritated further from soft lens wear. Therefore, the bulbar conjunctiva and peripheral cornea need to be monitored in these patients. In addition, as a result of the reduction in elasticity of the conjunctival tissue, "conjunctival drag" is more apparent, making assessment of soft lens movement with the blink misleading if not carefully evaluated (that is, the lens appears to be moving more than it actually is).

Cornea

With aging, the cornea also undergoes changes that can affect contact lens wear. As mentioned previously, decreased tear flow with age can result in corneal desiccation, notably manifested by a localized superficial punctate keratitis (SPK) with rigid lens wearers. The drying of the soft lens surface in conjunction with reduced tear flow also can promote mucoprotein and lipid lens deposition and contamination, and diffuse epithelial staining is possible due to the trapped debris. It is very important to perform a fluorescein evaluation of the cornea under filtered (cobalt blue), slit-lamp magnification before and during the fitting process with all contact lens-wearing patients, especially the elderly.

A second corneal change with age is a decrease in corneal sensitivity resulting from a loss in nerve elements; this process is accelerated greatly following cataract surgery. Reduced corneal sensitivity can be beneficial in some cases; for example, as a nervous, elderly, first-time wearer who discovers that new rigid contact lenses are not as "painful" as feared. Conversely, reduced corneal sensitivity may be detrimental in not alerting the patient early in the event of an ocular complication that requires prompt medical treatment. A third change pertains to decreased oxygen transmission to the superior cornea as a result of the aforementioned possibility of lid ptosis (Benjamin and Borish, 1991; Benjamin and Rasmussen, 1988). This can be clinically significant because most bifocal designs and all aphakic lenses are much thicker than conventional, or non-aphakic lenses; therefore, the role of oxygen transmission is even more important. Finally, the degeneration of subepithelial tissues, including Bowman's membrane, and their replacement by other connective-like tissue, can result in pterygia. It can be stated that, unless absolutely necessary, contact lens wear should be contraindicated in cases where rigid or soft lenses can aggravate an existing corneal condition.

The aforementioned corneal changes make it imperative to select a highly oxygen-transmissible contact lens and to fit it with sufficient lens lag movement and to maximize tear interchange and flushing. Higher oxygen transmissibility can be achieved better with a rigid lens than with a soft because of the "metabolic pumping" action of RGP lenses, especially if extended wear is deemed necessary. If the patient can handle the lenses and is motivated to do so, a daily-wear schedule should be recommended rather than overnight wear, except for special therapeutic indications, to be discussed below.

Visual Function

Not only does the elderly patient have to adjust to the loss of accommodative amplitude, but a reduction in retinal luminance and contrast sensitivity also occur over time. it has been found that contrast must be increased by a factor of approximately 3 in order for 70% of a 60-year-old population to restore visual performance of their eyes to that equivalent at age 20 (Blackwell and Blackwell, 1971). In addition, as a result in part of reduced pupil size and opacification of the ocular media with age, elderly patients require more illumination to perform near visual tasks. Target illumination may need to be doubled every 13 years over the age of 20 to achieve equivalent dark-adapted vision (Guth, 1957). This effect is compromised even further by uncorrected errors of refraction. For mesopic vision, one diopter out of focus may require two to three times the amount of light, whereas a two diopter uncorrected error may necessitate five to six times the light (Benjamin and Borish, 1991). Precise optical correction, therefore, becomes most important in the older patient in order to minimize the effect of the reduced visual functions.

For these reasons, it is first important to perform an accurate refraction in elderly contact lens candidates and, upon diagnostic fitting with a contact lens, perform a careful over-refraction that should be fully incorporated in the proposed contact lens. In addition, presbyopic contact lens wearers should be advised to increase the normal level of background illumination used in near tasks, especially if simultaneous vision bifocals (to be discussed) have been fitted.

Presbyopic Patients

The largest proportion of older, potential contact lens patients are presbyopes who require optical correction at distance and near. It is a rapidly growing and currently the largest segment of the population in the United States as the so-called post-war baby-boomers reach presbyopic age. With 43 million 40- to 50-year-old individuals in 1990 and an expected 60 million by the end of the century, a large group of potential bifocal contact lens wearers will exist (Barr and Bailey, 1991). As 40% of these individuals require *spherical* (bifocal) corrections, this age group definitely represents the largest untapped segment of the soft contact lens market (Hansen, 1989). Manufacturers are attempting to meet this anticipated demand by introducing many new rigid and soft bifocal designs with many others being patented and under clinical investigation. As a result of such factors as cost, perceived design and fitting complexity, limited success, and the wealth of spectacle lens advertising, the numbers of bifocal or multifocal contact lenses fitted up until now has been low. However, this should change as new and better lenses replace older ones, and consumer confidence in the improved lenses and fitting skills of practitioners is established.

There are several contact lens options for the presbyope. These include (1) single-vision contact lens wear and over-reading glasses, (2) monovision, (3) modified monovision, and (4) bifocal contact lenses, of which there are many, both in RGP and hydrogel materials.

SINGLE-VISION CONTACT LENS WEAR AND READING GLASSES

The use of single-vision lenses (hydrogel or RGP) in combination with reading glasses affords the benefits of simplicity of fit, optimum vision at distance and near, and limited expense. The overspectacles are usually single-vision plus add lenses, but may be progressive addition type, and, in some cases, minimal add powers are used only as needed to enhance the reading ability of emerging presbyopes. However, patients with varied near and distance tasks will complain of the inconvenience of frequently putting on and removing their spectacles. In addition, many patients choose contact lenses with the intent or wish of eliminating the need for spectacles. Nevertheless, it is important that the single vision/overspectacles option be presented to all potential presbyopic contact lens wearers. Some patients will prefer to begin with this most basic option; however, at a later date, they will change to one of the other presbyopic contact lens systems mentioned to them at the original fitting/consultation visit.

MONOVISION

Monovision is defined as contact lens correction of one eye for distance vision and the other eye for near vision. Currently, it represents the most commonly used method of presbyopic contact lens correction, being used in approximately 70% of all presbyopic fittings (Josephson and Caffrey, 1991). This form of correction has many advantages when compared to bifocal contact lenses including: (1) conventional lenses are used, and special lens designs are not necessary; (2) it is less time-consuming; (3) it is less expensive; (4) thinner lenses may be used, which are more physiologically acceptable to the cornea; (5) only one contact lens need be changed for present wearers; and (6) many of the patient symptoms/compromises present with bifocal contact lenses, including ghost images, reduced illumination, reduced contrast sensitivity, or fluctuating vision related to pupil size changes are avoided.

There are, however, several possible problems that are observed and reported from this mode of presbyopic contact lens correction. These include reduced stereopsis, spatial disorientation, decreased contrast sensitivity, difficulty in resolving critical distance vision tasks, and possible liability considerations (Josephson et al., 1991). Although it has been found that reduced measurable stereopsis is present as a result of monocular blur (McGill and Erickson, 1988), it is arguable whether this effect is often transferred into subjective problems with depth perception. Therefore, it has been recommended that any reduced stereopsis compromising contact lens performance would be contraindicated if stereoacuity is very important occupationally (Josephson et al., 1991). Some monocular suppression of blur occurs in monovision, which is desired; however, the blurred eye will still contribute to binocular summation (Westendorf et al.,

1982). The degree of suppression usually increases as the add increases. Contrast sensitivity function is reduced in monovision and, in high adds, binocular summation is difficult to achieve (Loshin et al., 1982; Collins et al., 1989). However, this visual compromise is not dissimilar to that resulting from simultaneous vision bifocal lens designs. Simultaneous vision will be discussed elsewhere. Blurring one eye for distance, especially in advanced presbyopia, can result in significant compromise in critical distance vision-related tasks, including night driving and some occupations. Finally, it is certainly possible that a practitioner could be liable for any injury for which a monovision prescription could be a contributing factor (Harris and Classe, 1988).

The philosophy of monovision must first be discussed with the patient. Some patients require assurance that no damage to their sight will occur. The likelihood of the need for supplementary forward spectacles, as will be described, also should be emphasized to prevent later misunderstandings.

Some fitting and prescribing considerations for monovision include the following (Bennett et al., in press):

1. Fit patients who do not require long periods of critical distance vision.
2. Perform binocular function testing to determine the effect of monovision on stereopsis.
3. Demonstrate the add power effect to the patient; the patient could actually wear a trial frame to simulate this effect on vision. Subjective reaction to plussing one eye at times helps determine the preferred distance corrected eye.
4. Select the proper eye for near; as it is most important for distance vision to be less impaired, the near eye typically represents the non-dominant and/or the eye in which vision is reduced relative to the other eye. Often, but not always, this is the left eye. This may be reversed if the patient's job involves prolonged close work, or if a subjective preference indicates this during the diagnostic visit. If the patient is anisometropic, the higher myopic eye should be considered for near, all other factors being equal.
5. Prescribe the full amount of correction; it is tempting to underplus the near eye and overplus the distance eye to lessen the anisometropia. However, for optimum near and distance vision, it is preferable to prescribe the full add amount.
6. Strongly encourage (if not require) monovision patients to either purchase a pair of "driving" spectacles (that is, minus power over near eye) or a second distance contact lens for use while driving.
7. An informed consent that discusses the benefits and limitations of monovision in addition to discussing alternative forms of presbyopic correction (contact lens and spectacle) should be reviewed and signed by the patient.
8. A handling tint in the contact lenses also is recommended to aid lens location and application..

9. Although most patients adapt to monovision within 2 weeks, they nevertheless should be told it could take up to 4 to 6 weeks for complete adaptation.

BIFOCAL CONTACT LENS DESIGNS
Definitions

Bifocal contact lenses provide a multifocal optical effect, use either the simultaneous vision or alternating vision technique, and are available in soft and rigid lens materials.

Simultaneous Vision

Simultaneous vision (also termed "bivision" and "selective image") pertains to the vision achieved when the distance and near-power elements are positioned within the pupillary opening at the same time; therefore, light rays from both distance and near targets are imaged on the retina. The patient will selectively suppress the most blurred images that are not desired for a given visual task. This concept functions on the basis of blur interpretation and/or blur tolerance of superimposed multiple images on the retina, which are formed by the various powers of the lens (Benjamin and Borish, 1991). For true simultaneous vision, the two primary segments must remain within the pupillary boundary in all positions of gaze and, in order to give equally bright images, the distance and near areas of the lens should cover nearly equal areas of the pupil. Three designs using the simultaneous vision concept are (1) aspheric, (2) concentric/annular (or target), and (3) diffractive. *Aspheric* lens designs have a gradual change of curvature along one of their surfaces based on the geometry of conic sections. This rate of flattening (or eccentricity) is much greater than with aspheric single vision lenses and creates a plus add power effect. In some aspheric multifocals, eccentricity is located on the posterior surface and increases in plus power from the center to the periphery. Conversely, center-near aspherics have their maximum plus power at the center, which then gradually decreases away from the geometrical center. *Concentric or annular* lens designs are structured with a small (typically two-thirds to three-fourths the size of the pupil in normal room illumination) annular central zone which, in most designs, provides the distance vision correction; the near correction is ground on the annulus that surrounds the distance zone. Reverse centrad concentric bifocals are constructed so that the *near add* occupies the central 2- to 3-mm segment portion of the lens. *Diffractive* lenses function through a central diffractive zone plate that focuses images at distance by *refraction* of light and near through *diffraction* principles created by the zone eschelettes. This design is *pupil independent* as equal amounts of light pass through both the distance and near-power elements of the lens for all normal pupil opening diameters. All three of these "simultaneous vision" lens designs must center reasonably well and not exhibit excessive movement with blinking or with shifts of gaze (Bennett et al., in press). For that reason, soft lenses, which traditionally center well and fit with minimal blink-induced lag, perform better than the more mobile similar rigid lenses in simultaneous vision multifocal fitting.

Alternating Vision

Alternating vision pertains to lens designs and function in which vertical movement or *translation* results in only one power zone to position in front of the pupil (or visual axis) at any one time (that is, ideally the distance zone is in front of the pupil when viewing at a distance and the near zone when viewing at near). Essentially there is an intentional shifting of lens position in which separate, discrete images formed by the two power segments in the lens focus on the retina with a change of gaze from distance (up) to near (down) or vice versa. Typically these designs are non-rotating by prism ballast construction, sometimes in combination with inferior truncation, which stabilizes the lens and allows a smooth translation from the superior distance zone to the inferior near zone when lowering the gaze in order to read. Several types of rigid prism ballast lenses have been developed through the years, including *decentered concentric, one-piece segmented,* and *fused crescent and segmented.* These non-rotating segmented designs are similar to spectacle bifocals as executive and flat-top segments are used. They are most commonly used with rigid lens materials, although several attempts have been made to create translating ballasted hydrogel bifocals with limited success, however. It is imperative for alternating bifocal lenses to translate sufficiently when the patient shifts gaze from one distance to another, and this translation is attained much more easily with rigid lenses than with hydrogels. For these reasons, simultaneous image designs have been more successful when incorporated in soft lenses, and alternating image designs have been more successful when incorporated in rigid ballasted lenses.

RIGID BIFOCAL DESIGNS
Simultaneous Vision

Three types of simultaneous image rigid bifocal designs are either available or soon to be available. These include aspheric, concentric, and diffractive lenses.

Aspheric

There are numerous presbyopic designs having an entirely (that is, not peripheral only) aspheric back surface geometry. The peripheral flattening of the back surface provides a continuously variable near addition. To provide the maximum near addition, a high degree of peripheral curvature flattening or asphericity must be used. This departure from spherical shape is known as eccentricity or e factor. These lenses are commonly fit as much as 2.5 to 5 D steeper than K. However, as a result of the aspheric geometry, fluorescein pooling will be present centrally and mid-peripherally (Figure 9.1). The best candidates for these lenses are individuals who are not good candidates for translating design bifocals. With aspheric RGPs, it is difficult to generate the necessary add power within the pupillary zone without inducing disturbing aberration effects on distance vision; therefore, early or emerging presbyopes are best candidates. Other candidates include any one having the following anatomic characteristics:

1. Average pupil size
2. Lower lid margin well above or below limbus
3. Steep corneal curvatures
4. Loose lids that will not support prism ballast lenses

The benefits of aspheric designs include the absence of prism and truncation in their construction. Therefore, the thickness profile is similar or better than conventional single-vision lenses. In addition, no image jump or flare from a segment line is present. Good intermediate vision is often obtainable because of the progressive add feature.

The major disadvantage with this design is decentration, often difficult to attain with RGP lenses. If this lens does not exhibit optimum and consistent centration, blurred distance vision will result. Likewise, less lens movement with the blink is desirable, preferably about 1 mm. Limited success with fitting the advanced presbyope is also a disadvantage.

After fitting the lens, the following problems may occur; the management option(s) are provided as well:

1. *Excessive lens lag* — select a steeper base curve radius.
2. *Poor centration* — select a steeper base curve radius or larger diameter; if no improvement is present, use another design.
3. *Adherence* — select a flatter base curve radius; flatten peripheral curve.

Annular/Concentric
The front or back surface concentric designs, also known as "target" bifocals, which have either distance or near power in the central annular zone; thus the terms "center-near" or "center-distance" multifocals. Usually, the diameter of this central zone is equal to approximately two-thirds to three-fourths of the size

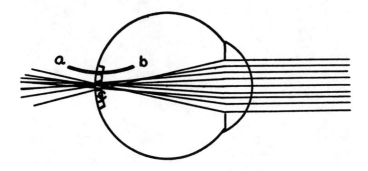

Figure 9.1 Ray tracing diagram showing the optical caustic formed on the retina by central and paraxial rays passing through an aspheric contact lens on the cornea.

of the pupil in normal room illumination, so that nearly equal amounts of light enter from both power zones simultaneously.

This is the oldest and least commonly used bifocal RGP design. Candidates for these type of lenses are similar to those suitable to aspheric design. The advantages and disadvantages are similar as well, except that the quality of vision attainable with concentrics is very dependent on pupil size (and the level of illumination) at any given time. The importance of good centration and limited lens lag is also very evident in these cases.

When problem-solving with this lens, the following examples may be useful:

1. Poor distance vision – order larger distance zone (or smaller near zone)
2. Poor near acuity – options include either selecting a flatter base curve radius, reducing the overall diameter, or increasing the add power
3. Flare at night – select a larger distance seg diameter

Diffractive

Diffractive lenses, the newest concept of bifocal contact lens correction, have been available in a soft lens form since 1989, but were only recently introduced in rigid lens form. As with other simultaneous vision bifocal designs, good centration relative to the visual axis is important (Figure 9.2). Therefore, this type of lens is fitted approximately 1 D steeper than K. Minimum movement with the blink is also desirable. Patients with these lenses need to be educated about possible adaptation problems inherent in these diffractive lenses, which may include ghost images around reading material, and reduced luminance

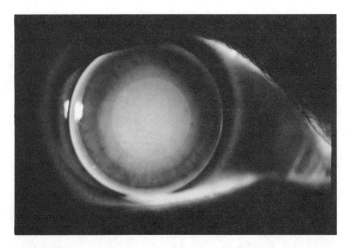

Figure 9.2 Flourescein fitting pattern of the Diffrax bifocal RGP. Note the diffractive zone confined to the center of the lens.

as a result of the loss of light to higher orders of diffraction with this design (Loshin, 1989; Bennett et al., 1990). Patients should be told that it may take up to 2 months to adapt.

The best candidates for rigid diffractive (Diffrax) lenses are similar to those eligible for other simultaneous vision designs described above. However, diffractive designs have an important advantage; they are pupil *independent*. Light entering through diffractive zone areas is divided equally for distance and near throughout the diffractive zone plate of the lens. The concentric simultaneous vision designs typically have near and distance zones representing unequal areas within the pupillary borders at any given time, which results in a difference in image brightness between the distance and near viewing areas (Figure 9.3 and Figure 9.4). In contrast to other simultaneous vision bifocals, diffractive designs are recommended in moderate to advanced presbyopia, not the beginning presbyope as the latter may experience a rivalry between the distance and near images that are superimposed on the retina. Disadvantages that may occur with diffractive RGP lenses include the need for good centration, reduced illumination, possibility of glare (similar to other simultaneous vision bifocals), and reduced contrast sensitivity (Bennett et al., 1990).

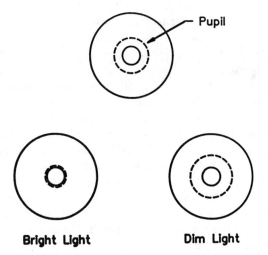

Concentric Bifocals

Pupil

Bright Light

Dim Light

Figure 9.3 Diagram demonstrating the relation of the pupil, in bright and dim illumination, to the fixed distance segment zone of a concentric bifocal, making this bifocal "pupil dependent."

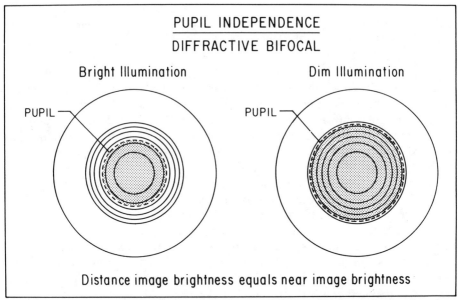

Figure 9.4 Diagram demonstrating the relation of the pupillary opening to the phase plate zone of a diffractive bifocal, creating a "pupil independent" optical effect and providing equal retinal image luminance from both powers of the lens.

Alternating Vision

There are two types of alternating (translating) bifocal RGP designs. These are more commonly used than the simultaneous type bifocals just discussed. These include concentrics, the translating (early), and segmented, more recently developed.

Annular/Concentric

These designs differ from their simultaneous vision counterparts in several ways. Typically, the central distance zone is larger, often 3.5 to 5 mm, it is decentered to the superior part of the lens, and prism and truncation are present to prevent lens rotation and to facilitate translation when shifting gaze. One commonly used alternating concentric design (VE-ACC, Salvatori Ophthalmics) incorporates 1 to 1.5 Δ with a small amount of truncation. The distance zone is decentered 1 to 2 mm superiorly (Figure 9.5). When the patient shifts gaze inferiorly to read, the near zone of the lens should translate into the proper position in front of the pupil as the lens is held by the lower lid margin and the eye rotates downward. Thus, the term "alternating" vision is used. This is the mechanism by which all translating lenses function.

Good candidates for this design, as well as for all other prism ballast segmented bifocals, include patients having a lower lid margin tangent to, or slightly above, the limbus, an 8.5-mm or larger vertical fissure size, normal (not loose) lid tension, and myopic/low hyperopic refractive powers. The benefits of these lenses include the ability to achieve precise correction and good vision at distance and near uncompromised by secondary images, assuming proper fit, minimal lens rotation, and consistent translation. In addition, any amount of presbyopic adds can be corrected successfully. The disadvantages may include the increased center thickness required with a prism ballast, although the translating concentrics are the thinnest of the prism ballast bifocals. The thicker inferior edge may result in temporary lid awareness. With annular segments, it is important to specify a distance zone large enough (>4.0 mm) to minimize distance flare. Finally, image jump, due to prismatic effects resulting from the bicentric construction of these lenses, can result in patient problems during gaze shift with concentric, translating bifocals. Some representative fitting problems and methods of managing them are listed below. These are applicable to all types of prism ballast including segment type bifocal RGPs.

1. Poor distance acuity:
   a. If seg is too high — truncate or increase existing truncation
   b. If seg is too low — use a larger overall diameter; order higher seg position
   c. Lateral decentration — thin anterior edges, steepen base curve, or consider another design
2. Poor near acuity:
   a. If seg is too low — consider smaller distance seg or steeper base curve radius or both
   b. Lens going underneath lower lid — use additional truncation, square its shape, or order more prism
   c. Insufficient add power — increase add to the patient's best working distance

Segmented

The most popular and perhaps the most successful bifocal contact lenses are the rigid *segmented* translating designs. These lenses have had a long history of development and refinement during the "PMMA" years — 1960–1980. Segmented bifocals can be divided into two types: one-piece and fused. The primary benefits of these lenses are absence of image jump and no "boundary diplopia" during translation because of the unique *monocentric* construction of the newer lenses. Monocentric means that the optical centers of the lens power zones are coincident. Fused bifocals, which consist of fusing or encapsulating a higher index material for the near segment into the distance button, may be manufactured thinner than the "one piece" bifocals; therefore, they have the advantages of a thinner profile in addition to the absence of image jump. Various fused segmented bifocals in PMMA material, pioneered by George Tsuetaki and Charles Neefe, were once popular; however, fusing a bifocal segment into the silicone-containing RGP polymers has been difficult to achieve; therefore, one-piece, non-fused bifocal designs have been the most frequently used to date.

The most commonly used segmented bifocal and the first to receive FDA approval is the Tangent Streak (Fused Contacts). This is the only approved mono-centric (that is, near and distance optical centers are coincident at the segment line), one-piece segmented bifocal. As the near and distance optical centers meet at the geometrical center of the lens, the potential problem of image jump and resulting boundary diplopia as the patients shift gaze is eliminated. This lens is available in a series of fluoro-silicone/acrylate (that is, Fluorex 300, 500 and 700 with Dk values of 30, 50, and 70, respectively) lens materials. A full range of powers and geometries are also available because the lenses are custom designed by the clinician. It is heavily prism ballasted (1.75–4.00 Δ available) and trun-cated. The segment shape is similar to an "executive" bifocal; the seg can be ordered at any height, and a trifocal version of this lens is also available.

The following diagnostic lens specifications are recommended (20 lenses) by the manufacturer:

BCR: 41.00–45.50 D
Seg Height: 4.2 mm
Power: $+/-2.00$ D
Add: $+2.00$ D
OAD: 9.4/9.0 mm

The lens diameter and seg height are determined from the following measure-ments:

1. The vertical lens size = lower lid to superior limbus minus 2 mm
2. The seg height = lower lid to visual axis minus 1.3 mm

Recommended lens dimensions based upon the lower lid to limbus position are provided in Table 9.1. The amount of prism to insure non-rotation and proper

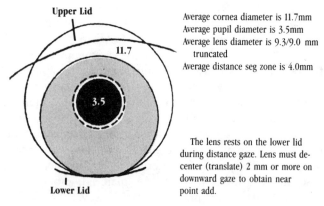

Upper Lid

11.7

3.5

Lower Lid

Average cornea diameter is 11.7mm
Average pupil diameter is 3.5mm
Average lens diameter is 9.3/9.0 mm
   truncated
Average distance seg zone is 4.0mm

The lens rests on the lower lid during distance gaze. Lens must de-center (translate) 2 mm or more on downward gaze to obtain near point add.

Figure 9.5 Representation of a correctly positioning ACC-translating rigid bifocal on an average eye at primary distance gaze.

Table 9.1 Parameters of approved therapeutic hydrogel contact lenses

Lens Designation /Source	Water Content (%)	Posterior Curve(s) (mm)	Central Thickness (mm)	Overall Diameter(s) (mm)
Low Dk/L				
Sofcon/Ciba	55	8.1, 8.4	0.35	14.0, 14.5
Plano T/B&L	39	8.1	0.17	14.7
Plano B4/B&L	39	8.8	0.12	14.5
High Dk/L				
Permalens/Cooper	70	9.0	0.26	15.0
Plano U/B&L	39	8.5	0.07	12.5
Plano U3/B&L	39	8.6	0.07	13.5
Plano 04/B&L	39	8.8	0.03	14.5
CSIT/SBH	39	8.6, 8.9, 9.4	0.03	14.8
		8.6, 8.9	0.03	13.8

position typically varies between 1.75 to 3.00 Δ and increases with increases in minus power and increased add power.

An "On K" to slightly flatter than K lens is recommended. A steeper than K lens often results in insufficient translation and excessive rotation (Figures 9.6 and 9.7). A flat lens may result in excessive "lifting" and/or decentration.

When the eye is in the primary position, the upper edge of the lens should be about 0.5 mm above the superior border of the pupil. The segment line is

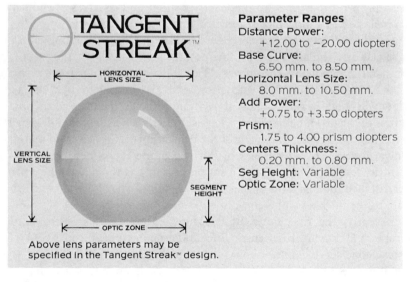

Figure 9.6 Parameter ranges of the Tangent Streak bifocal contact lens (courtesy of Fused Contacts).

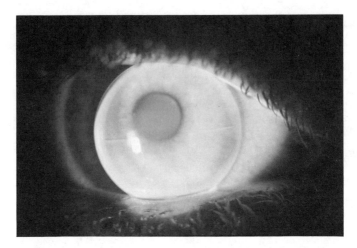

Figure 9.7 Fluorescein pattern of a well-fitting and positioning Tangent Streak lens. Note that the segment line is slightly above the lower pupillary border.

observed easily by fluorescein, which collects at the junction of the distance and near sections. When the patient looks straight ahead, and the lens is in its lowest riding position, the top of the segment can be as high as 1.0 mm above the inferior pupil margin in room illumination without disturbing distance vision. The lens should ride with its lower edge supported by the lower lid margin. With the patient fixating straight ahead, the lens is usually picked up 1 to 2 mm on the blink, and then drops back to the lower position quickly. This phenomenon of prism ballasted lens movement is termed lens "lift and recovery."

Good candidates for this design are similar to other translating bifocals and include (1) early and advanced presbyopes; (2) lower lid above, tangent to, or no more than 0.5 mm below the limbus; (3) myopia and low hyperopic powers; (4) normal to large palpebral fissure sizes; and (5) normal to tight lid tension. Patients with high hyperopia may have more difficulty because of the increased thickness of the prism ballasted plus lenses. Individuals with loose lids may not be able to maintain proper alignment of the truncation on the lower lid margin with downward gaze. The advantages of this design are the same as the translating concentric designs; however, the Tangent Streak has the advantages of having larger distance zones and the absence of image jump. The disadvantages primarily pertain to the thickness inherent in their construction.

Recently, the first *fused* RGP segmented bifocal was introduced. The Fluoroperm 60 Fused Monocentric Bifocal (Paragon Optical) consists of a 60-Dk fluoro-silicone/acrylate button into which an encapsulated higher index segment is fused (Figure 9.8). A three-step molding process is used; the final step involves casting the Fluoroperm 60 material to totally "bury" the high index bifocal segment. Prism ballast and truncation are used for stabilization; however, the

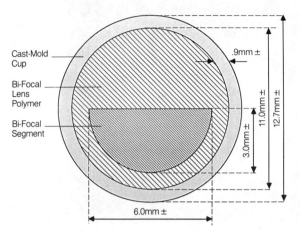

Cast-Mold Cup

Bi-Focal Lens Polymer

Bi-Focal Segment

.9mm ±

11.0mm ±

12.7mm ±

3.0mm ±

6.0mm ±

Figure 9.8 Construction of the Paragon ST Fused Monocentric Bifocal RGP showing dimensions of the lens button. (courtesy of Paragon Optical).

amount of prism required is less (that is, 1.25 to 1.75 Δ in plus powers; 2.00 to 2.50 Δ in minus powers) than with the Tangent Streak lens because this lens design may be lenticulated, and truncation may not always be necessary with minus lens powers.

Similar to the Tangent Streak, the diagnostic set consists of +/− 2.00-D distance powers, a + 2.00 D add, 9.4/9.0-mm overall diameters, and 1.5 Δ. The initial base curve selection depends upon the amount of corneal toricity. Typically, in spherical and low astigmatic corneas, fitting 0.25 to 0.50 D flatter than K is recommended. Moderate to high astigmatic patients should be fitted 0.25 to 0.75 D steeper than K (Hansen, 1992). As with other bifocal designs, power determination is very critical. The use of trial lenses for refining the distance power and determining the add power is important. To confirm proper fit, the fluorescein pattern should exhibit apical alignment to minimal apical touch (Figure 9.9).

The segment top should be positioned at, or slightly below, the inferior pupillary margin in normal room lighting. High slit-lamp illumination while viewing lens position will lead to ordering segments artificially low because of pupillary constriction. A minimum of 2 mm translation from primary to down gaze is required for proper segment function, with 3 mm being ideal.

This lens design is recommended for the same candidates as the other translating RGP bifocals. The primary advantages of the fused segment bifocal over the one-piece annular or crescent bifocals are: (1) monocentric optics resulting in an absence of image jump (the exception to this would be the Tangent Streak design), and (2) a 25% to 40% thinner and tighter lens profile. The problems present with this lens and their management options are similar to the Tangent Streak, and some patients report a disturbing peripheral glare, probably due to the internal reflection caused by the seg-lens interface.

Translating RGP lenses yield the highest success rate of any contact lens bifocals available today, but their fitting requires precise measurement of anterior eye anatomy, familiarity with the translating concept, use of a reliable diagnostic

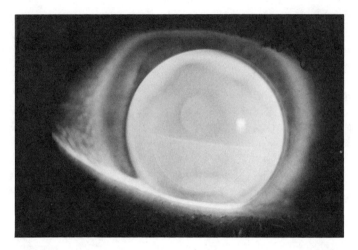

Figure 9.9 Fitting pattern of a properly positioned Paragon ST bifocal lens. Note fluorescence in the segment, which is correctly positioned slightly below the inferior pupillary margin.

lens, and a commitment to manage a specialty, complex lens that is custom designed by the clinician.

SOFT BIFOCAL DESIGNS
Simultaneous Vision

Simultaneous vision soft bifocals are similar in basic design to their rigid counterparts. These multifocal lenses include center-distance and center-near aspheric designs, center-distance and center-near concentric (target) designs and a diffraction bifocal. Centration is easier to obtain with soft lenses than with RGPs; therefore, the simultaneous image designs discussed below are easier to fit, but even with an ideal physical fit, they may not be as optically effective as similarly designed rigid lenses because of optical characteristics unique to soft lenses.

Aspheric
Center-Distance There are several available lens designs in which the center of the lens contains the distance correction, while the *posterior* aspheric surface flattens progressively toward the periphery, thus creating a gradual increase in plus power. These lens designs vary in their eccentricity or rate of posterior curve flattening, but even with the highest practical eccentricity, a +1.50 D add is the expected maximum add power for these aspherics.

These lenses are relatively easy to fit. Typically, only one or two "universal" base curve (often termed "shape factor") is available with a fixed progressive near add. As with rigid aspheric designs, good centration is imperative, as is adequate (but not excessive) lens movement with the blink.

The best candidates for these lenses include the early emerging presbyope, especially the first-time wearer who has never worn any correction and is now complaining of nearpoint problems. Because this design tends to provide good intermediate vision for the moderate presbyope, it often is fit unilaterally in combination with another form of bifocal design in a modified monovision correction. Patients exhibiting an average pupil size are preferable for this type of aspheric center-distance multifocal, as blur at distance is probable with large pupils, and inadequate vision at near is often reported with small pupils.

In problem-solving with this lens the following information may be beneficial:

1. Slight decentration — increase minus distance power
2. Excessive decentration — select another type of bifocal design
3. Blur at distance — re-evaluate such factors as pupil size, refractive cylinder, residual astigmatism, and centration
4. Blur at near — same as 3; in addition, if a higher add is required, changing to either a higher eccentricity or another type of bifocal would be indicated

Examples of this lens design are PA-1 (B & L), the Hydrocurve Bifocal (SBH), Allvue (Salvatore), and VX (CBF Laboratories).

Center-Near   The center-near design, more recently introduced, consists of a *front surface* aspheric in which the rate of curvature steepening or eccentricity decreases at a constant rate from the center to the edge of the optical zone, creating more minus power at the periphery. Therefore, the most plus (or add) power is central, and distance power increases as the distance from the optical center increases. It is also claimed that some of these lenses will correct up to 1 D of refractive with-the-rule astigmatism as a result of the aspheric optics (Bennett et al., 1990).

The initial lens power is determined by taking the best spherical refraction, dropping the cylinder, and adding one-half of the necessary add power. Another method for the initial trial lens is simply to add + 1.25 D to the distance spherical refraction. A binocular over-refraction using trial lenses is by far the best method of power determination and should be performed in normal room illumination. Distance clarity of vision should be emphasized in the dominant eye, and maximum plus near power should be prescribed for the non-dominant eye. Examples of this lens type are the Unilens and PS-45 (Nissel). Some of the problems of aspheric multifocal soft lenses relate to unpredictable lens draping and flexure on some corneas, which affects the in-situ power of the lens, and the angle Kappa (visual axis and its relation to the geometric center of the pupil).

Concentric/Annular

Center-Distance   Most of the concentric soft bifocals are center-near in design, although one center-distance design is presently available. Some are available in multiple base curve radii, and all have a range of add powers. These lenses are known as "pupil dependent" bifocals, using "shared simultaneous imagery" (Josephson and Caffery, 1991).

Good centration is imperative for successful adaptation. As pupil size varies, both between individuals as well as resulting from change in illumination, it is difficult to maintain the necessary parity of near and distance focus light reaching the retina. In particular, for individuals with small pupils performing near work with a high-intensity light source, it is possible that essentially none of the near zone will be located within the pupil. Therefore, normal to slightly large pupil sizes are recommended for this lens type. The availability of high add powers makes these concentric lenses a possible alternative to aspheric simultaneous vision lenses in advanced presbyopia. It has been used effectively in combination with aspheric soft lenses to provide a "modified" monovision correction in some patients (Herndon et al., 1984), using two different types of bifocal lenses on each eye.

Center-Near As with rigid concentric bifocal lenses, the rationale for this type of design is that pupil constriction will maximize near vision, assuming high illumination conditions, whereas distance vision will be optimized in lower illumination conditions as the pupil enlarges. There are several of these designs currently available (e.g., Alges [Universal], Spectrum [Ciba]).

Typically, these lenses are available in multiple add diameters and powers. The ability to vary the size of the near zone is a major advantage of this lens design and, for that matter, with any multifocal lens. To balance the near and distance vision, the center add diameter is selected to achieve approximately 50% area coverage of the pupil when in illumination levels appropriate for reading (Baldwin, 1988). In addition, unequal add diameters often are used to optimize distance vision in one eye and near in the other eye. The ability to vary the add diameter in combination with the availability of both low and high add powers increase the chances of patient acceptance and success. However, as with aspheric and other simultaneous vision concentric designs, vision at distance and near may vary because of the pupil size dependence. Patients with small pupils (that is, 2 to 3 mm), in particular, may not be good candidates for center-near bifocals because of compromised distance vision. For example, while a person is driving a car during daylight hours or participating in outdoor sports, blurred vision at distance caused by a combination of small pupil size and pupil constriction can severely affect performance (Josephson and Caffery, 1991).

Some representative problems and management alternatives include:

1. Blur at near — increase add diameter in non-dominant eye
2. Blur at distance — decrease add diameter in dominant eye
3. Poor intermediate vision — change to aspheric design

Diffractive Bifocals

Diffractive bifocals, which are a recently developed and different lens design and concept, called Echelon (Allergan) are cast molded and, as with the rigid diffractive lens (Diffrax), use a diffraction zone plate to equally separate light rays to both the distance and near focal images. The distance power is *refracted,* and the near power is achieved by the diffractive principles. The major advantage of this design is pupil size *independence.* The near diffractive power is achieved through the circular annular grooves (echelettes) on the back surface of the lens and the refractive index of the tear layer that pools behind the grooves. The radii and spacing of the annular grooves determine the add power of the lens. This posterior diffractive zone is approximately 4.00 to 4.5 mm in diameter, located at the center of the line, and the entire lens contains the distance power. The central zone plate can easily be observed against the dark background of the pupil with biomicroscopy. When fitting this lens, the use of trial lenses to assess fit, centration, and power determination by over-refraction is essential (Figure 9.10). If only slight decentration is present, the patient can still be successful with the Echelon lens; however, more add power may be required in this case.

Patient education is very important to the eventual success of this lens and, for that matter, for most multifocal contact lenses. There is typically as long as a 1-month adaptation period. Patients must be informed that a glare or ghosting of images effect is often present initially. For this reason, driving at night is not recommended for the first several days when initial adaptation is occurring. In addition, a "3-D" effect, in which a shadow-like ghost image is present around printed letters, is often reported (Herrin, 1989). These optical disturbances often dissipate with adaptation. Finally, patients must be aware that there will be reduced retinal luminance at all distances, and high ambient illumination will be necessary for many visual tasks, especially those involving critical near work.

Both moderate and advanced presbyopes are candidates for this design if they react favorably to the visual compromises discussed above during the trial fitting evaluation. A benefit of this design is often that the optometrist can

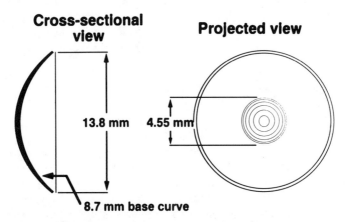

Figure 9.10 Diagram of the Echelon soft bifocal contact lens.

determine if the patient is going to be successful or not during the trial fitting process alone. If good centration is obtained without excessive lens lag (2 mm or greater) with the blink, and the patient does not complain of "darkness," then this patient probably will be successful. In theory, this pupil-independent bifocal concept provides two discrete, focused images on the retina (distance and near), which are more competitive with each other than in the case of other simultaneous image bifocals; therefore, one can be more readily suppressed for a given visual situation.

Problem-solving with the Echelon is similar to the Diffrax lens and is based upon recommendations provided in the literature (Bennett et al., 1990; Vehige, 1992).

Alternating Vision

One alternating vision soft bifocal (Bitech [Bausch and Lomb]) is currently available. This is a periballasted truncated, non-rotating lens that has an executive style segment. It is available in multiple base curve radii and several seg heights. It is of monocentric design; therefore, no image jump occurs when the patient views from distance to near. It is cast molded on the anterior surface and lathe cut posteriorly and has good optics.

The flattest base curve with the highest seg should be fitted initially as comfort and distance vision are often good with this lens, but adequate near vision may be a problem because of incomplete or inconsistent upward translation of the near seg. Obviously, it is desirable to have the segment near the inferior pupillary margin during distance gaze, and attain 2–3 mm upward translation of the lens with downward gaze for optimum near vision.

The benefits of this lens are identical to rigid monocentric ballasted translating designs, albeit with astigmatic restrictions of hydrogel lens correction. Early and advanced presbyopes of any pupil size may be fitted with this lens. If it translates properly during near gaze, the vision should be quite good at both distances. However, it is important to carefully evaluate the position of the near segment when viewing inferiorally with the aid of a dental mirror. Unfortunately, too often there is a tendency for the lens truncation to slip under the lower lid, thereby losing the add effect. In this case, this lens design is not recommended.

LENS SELECTION
Success Rates

The low lens cost, ease of fitting, and relatively high success rates (often 70% to 90%) achieved with monovision have made it a popular technique for presbyopic contact lens correction among practitioners (Josephson et al., 1991). In a large population study comparing monovision to both a small (2-mm) zone center-near bifocal lens and a similar size zone in a center-distance lens design, monovision was preferred in about 70% of the cases (Back et al., 1987). However, several comparison studies (Josephson and Caffery, 1987; Pence et al.,

1986) have resulted in slight patient preference for center-distance aspheric bifocal designs versus monovision. In another comparative study, a high but similar patient preference was found for monovision and a hydrogel diffractive lens, versus a low patient preference for a concentric zone bifocal (Molinari, 1989). Published soft bifocal success rates have varied considerably depending on the study design, the definition of "success," the length of the study (that is, one-year would be preferable to 3- or 6-month studies), how patients were screened, and acceptance criteria. Most soft bifocal studies result in only a 40% to 50% success rate (Donshik and Luistro, 1987; Hanks, 1984; Edwards and Haig-Brown, 1987; Herrin, 1989). Therefore, the need to screen patients and use an adequate and reliable diagnostic set of the desired bifocal lens design is imperative. Clinical success rates have been reported to be much higher with rigid bifocal lenses, especially translating designs such as the Tangent Streak in which success rates have varied from 52% to 91% (Josephson et al., 1989; Remba, 1988; Kirman and Kirman, 1990). Research with 200 patients enrolled in the Diffrax RGP investigation resulted in 79% of presenting patients being acceptable to fit; of these patients, 75% achieved successful wear (Walker and Churms, 1987).

Extended wear is not recommended for older patients, particularly as complication rates for all extended wear soft lenses is approximately four to six times that of daily wear (Poggio et al., 1990). Aphakic extended wear is discussed in Chapter 11.

Factors Important to Patient Success

A summary nomogram of lens — eye matching outlining which bifocal lens should be fit to a given patient based on such factors as refractive error, add power, lid position, pupil size, and oxygen need is presented in Figure 9.11. The most important considerations, however, are the visual demands and expectations of the patient (Caffery and Josephson, 1991). The first lens of choice for those individuals who lower their gaze to perform their work is a translating RGP segment design. Patients who need intermediate and/or near vision while viewing in the primary position of gaze would benefit from a simultaneous bifocal such as an aspheric, or annular design. Annular and diffractive bifocals would benefit the advanced presbyope, and aspheric multifocals often are used in a modified monovision technique for emerging presbyopes. Therefore, such individuals as video display terminal operators, plumbers, electricians, and draftsmen can be considered for these simultaneous image type lenses. It is preferable to attempt to simulate the patient's working environment during the screening visit when determining the type and powers of a presbyopic contact lens correction with the aid of trial lenses. At minimum, one translating RGP trial set, one aspheric RGP trial set, and two to three different soft simultaneous design trial sets should be sufficient for good patient screening and success assessment. Initially, it is desirable to order lenses on a warranty basis; once experience has been gained with a particular bifocal lens, the additional fee for a warranty may not be necessary. For the many patients who are entering presbyopia and are long-term successful single-vision

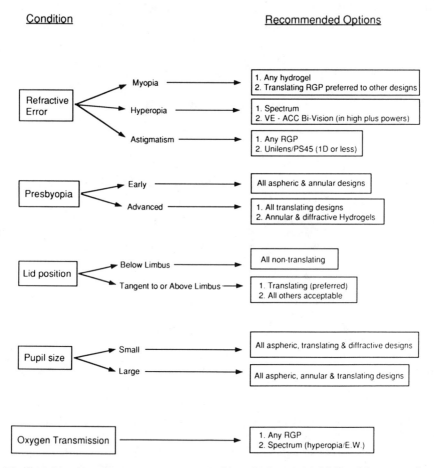

Bifocal Contact Lens Selection Nomogram

Figure 9.11 A summary monogram matching the best initial bifocal lens type for specific ocular characteristics.

contact lens wearers, it is best to stay with the same lens material, rigid or soft, when refitting with a multifocal lens.

What about the role of monovision? Certainly, the controversy continues as to how monovision should be positioned in the practice, whether as a first or last choice. Although monovision is a viable option, unless definite contraindications are found, it is a good idea to assess patient response to a bifocal diagnostic lens fitting prior to choosing monovision empirically as the first presbyopic contact lens option.

PATIENT EDUCATION AND LENS CARE

Presbyopic patients, especially new contact lens wearers, need to be thoroughly educated about proper lens care and handling. Contact lens wear can be intimidating for the patient who has not only experienced 45 or more years of non-lens wear but who also may have been exposed to negative experiences/complications from friends and relatives. In addition, these individuals need to be monitored closely, as a result of possible complications that may arise from the aforementioned physiologic changes of the aging eye, as well as to reinforce compliance to lens care procedures.

Care and Handling

The keys for successful handling of contact lenses by the presbyopic patient is patience and *reassurance*. These older individuals — especially the novice wearer — will be apprehensive, and lack confidence. No matter how frustrating it is to the individual performing the instruction, that feeling of frustration must not be conveyed to the patient. The instructions must be provided slowly and on a one to one basis. The patient should never have the perception that the optometrist has lost confidence in his or her ability to handle the lenses properly; otherwise, feelings of failure and surrender may result. Conversely, if the patient feels confident about handling the lenses, the feeling of accomplishment improves the motivation to succeed.

The key to successful insertion and removal of both soft and rigid lenses is proper manipulation of the lid. For insertion, the fingers are positioned over the lashes, or close to the lid margins while retracting the lids, the lenses can be inserted easily, no matter how much resistance is initially present. This is especially important with the older patient who usually has loose lids. If improperly performed, the lids may evert, resulting in insufficient pressure to either insert or remove the contact lens. The customary lid pull "scissors" technique is used in removing rigid lenses. Both hands should be used to execute a lens ejection technique. The middle and index fingers of the same hand (as eye) are positioned over the lower lid; the middle and index fingers of the opposite hand hold up the upper lid (Figure 9.12a). The lids are then pulled laterally and, while the patient blinks, the lens is ejected (Figures 9.12b and 9.12c). The lid margins are responsible for the lens ejection. Some difficulty can be present in full opening of the lid aperture when inserting a soft lens because of the larger diameter. Once again, it is important to use both hands to fully retract the lids for soft lens insertion. The middle finger of the opposite hand should be placed underneath the upper lashes; with the lens on the forefinger of the same hand as the eye, the middle finger of this hand is placed over the lower lashes (Figure 9.12). This should create a sufficient aperture for direct lens placement on the eye. Soft lens removal may be accomplished by the usual decentration and "punching" method or by "ejection" using pressure of upper and lower lid margins against the lens edges, pressing into the globe.

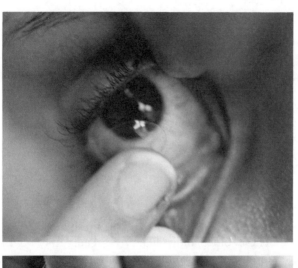

A

B

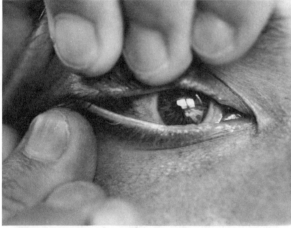

C

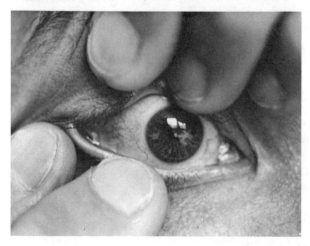

Figure 9.12 (a) Method of lid retraction and contact lens insertion best suited for most presbyopic contact lens users. (b) "Scissors" method of rigid lens removal. (c) "Squeeze" or ejection method of rigid lens removal.

During the training visit, a minimum of three successful insertions and removals is recommended, although the number depends on the level of the patient's confidence. It may require two or three visits (closely spaced to maximize memory of techniques and to minimize further anxiety) for the patient to master lens handling. This is occasionally necessary with the presbyopic hyperopic patient who is not only apprehensive but may experience difficulty seeing the lens because of the short working distance involved in lens preparation. To assist with this problem — especially with the absolute presbyope — ordinary reading spectacles can be worn up to the time of lens insertion. In addition, special magnifying lens insertion aids are available, or an illuminated makeup mirror may be useful.

Educational Methods

Comprehensive education of the presbyopic patient is mandatory. A four-step process has been recommended (Bennett and Grohe, 1991; Bennett, 1991). This should include (1) a written manual, (2) verbal, (3) video, and (4) re-education.

Separate *instructional manuals* for soft and rigid lenses are available from all manufacturers and other sources. A patient instructional manual should be comprehensive and written in layman's language with print quality that makes it easy to read, understand, and comply with the information presented. This manual should include the following information:

1. Benefits of contact lens wear (rigid or soft)
2. Insertion and removal
3. Cleaning techniques
4. Normal and abnormal adaptation symptoms
5. Importance of adhering to prescribed wearing schedule
6. Causes of reduced wear
7. Importance of using recommended care regimen
8. Spare pairs, spectacles
9. Service agreement
10. Cosmetic use
11. Caring for the lens case

It also can contain a patient agreement that has the individual office policy on issues such as the payment and refund policy, care regimen, and what to do in case of an emergency. This should be signed in duplicate by the patient. It cannot be expected that the patient will read and understand the entire document; therefore, this agreement can serve as an informed consent for medico-legal purposes. A special informed consent for monovision patients has been recommended (Harris and Classe, 1988). This should indicate the benefits and possible hazards with monovision in addition to mentioning that alternative forms of vision correction were discussed with the patient. The instruction manuals may be customized by the practitioner and should be printed professionally or by a desktop publishing system. Graphics showing how to handle the lenses are beneficial. These can be provided by a graphic artist or can be obtained on an Apple or IBM floppy diskette from Anadem Publications, Inc. (P.O. Box 14385, Columbus, OH 43214). The standard educational booklets from Anadem can be customized to the practitioner's satisfaction. Additional patient educational material is available from manufacturers of presbyopic lenses and are useful.

In addition to instructions on handling, the patient needs to be instructed on the functions of the various solutions and how to properly use them. The most important information contained in the manual or patient brochure should be discussed with the patient, and the patient can be encouraged to ask questions. In fact, the patient should be asked to review how to use the solutions to ensure compliance of cleaning, rinsing, and disinfection steps. It should be emphasized that the *verbal* and *visual* (demonstrated) educational process is much more important than the written because patients cannot be expected to understand all of the information provided and, on occasion, the manual may not be read at all.

A more innovative and effective method of patient education is the use of *videotapes* on care and handling to supplement the instructional manual and verbal information. A generic rigid lens care and handling videotape is available from the RGP Lens Institute/CLMA (1-800-343-5367). If any reservations exist pertaining to a patient's ability to handle or care for contact lenses, a videotape reviewed together in the office or for frequent viewing at home would be an excellent supplement to the instruction manual.

Finally, lens care instructions and care compliance should be reinforced at every follow-up visit. For example, patients should be asked to repeat the name and use of the solutions they are currently using, if they have any questions about handling, the condition of their case if available (the optometrist may want to replace the case at regular intervals such as every 3 months), how they are caring for the lenses, and the wearing schedule. It has been found that if the manufacturer's recommended care instructions are reinforced at every progress visit, only 6% of the solution samples were contaminated; if the care instructions were not reinforced, more than 50% of the samples were contaminated (Wilson, 1991). All of these suggestions become more important for the aging patient, who is more likely to forget.

The Care Regimen

Every product in the care kit provided to a new RGP or soft lens patient should be explained because each component is part of a system. It cannot be assumed that every patient will carefully read and understand product labels and care instructions. It is not uncommon to have patients who believe that their wetting/soaking solution also cleans the lenses, or that their cleaning solution is also used for wetting and soaking. If each product is explained and the patient still appears to be confused, the specific care instructions for each care product can be provided in written form. In addition, a large label can be placed on each bottle specifically indicating its function.

The decrease in tear quality and volume occurring with age, which contributes to lens deposits, makes it imperative to carefully explain the importance of proper and regular cleaning and enzyme use to minimize deposit-related problems. Rewetting drops are frequently prescribed, and their proper application should be reinforced.

Follow-up Care

Presbyopic contact lens patients should be regularly monitored, preferably every 6 months. As a result of their predisposition for dryness-related problems, a careful slit-lamp evaluation with contact lens wear is important. The surface condition and wettability of the worn lens should be carefully evaluated and aging, deposited lenses must be replaced. If feasible (that is, monovision), a one- to three-month planned replacement program should be used with soft lens wearing patients. With lenses off, the cornea should be evaluated with fluorescein dye and the upper eyelids should be everted to rule out papillary changes. In addition, as the bifocal lens designs are often thicker than their single-vision counterparts, the cornea should be evaluated for the presence of corneal edema resulting from possible hypoxia. If straie, central corneal clouding, or another form of edema is present, a thinner design and higher oxygen transmissible material are indicated. Keratometry and refraction also should be performed during follow-up visits, notably with patients wearing the thicker bifocal designs, in which undesirable curvature and refractive changes may occur.

PRESBYOPIA SUMMARY

The presbyopic contact lens market is growing every year. It appears that numerous companies are developing new multifocal lenses in hopes of capturing the "baby-boomers" who have, or are reaching, presbyopic age. The cosmetic and sometimes functional benefits of contact lenses should make them a recommended option for every contact lens-using presbyopic patient and for the many who are becoming aware of multifocal contact lenses. Every presbyopic patient should not automatically be considered for monovision; in fact, a bifocal diagnostic fitting should be considered as the first option for most presbyopes. Finally, comprehensive education and follow-up care should be performed to ensure patient confidence with care and handling, verify compliance with the care regimen, and minimize the risks that are associated with contact lens wear.

THERAPEUTIC/BANDAGE CONTACT LENS*

When a contact lens is applied to heal or protect the eye, as opposed to use for either refractive correction or as a cosmetic aid, it is considered a therapeutic or "bandage" contact lens. This is not a new concept; contact lenses have been used to protect eyes for almost 100 years, beginning with scleral shells (Obrig, 1942) and continuing through the early use of hydrogels (Gasset and Kaufman, 1970).

Hydrogel contact lenses, in particular, have emerged as valuable devices in managing many corneal diseases over the last several decades, with the following broad clinical goals (Mondino et al., 1987):

1. Reduction of pain from corneal epithelial defects;
2. Facilitation and maintenance of corneal epithelial healing;
3. Protection of the cornea from desiccation (drying);
4. Protection of the cornea from mechanical damage secondary to entropion and trichiasis; and
5. Restoration of the anterior chamber following collapse from small corneal perforations.

The majority of patients aided by the use of these bandage hydrogel contact lenses are elderly. The diseases tend to be chronic, usage of these lenses is often on an extended wear basis, and because of this use and the co-existence of often multiple disease processes, both ocular and systemic, these patients are known to be more at risk for corneal infection (Brown et al., 1974; Donnefield et al., 1986; Kent et al., 1990).

Available Lens Designs

Several hydrogel contact lenses have received specific FDA approval for use in a therapeutic mode; these are listed in Table 9.1. These lenses are usually prescribed plano in optical power, so as to provide a parallel-sided uniform thickness shell of hydrophilic plastic to maximize oxygen flux (Weissman, 1982).

Clinicians, however, do not restrict themselves solely to these designs, but often use any of the many different types of "conventional" contact lenses available to meet the specific clinical needs of the patient, almost always using soft rather than rigid contact lenses. Although it is best from the standpoint of maintaining oxygen supply to the cornea to use essentially plano-powered lenses, occasionally the specific needs of a particular patient also must be considered, and powered lenses are occasionally applied for dual use as both a therapeutic bandage and a refractive device. In either case, vision is often optimized with forward overspectacles, as excessively high power, thick lenses should be avoided if possible.

Therapeutic Hydrogel Contact Lens Fitting Principles

The first principle is that *corneal protection demands full corneal coverage.* To this end, most hydrogel contact lenses employed as bandages will have larger (14.5–15.5mm), rather than smaller overall diameters (13.0–14.0mm).

*This part of the chapter was written by Barry A. Weissman, O.D., Ph.D., of the Jules Stein Eye Institute, UCLA School of Medicine. The authors gratefully acknowledge the assistance of Bartley Mondino, M.D., of the same institution in the preparation of this section.

Lens thickness should be minimized to maintain oxygenation both for the maintenance of corneal physiology, especially if extended wear lenses are used, and to promote epithelial healing (Mauger and Hill, 1987).

Lenses should be applied, with the proper selection of base curve and diameter, to *maintain lens centration and stability*; movement of the lens on the anterior ocular surface should be somewhat less than required for a cosmetic application, but not so tight as to totally restrict movement. Minimization of lens movement facilitates patient acceptance by decreasing lid sensation and is helpful in decreasing mechanical trauma to healing epithelial cells. Lenses should not be so steep, however, that indentation of the sclera, conjunctival vascular blanching, central air bubbles, or rippling of the conjunctiva (Mobilia et al., 1980) occur; in themselves, these may not be serious problems, but hydrogel lenses, especially if used for extended wear, may steepen with dehydration or changes in pH or aging, and then may induce a "tight lens syndrome," where the eye becomes painful and inflamed, and the epithelium may even slough (Murphy, 1981; Snyder et al., 1982).

Optimum water content is an area of some controversy. Some authors suggest that the higher water content hydrogel lenses are effective in dry eye situations by providing a reservoir for fluid (Thoft, 1983). Others propose that evaporation from the anterior surface of high water content hydrogel lenses draws water from the precorneal tear film and epithelium, perhaps then further dehydrating the anterior surface of the eye (Baldone and Kaufman, 1983). This effect, if it exists, may be helpful in managing bullous keratopathy but problematic in cases of dry eye.

In addition, if it is at all possible for the patient to manage a therapeutic lens on a daily wear basis, and if the disease being managed allows such use (as opposed to requiring continual overnight wear), such a mode is preferable to reduce the risk of infection and neovascularization and to facilitate the installation of medication. The thinner, lower Dk/L lenses are ideal for such use. Lens maintenance and cleaning should be with heat, chemical agents, or peroxide as appropriate for the contact lens material and patient situation. The higher Dk/L lenses should be used when extended wear is elected or necessitated. Disposable or frequent replacement hydrogels might be ideal in this use. Cleaning routines as appropriate should be employed as frequently as the disease process and the patient's particular situation and removal cycles will allow.

Frequent professional evaluations are essential in the continuing management of therapeutic contact lens patients, especially if the lenses are used under extended wear conditions. The initially fitted patient should be seen one to two hours after the first lens application to confirm the continued proper fit of the lens and to observe any acute physiological or physical response. Lens changes are not uncommon at this point in order to refine the fit. The progress schedule beyond this evaluation varies with the precise situation, but in general patients should be seen the day after application, the day following the first night lens wear, and at intervals ranging from weekly to monthly or perhaps — when the patient's situation is stable and if the clinician considers risks minimum (e.g., the lens is used for daily wear) — at even 3-month intervals. Some situations suggest therapeutic lens management only for short intervals, days or weeks, while healing occurs, and others require maintaining the lens on the eye for months or even years to manage chronic and/or unresponsive problems. In many such cases, patients who are unable to handle their lenses visit the clinician's office periodically for lens cleaning, inspection, and reinsertion. Coordinated co-management of most of these patients with both a contact lens provider and corneal specialist is considered ideal. Concomitant aggressive medical (e.g., antibiotics, cyclopegics, steroids) and perhaps surgical treatment is often required for best patient care.

Indications for therapeutic hydrogels:

1. Corneal dystrophies that result in epithelial irregularity and erosion, such as map-dot-fingerprint, Meesman's, Reis-Buckler's, lattice, granular, and macular dystrophies. Hydrogel lenses decrease recurrent breakdown of the epithelium, minimizing pain, foreign-body sensations, photophobia and tearing.
2. Other recurrent or chronic epithelial erosions or healing disorders, perhaps due to trauma, metaherpetic disease, chemical (especially alkali) burns or surgery, where the lens is an alternative to pressure patching the eye to promote re-epithelialization of a surface defect.
3. Protection from corneal damage due to rubbing of inwardly directed eyelashes in entropion with trichiasis, or from the inflammation and mechanical abrasion of the large papillae of the upper tarsal conjunctiva in vernal keratoconjunctivitis.
4. Improving patient comfort and healing with Thygeson's superficial punctate keratitis (Forstot and Binder, 1979; Goldberg et al., 1980).
5. Maintaining comfort for patients with endothelial failure and corneal edema from Fuch's dystrophy, or aphakic or pseudophakic bullous keratopathy. The related severe epithelial and stromal edema leads to large epithelial blisters that produce photophobia, foreign-body sensation, and pain when they rupture. The presense of a hydrogel bandage lens reduces these problems, perhaps by mechanically reinforcing the damaged tissue, by reducing the occurrence of ruptures, or by covering the otherwise exposed nerve endings from the rubbing action of the lids.
6. Relief of pain associated with superior limbic keratoconjunctivitis (Mondino et al., 1982).
7. Protecting the cornea in cases of dry eye, with additional artificial tears and ocular lubricants. This use is somewhat controversial (see above) and, again, patients are often at greater risk of infection (Dohlman et al., 1973) and should be managed very conservatively.
8. Bullous diseases of the conjunctiva, such as ocular cicatricial pemphigoid and the Stevens-Johnson syndrome, may be partially managed with therapeutic hydrogels (Mondino et al., 1987). The lenses protect the corneal epithelium from drying and from mechanical damage from eyelid abnormalities such as entropion with trichiasis.

9. Protecting the corneal surface after neurological damage to cranial nerve V or VII to facilitate and maintain the epithelial cells. Because of the very high risk of infection (lesions to cranial nerve V result in anesthesia, and lesions to cranial nerve VII lead to abnormal blinking and secondary hydrogel lens dehydration), this should be considered only after other methods, such as pressure patching, tarsorraphy, and conjunctival flap, cannot be considered or have failed.

10. Structural reinforcement and promotion of healing and vascularization of weakened sites in the cornea: reforming the anterior chamber following a small perforation or wound dehiscence (Mannis and Zadnik, 1988) where the contact lens functions as a temporary splint, sometimes concomitant with the use of tissue adhesives, to seal the perforation; or supporting descemtoceles, and other stromal thinning disorders (e.g., Mooren's ulcer [Leibowitz and Rosenthal, 1971; Arentsen et al., 1984]), perhaps to temporize patient care while waiting for definitive surgical treatment (Leibowitz and Berrospi, 1975).

11. Filimentary keratitis, especially if associated with blinking abnormalities.

Contraindications

Therapeutic hydrogel contact lenses should not be used in the presence of active microbial infection of the eye. When the contralaterial eye is infected, lens wear should be discontinued, if at all possible, until the infection has cleared to preclude the possibility of it spreading to the second eye.

A therapeutic lens should not be used when a patient is unwilling or unable to return for progress evaluations or unwilling or unable to comply with reasonable care guidelines. Not only should patients present for their scheduled visits, they also should be advised to return immediately if they should experience any pain, injection of the conjunctiva, or reduced vision. The participation of family members in their lens handling and follow-up compliance is very helpful and should be encouraged.

Additional contraindications include all of those that apply to all potential hydrogel lens users: dusty, polluted environments, poor personal hygiene, concomitant lid diseases like blepharitis; obstructions or infections of the lacrimal drainage system; or filtering blebs, which can serve as a pathway for infection to spread from the surface of the globe to become endophthalmitis. In general, any actively inflamed eye, with lid and conjunctival chemosis, is difficult to manage and more likely to develop infectious and inflammatory complications. Most corneal topographies and curvatures, however, may be fitted with today's wide range of available lenses.

Contact Lens Complications

All of the known complications of contact lens wear can occur with therapeutic lens use, but they are likely to be both more severe and more prevalent in this setting with the elderly patient. Of greatest concern is infectious keratitis, which tends to be associated with gram positive and fungal microbes (rather than gram negative as found in cosmetic contact lens wear (Schein et al., 1989), and corneal neovascularization, which is probably stimulated by both a concomitant corneal disease and the extended wear of such lenses and, although desirable in some cases to promote the healing process, may result in visual loss from corneal opacification (Cogan and Kuuwabara, 1955) in others. The clinician should also be alert to sterile infiltrates, hypopyon, corneal staining, GPC, and so forth.

Collagen Shields

Contact lens type devices, made from biodegradable collagen, have recently been introduced to be used in a therapeutic contact lens format. These all dissolve while on the eye over an imprecisely defined time period of hours to days and may be best employed in a drug (principally antibiotic) delivery rather than protective mode, although the lubricant value of the dissolving device in wound healing may be helpful as well.

Success

Zadnik concludes that therapeutic hydrogel contact lenses are a valuable tool in managing the compromised corneal surface, although they are not universally efficacious (Zadnik, 1990). Because the eyes are diseased and the anterior segments compromised prior to the application of the contact lens, the failure of the device to achieve the therapeutic outcome desired may have been preordained. Such events should not discourage the contact lens practitioner; management of disease is not always successful.

REFERENCES

1. Arentsen, J.J., P.R. Laibson, and E.J. Cohen. "Management of corneal descemetoceles and perforations." *Trans. Am. Ophthalmol. Soc.* 82 (1984): 92–105.
2. Back, A.P., R. Woods, and B.A. Holden. "The Comparative Performance of Monovision and Various Concentric Bifocals." *Trans. BCLA Conference* (1987): 46–47.
3. Baldone, J.A., and H.E. Kaufman. "Soft contact lenses in clinical disease." *Am. J. Ophthalmol.* 95 (1983): 851.
4. Baldwin, J.S. "Fitting a Reverse RGP Bifocal." *Contact Lens Forum* 12, no. 2 (1988): 62–65.
5. Barr, J.T., and N.J. Bailey. "1990 Annual Report." *Contact Lens Spectrum 5*, no. 1 (1991): 32–39.
6. Benjamin, W.J., and I.M. Borish. Presbyopia, and Influence of Aging on the Contact Lens Prescription. In: Guillon, M., and C.M. Ruben (eds.). *A Textbook of Contact Lens Practice*. London: Chapman & Hall, in press.
7. Benjamin, W.J., and I.M. Borish. "Physiology of Aging and Its Influence on the Contact Lens Prescription." *J. Am. Optom. Assoc.* 62, no. 10 (1991): 743–752.
8. Benjamin, W.J., and M.A. Rasmussen. "Oxygen Consumption of the Superior Cornea following Eyelid Closure." *Acta Ophthalmol.* 66 (1988): 309–312.

9. Bennett, E.S., P.D. Becherer, R. Shaw, and V.A. Henry. "Bifocal Contact Lenses in the 1990s." *Contact Lens Forum* 15, no. 4 (1990):33–48.
10. Bennett, E.S., P.D. Becherer, R. Shaw, et al. "Bifocal Contact Lenses." In: Bennett, E.S. and V.A. Henry (eds.). *Clinical Manual of Contact Lenses.* Philadelphia: J.B. Lippincott, in press.
11. Bennett, E.S. "Contact Lens Care Systems." Presented at the Annual *National Research Symposium.* Toronto, Canada, August, 1991.
12. Bennett, E.S., and R.M. Grohe. "Lens Care and Patient Education." In: Bennett, E.S., and B.A. Weissman (eds.). *Clinical Contact Lens Practice.* Philadelphia: J.B. Lippincott, 1991: pp. 25–1 to 25–12.
13. Bennett, E.S., V.A. Henry, and B.W. Morgan. "The Diffrax™ Bifocal." *Contact Lens Forum* 15, no. 3 (1990): 31–35.
14. Blackwell, O.M., and H.R. Blackwell. "Visual Performance Data for 156 Normal Observers of Various Ages." *J. Illuminating Engineering Society* 1 (1971): 3–13.
15. Brown, S.I., S. Bloomfield, D.B. Pierce, and M. Tragakis. "Infections with therapeutic soft contact lens." *Arch. Ophthalmol.* 91 (1974): 274–277.
16. Caffery, B.A., and J. Josephson. "Rigid Bifocal Lens Correction." In: Bennett, E.S., and B.A. Weissman, (eds.). *Clinical Contact Lens Practice.* Philadelphia: J.B. Lippincott, 1991: 42–1 to 42–11.
17. Cogan, D.G. and T. Kuuwabara. "Lipogenesis of cells of the cornea." *Arch. Ophthalmol.* 59 (1955): 453–456.
18. Collins, M.J., B. Brown, and K.J. Bowman. "Contrast Sensitivity with Contact Lens Corrections for Presbyopia." *Ophthalmic. Physiol. Opt.* 9 (1989): 133–138.
19. Dohlman, C.H., S.A. Boruchoff, and E.F. Mobilia. "Complications in use of soft contact lenses in corneal disease." *Arch. Ophthalmol.* 90 (1973): 367.
20. Donnefield, E.D., E.J. Cohen, J.J. Arentsen, et al. "Changing trends in contact lens associated corneal ulcers." *CLAO J.* 12 (1986): 145–149.
21. Donshik, P.C., and A. Luistro. "Soft Bifocal Contact Lens Fitting with the Alges Lens." *CLAO Journal* 13, no. 3 (1987): 174–176.
22. Edwards, K., and G. Haig-Brown. "An Evaluation of Bifocal Lens Performance and the Design of a New Fitting Protocol." *Transactions of the BCLA* (1987): 30–34.
23. Forstot, S.L. and P.S. Binder. "Treatment of Thygeson's superficial punctate keratopathy with soft contact lenses." *Am. J. Ophthalmol.* 88 (1979): 186.
24. Gasset, A.R. and H.E. Kaufman. "Therapeutic uses of hydrophilic contact lenses." *Am. J. Ophthalmol.* 69 (1970): 252.
25. Goldberg, D.B., D.J. Schanzlin, and S.I. Brown. "Management of Thygeson's superficial punctate keratitis." *Am. J. Ophthalmol.* 89 (1980): 22.
26. Guth, S. "Effects of Age on Visibility." *Am. J. Optom.* 34, no. 9 (1957): 463–476.
27. Hansen, D. "Rigid Bifocal Contact Lenses." Presented at the *Annual Meeting of the American Academy of Optometry,* New Orleans, LA, December, 1989.
28. Hansen, D.W. "Current concepts of RGP multifocal lenses." *Practical Optom.* 3 (1992): 70–78.
29. Hanks, A. "Contact Lenses for Presbyopia." *Eye Contact* (1984): 9–14.
30. Harris, M.G., and J.G. Classe. "Clincolegal Considerations of Monovision." *J. Am. Optom. Assoc.* 59, no. 6 (1988): 491–495.
31. Herndon, L.A., D.J. Egan, and E.S. Bennett. "Case History: A Modified Approach to Hydrogel Bifocal Fitting." *Contact Lens Journal* 12, no. 6 (1984): 15–16.
32. Herrin, S. "How to Fit the New Bifocal Soft Lenses." *Rev. Optom.* 126, no. 6 (1989):57.

33. Josephson, J.E., and B.E. Caffery. "Monovision vs. Bifocal Contact Lenses: A Crossover Study." *J. Am. Optom. Assoc.* 58, no. 8 (1987): 652–654.
34. Josephson, J.E., and B.E. Caffery. "Hydrogel Bifocal Lenses." In: Bennett, E.S., and B.A. Weissman (eds.). *Clinical Contact Lens Practice.* Philadelphia: J.B. Lippincott: 43–1 to 43–20.
35. Josephson, J.E., P. Erickson, and B.E. Caffery. "The Monovision Controversy." In: Bennett, E.S., and B.A. Weissman (eds.). *Clinical Contact Lens Practice.* Philadelphia: J.B. Lippincott: 44–1 to 44–6.
36. Josephson, J.E., M. Wong, and B.E. Caffery. "Clinical Experience with the Tangent Streak RGP Bifocal Contact Lens." *J. Am. Optom. Assoc.* 60, no. 3 (1989): 166–170.
37. Kent, H.D., E.J. Cohen, P. Laibson, and J.J. Arentsen. "Microbial keratitis and corneal ulceration associated with therapeutic soft contact lenses." *CLAO J.* 16 (1990): 49–52.
38. Kirman, S.T., and G.S. Kirman. "Tangent Streak Bifocal Contact Lenses." *Contact Lens Update* 9, no. 5 (1990): 65–69.
39. Leibowitz, H.M. and A.R. Berrospi. "Initial treatment of descemetocele with hydrophilic contact lenses." *Ann. Ophthalmol.* 7 (1975): 1161–1166.
40. Leibowitz, H.M. and P. Rosenthal. "Hydrophilic contact lenses in corneal disease. I. Superficial sterile, indolent ulcers." *Arch. Ophthalmol.* 85 (1971): 163–166.
41. Loshin, D.S. "The Holographic/Diffractive Contact Lens." *International Contact Lens Clinic* 16 no. 3 (1989): 77–86.
42. Loshin, D.S., M.S. Loshin, and G. Comer. "Binocular Summation with Monovision Contact Lens Correction for Presbyopia." *International Contact Lens Clinic* 9 (1982): 161–165.
43. Mannis, M.J., and K. Zadnik. "Contact Lenses in the Elderly Patient." *Geriatric Opthalmology* 2, no. 6 (1986): 23–27.
44. Mannis, M.J. and K. Zadnik. "Hydrophilic contact lenses for wound stabilization in keratoplasty." *CLAO J.* 14 (1988): 199–202.
45. Mauger, T.F. and R.M. Hill. "Corneal epithelial healing in hypoxic environments." *Invest. Ophthalmol. Vis. Sci.* 28 (ARVO Suppl. 1987): 2.
46. McGill, E. and P. Erickson. "Stereopsis in Presbyopes Wearing Monovision and Simultaneous Vision Bifocal Contact Lenses." *Am. J. Optom. Physiol. Opt.* 65 (1988): 612–626.
47. Mobilia, E.F., G.K. Yamamoto, and C.H. Dohlman. "Corneal wrinkling induced by ultrathin soft contact lenses." *Ann. Ophthalmol.* 12 (1980): 371.
48. Molinari, J.F., and L. Caplan. "Clinical Evaluation of Two Soft Lens Bifocals." *J. Am. Optom. Assoc.* 57, no. 9 (1986): 484–487.
49. Mondino, B.J., B.A. Weissman, and R. Manthey. Therapeutic Soft Contact Lenses. In: Stenson, S.M. (ed.): *Contact Lenses: A Guide to Selection, Fitting and Management of Complications.* Norwalk: Appleton & Lange, 1987: 155–183.
50. Mondino, B.J., G.W. Zaidman, and S.W. Salamon. "Use of pressure patching and soft contact lenses in superior limbic keratoconjunctivitis." *Arch. Ophthalmol.* 100 (1982): 1932.
51. Murphy, G.E. "A case of sterile endophthalmitis associated with the extended wear of an aphakic soft contact lens." *Cont. Intraocul. Lens Med. J.* 7 (1981): 5.
52. Obrig, T.E. *Contact Lenses.* Philadelphia: Chilton, 1942: 41–92.
53. Pence, N.A., S. Polling, and P.S. Soni. "Progressive Soft Bifocal Lenses: A Comparative Study of Bausch & Lomb Versus Hydrocurve." Presented at the *Annual Meeting of the American Academy of Optometry,* Toronto, Canada, December, 1986.

54. Phillips, A.J. "Contact Lenses and the Elderly Patient." In: *Vision and Aging General and Clinical Perspectives*. Rosenbloom, A., and M. Morgan (eds). New York: Professional Press, 1986: pp. 267–300.
55. Poggio, E.C., R.J. Glynn, O.D. Schein, et al. "The Incidence of Ulcerative Keratitis among Users of Daily-Wear and Extended-Wear Soft Contact Lenses." *New Eng. J. Med.* 321, no. 12 (1989): 779–783.
56. Remba, M.J. "The Tangent Streak Rigid Gas Permeable Bifocal Contact Lens." *J. Am. Optom. Assoc.* 59, no. 3 (1988): 212–216.
57. Schein, O.D., L.D. Ormerod, E. Barraquer, et al. "Microbiology of contact lens-related keratitis." *Cornea* 8 (4) (1989): 281–285.
58. Snyder, D.A., S.M. Litinsky, and H. Calender. "Hypopyon iridocyclitis associated with extended wear soft contact lenses." *Am. J. Ophthalmol.* 93 (1982): 519.
59. Thoft, R.A. Therapeutic Soft Contact Lenses. In: Smolin, G. and R.A. Thoft, (eds.). *Cornea*. Boston: Little, Brown, 1983: 477–487.
60. Vehige, J.G. "Hydron Echelon Lens Fitting Guide: Part III Fitting Factors for Success." *Contact Lens Spectrum* 7, no. 2 (1992): 39–46.
61. Walker, P., and P. Churms. "The Diffractive Bifocal Contact Lens." *Optician* 194 (1987): 21–24.
62. Weale, R.A. *A Biography of the Eye: Development, Age, and Growth*. London: H.K. Lewis, 1982.
63. Weissman, B.A. "Designing uniform thickness contact lens shells." *Am. J. Optom. Physiol. Opt.* 59 (1982): 902.
64. Westendorf, D.H., R. Blake, M. Sloane, and D. Chambers. "Binocular Summation Occurs during Interocular Suppressions." *J. Exp. Psych.* 8 (1982): 81–90.
65. Wilson, L.A., A. O. Sawant, R.B. Simmons, and D.G. Ahearn. "Microbial Contamination of Contact Lens Storage Cases and Solutions." *Am. J. Ophthalmol.* 109, no. 2 (1990): 193.
66. Zadnik, K. Therapeutic Soft Contact Lenses. In: Harris, M.G. *Contact Lenses and Ocular Disease*. Philadelphia: J.B. Lippincott, (1990): 632–642.

10

Functional Therapy in the Rehabilitation of Elderly Patients

Bruce C. Wick

Vision is a complex synkinesis of biochemistry, neural structures, physiology, and learning. The interrelationships are often not well understood but aging causes major changes in visual performance and, as is true in youth, specific deficits frequently do not account for overall performance decrements. The decline of visual abilities with age is a fact of mature life and ranges from severe deterioration to minor reductions in visual function. For most mature adults, the loss of visual sensory and motor abilities impairs performance of all perceptual tasks.

Perception of the environment through vision requires that the visual system be able to effectively gather information. Generally, people do not experience severe visual acuity impairment with increasing age (Weymouth, 1960); however, most suffer from decreases in oculomotor function. Losses of accommodative ability (presbyopia), field of vision, and eye movement speed and accuracy can cause profound difficulties in binocular information gathering and processing.

These losses often can be remedied by selective rehabilitative techniques. Although perceptual aspects of vision care are very important, these aspects will be dealt with only partially. The primary emphasis of the material in this chapter will be the functional rehabilitation of vision problems, with emphasis on motor aspects of binocular vision for patients with normal, static visual acuity.

OCULOMOTOR FUNCTIONS

A thorough understanding of the basis and development of normal oculomotor function is necessary before any rehabilitation can begin. Equally important is an understanding of the changing normals of age that occur in all individuals. For example, losses in vergence ability and changes in tonic vergence accompany presbyopia and the normal aging process. (Chapter 6 of this book discusses normal changes in visual function with aging.) Rehabilitative techniques should be considered when normal aging changes cause individuals to depart from required abilities to perform adequately.

VERGENCE EYE MOVEMENTS

The diagnosis and rehabilitation of oculomotor system dysfunction requires an understanding of pursuit, saccadic, and vergence eye movements (Schor and Ciuffreda, 1983). Vergence eye movements generally are considered to consist of four components: tonic, accommodative, disparity (fusional), and proximal (Maddox, 1893). In the diagnosis and treatment of visual motor problems, vergence magnitudes often are related to one another using various criteria to evaluate whether symptoms are likely to be caused by the findings present.

Components of the total vergence response depend on age and show specific decrements as time passes. There are especially dramatic decreases in accommodative function (Hamasaki et al., 1956; Sun et al., 1988) with a corresponding loss in accommodative vergence and, subsequently, near convergence ability (Sheedy and Saladin, 1975; Wick, 1985). In light of other decrements in motor and sensory ocular ability with age, it is not surprising that disparity vergence ability also decreases with age.

DIAGNOSIS OF OCULOMOTOR DYSFUNCTIONS

The proper diagnosis of visual problems of the aged is facilitated by taking a thorough, careful history. Patients usually have two or three main visual problems that they want solved. Careful listening by the examiner, combined with well-directed questions and a systematic approach to obtaining pertinent information, will improve the chances of an accurate history. The value of a complete, accurate history increases with the patient's age because ocular disease, systemic disease, side effects of medication, and accidental injury all have increased incidence. The history can be conveniently divided into two parts: general and visual.

General History

A general history should be taken prior to any examination, and it frequently indicates many tests that should be performed. During examination of elderly patients, pertinent visual complaints often are obscured by rambling, and sometimes incoherent, details. Often an accompanying member of the family can (or needs to) be consulted, because an aged patient may overlook key points of the history. In these instances, family members can be of great help, as well as prevent exasperation to the patient.

Visual History

Visual history taking should be continued throughout the examination. A fixed sequence of questions can be useful, but information volunteered by the patient during the examination often has the greatest value (Wick, 1960). Information gathered during the examination may lead to other areas that need to be explored and indicate ancillary tests that will facilitate an accurate diagnosis of the visual problem.

Determining the patient's occupation and hobbies is of the utmost importance for prescriptive purposes, including working distances, times, lighting conditions, and occupational requirements. Frequently, the aged are unaware that different types of lenses are needed or available for various visual tasks. Thus, in spite of a careful history, many visual requirements may be neglected because the patient is unaware of the visual requirements of specific tasks.

Specific questions related to binocular problems should be asked: When do symptoms occur? When do they start? How long do they last? What relieves the symptoms? With what tasks do they occur? And, is there any diplopia? When the patient complains of newly acquired diplopia, there is usually a paretic or restrictive etiologic factor involving oculomotor pathology. However, patients frequently confuse double vision with distorted or blurred vision, so it is important to be sure that diplopia truly exists. The following are nonpathologic causes of diplopia:

1. Strabismus/heterophoria
   a. *Fusional disturbances.* Intermittent diplopia may be associated with uncompensated heterophoria and comitant heterotropias with inadequate suppression.
   b. *Postoperative diplopia.* This is a complication of strabismus surgery that may persist for years. It frequently follows cosmetic operations in older patients.
   c. *Onset of comitant strabismus.* Diplopia is experienced briefly at the onset of a comitant deviation before suppression begins. These patients are typically young children who rarely describe their symptoms accurately.
   d. *Uncompensated congenital palsy.* In patients with congenital muscle palsies who have maintained single binocular vision by appropriate head posturing and fusional mechanisms, a breakdown in fusional ability may result in sudden diplopia. This occurs in particular with congenital superior oblique palsies in which fusional reserves are weakened (for example, following a long illness). A review of old photographs will reveal a head tilt that has been maintained throughout life.
   e. *Sudden onset of comitant strabismus.* Although almost all comitant strabismus develops insidiously, occasionally a comitant deviation appears suddenly and is accompanied by annoying diplopia. This is most common in patients with high heterophorias who have undergone an artificial interruption of binocular vision for several days (for instance, with unilateral patching for ocular injuries). When the patch is removed, fusion cannot be maintained, and there is constant diplopia. Although some cases resolve spontaneously, most require treatment in the form of prisms, lenses, or visual training.

f. *A and V patterns.* In these complex forms of horizontal strabismus, the deviation varies with vertical gaze. For example, in A exotropia, the exotropia increases on downgaze. Such patients frequently experience diplopia, especially with reading and other near tasks.

g. *Brown's superior oblique tendon sheath syndrome.* This condition involves a congenital superior oblique sheath defect that mechanically limits the eye's ability to elevate from an adducted position. Diplopia is noticed on upgaze.

2. *Physiologic diplopia.* Many patients are alarmed by a sudden awareness of normal physiologic diplopia experienced for objects off the singleness horopter.

3. *Anomalous prismatic effect of spectacles.* This occurs with poorly adjusted glasses, errors in spectacle fabrication involving the inclusion of unwanted prism, omission of previously worn prism, or the need for slab-off prism in anisometropia.

After it has been determined that diplopia does exist, a routine history is augmented with questions related to: (1) the duration of diplopia, (2) its first occurrence, (3) the location of diplopic images, and (4) the frequency and course of their occurrence.

TESTS AND MEASUREMENTS
Comitant Deviations

Once an accurate initial history has been completed, tests are done to thoroughly evaluate binocular function. Ocular health is evaluated (through fundus evaluation, biomicroscope examination, tonometry, visual field testing, the Amsler grid, and testing pupillary reflexes) to be sure that ocular, neurologic, or systemic disease is not causing the reported signs or symptoms. The analysis of binocular dysfunction in the aged is described in this section.

A thorough refraction, including tests of binocular and monocular visual acuity, should be performed. Monocular refraction under binocular conditions helps stabilize fusion and visual acuity. (American Optical vectographic slides or Turville's distance testing combined with the Borish or other binocular tests for near vision are recommended.) Fusional difficulties may cause binocular acuity to be less than the acuity of the better eye.

Obviously, plus additions are needed for the aged to maintain clear vision at near because of loss of accommodative ability. Proper history taking will help determine the best choice of near addition power and form (bifocal, trifocal, reading, or any other). Many tests can determine the addition. Excellent theoretical (Morgan, 1960) and test (Borish, 1970) descriptions are available. The basic premise is to prescribe the addition so that one-half of the accommodative amplitude is kept in reserve, or so that the desired working distance is in the central part of the range of clear vision through the near addition.

Heterophoria and binocular vision are evaluated at distance and near. Near evaluations are done through any plus addition indicated by refractive findings. Lateral heterophoria can be measured by various methods: objective and subjective cover tests, Maddox rod-flash and nonflash, and von Graeffe's technique-flash and nonflash (Hirsch and Bing, 1948). Tests in the natural environment are frequently superior to those made through the phoropter. A properly performed cover test (von Noorden, 1990) for assessment of phoria magnitude, as well as quality of fusional recovery, can be useful (Morgan, 1960). The cover test consists of two parts: the unilateral cover test (to detect strabismus) and the alternate cover test (to measure the angle of heterophoria or strabismus).

To perform the unilateral cover test, do the following:

1. Direct the patient to fixate a small, detailed target.
2. Closely observe one eye (the limbus may be used as a guide), and simultaneously occlude the other eye.
3. Note the direction and estimate the amount of movement required of the eye to fixate the target.
4. Immediately uncover the eye.
5. Repeat, if necessary.
6. Bring the occluder beneath the eyes to the opposite side. (*Be sure* the patient uses alternate fixation.)

If fixation is central for each eye, and there is no movement of either eye upon covering the opposite eye, there is heterophoria. Strabismus is indicated if there is movement of one eye upon covering the other. The test should be repeated in different fields of gaze to evaluate noncomitancy. For aged patients, the near cover test is done through any plus addition required.

To perform the alternate cover test, do the following:

1. Occlude one eye, and direct the patient to fixate a small target with the unoccluded eye.
2. Direct your gaze to the cover at a point where you assume the temporal limbus to be.
3. Quickly move the occluder to the fixating eye. Do not allow your gaze to follow the occluder.
4. Note the direction and estimate the amount of movement required of the uncovered eye to fixate the target. Movement of the eye with the occluder signifies an exodeviation, and movement opposite to the occluder indicates an esodeviation.
5. Return the occluder to the original position before the eye.
6. Between the occluder and the eye, orient a loose prism or prisms of sufficient power to neutralize the movement just seen.
7. Repeat the test, changing the power of the prism or prisms until just-perceptible movements of opposite direction are observed.
8. The midpoint of this pair of prism values represents the angle phoria or tropia.

The test is done in different fields of gaze to analyze noncomitancy. Occasionally, the alternate cover test will reveal a larger angle than did the unilateral cover test in the presence of strabismus. Such measurements are often evidence of unharmonious anomalous correspondence, although for exotropic patients (especially those with pseudodivergence excess), a properly performed (prolonged) near cover test will reveal more exodeviation than will just short, rapid occlusion.

Lateral Vergence Range and Fixation Disparity Testing

Disparity (fusional) vergence ranges are measured using loose or rotary prisms in free space and through the phoropter at distance and near. Because loose prisms are presented in discrete steps, they give good indications of the patient's fusional recovery ability. Measuring vergence ranges using rotary prisms through the phoropter frequently can be eliminated from the test sequence if forced vergence fixation disparity curves are measured at distance and near.

After determining lateral phorias, forced vergence fixation disparity curves are plotted at distance and near, and prism to reduce fixation disparity to zero is measured in all positions of gaze. Actual fixation disparity is only measured by instruments specifically designed for the task, for example, the Disparometer, and Woolf near card (Schor and Narayan, 1982). Most clinical tests (Mallett Distance and Near Fixation Disparity Tests, as well as Bernell lanterns) measure the prism to reduce fixation disparity to zero–the associated phoria.

Forced vergence fixation disparity curves (Disparometer and Wolff near card) are valuable for the analysis of binocular vision (Sheedy and Saladin, 1977). Figure 10.1 shows typical distance and near forced vergence fixation disparity curves for a symptomatic presbyopic subject with poor control of a near lateral phoria. Flat curves indicate better compensation for the phoria than do steep curves. For symptomatic patients, prism can be prescribed to approximately center the curve about the y-axis, or the center of symmetry (Schor, 1983). The associated phoria measurement (prism to reduce fixation disparity to zero) generally gives smaller prism prescriptions for symptomatic patients with steep curves than do other criteria for prescribing prisms, and the prescription found usually gives adequate relief of symptoms (Sheedy, 1980).

Vision therapy can be prescribed to improve binocularity and modify the curve shape. For the elderly patient, vision therapy progress can be followed using forced vergence fixation disparity curves. These curves generally flatten with successful therapy, just as do those of younger patients. After therapy, a small fixation disparity generally remains when the actual fixation disparity is measured (Schor, 1983).

Vertical Heterophoria and Fixation Disparity Testing

Arriving at the prism prescription for a vertical phoria frequently requires considerable clinical judgment. Various techniques have been recommended for prescription design, including equating vergence ranges, flip prism techniques (Eskridge, 1961), and fixation disparity tests (Morgan, 1949; Rutstein and Eskridge, 1986). Tests that measure prism to reduce vertical fixation disparities to

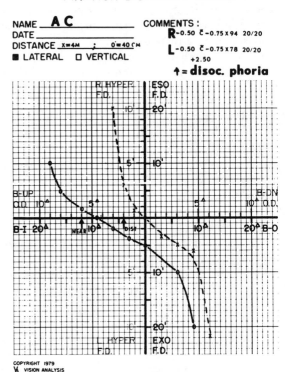

Figure 10.1. Fixation disparity curves measured at distance (x) and near (o) on patient with symptomatic near exophoria. There is a near exofixation disparity of 5′, and nearly 10Δ base-in is required to reduce the fixation disparity to zero. Source: Graph reprinted with permission from James E. Sheedy, University of California, Berkeley.

zero (measured clinically by American Optical vectographic slides, Turville's infinity balance, the Mallett distance and near unit, and the Borish near card) generally give vertical prism prescriptions that reduce symptoms. Nearly all patients can appreciate a difference of 0.5 Δ on vertical fixation disparity tests (Morgan, 1949).

Vertical heterophoria may be measured at distance and near by Maddox rods, a cover test, or prism dissociation. When a vertical heterophoria is present in an aged patient, comitancy should be evaluated carefully. Fixation disparity tests probably are the most accurate techniques for prism prescription. Fixation disparity measures have the added advantage that they can be conducted in all fields of gaze under more natural binocular viewing conditions.

When a lateral and a vertical fixation disparity exist simultaneously, the vertical fixation disparity should be corrected first. Then the horizontal fixation disparity curves should be measured. Correcting the vertical fixation disparity often will normalize (flatten) the slope found in horizontal fixation disparity curve measurement (Wick and London, 1987).

Vertical prism should not be prescribed for all vertical fixation disparities, but only when it gives improved visual performance (less suppression, increased fusion ranges, and flatter lateral forced vergence fixation disparity curves) and reduced symptoms. Generally, a reduction of vertical misalignment to zero under binocular viewing conditions (prism to reduce fixation disparity to zero) gives the most accurate prism prescriptions.

Stereopsis should be measured at distance and near. The stereoscopic threshold is relatively constant up to the ages of 45 to 50 years. After age 50, stereopsis declines gradually with increasing age (Pitts, 1982). However, there are large variations in individuals, and "normal" stereopsis may be found even in extremely aged persons.

Finally, the near point of convergence should be measured. In youth, the near point of convergence ranges from 1 cm to 4 cm from the spectacle plane (Cooper and Duckman, 1978). With the onset of presbyopia, there is a decrease of about 1 cm per decade, so by age 70, the normal convergence near point is 3 cm to 7 cm from the spectacle plane. Debility, systemic medication, and changes in binocular status can cause dramatic individual decrements.

Heterophoria, convergence, and binocular vision should be examined without the patient's wearing glasses if the patient does not normally wear them and with glasses (correct or not) if the patient does wear them. To evaluate the effects of lens prescriptions, and prism prescriptions, or both, the examination is repeated with the best possible correction and appropriate prescription modification.

Noncomitant Deviations

Deviations that vary significantly (greater than 5 Δ) when the eyes are directed into various fields of gaze are noncomitant (Griffin, 1976). These deviations also increase when an eye with one or more paretic muscles fixates; the secondary deviation is larger than the primary. Diagnosis is facilitated by taking a case history and performing tests to measure the amount and extent of diplopia, fusion, and noncomitancy. Noncomitant deviations are characterized by the following:

1. A limitation of monocular motility
2. A change in magnitude of the deviation in various fields of gaze
3. A change in diplopia with various fields of gaze
4. An increase in the angle of deviation when the eye with the paretic muscle fixates

Identification of the affected muscles begins with observation. The examiner looks for gross deviations in alignment, signs of lid abnormality, or an unusual head turn or tilt. Patients who have noncomitant deviations often adopt distinctive head positions to compensate for diplopia. Table 10.1 shows head positions adopted in noncomitancy and the extraocular muscles affected.

Noncomitancy generally is caused by three conditions:

1. Trauma, including head and orbital trauma
2. Neurologic disorders (disorders of gaze and muscle palsies caused by dysfunctions of cranial nerves III, IV, and VI)

Table 10.1 Abnormal head posture and affected extraocular muscle

Face Position			Muscle Affected
Turn	Chin Position	Tilt	
R	None	None	RLR
L	None	None	RMR
L	Down	L	RSO
L	Up	R	RLO
R	Up	L	RSR
R	Down	R	RLR
L	None	None	LLR
R	None	None	LMR
R	Down	R	LSO
R	Up	L	LLO
L	Up	R	LSR
L	Down	L	LLR

3. Muscle disorders, including orbital tumors and pseudotumors, which compromise muscle action; thyroid disease; and myesthenia gravis.

Tests to detect the affected muscle in noncomitancy must take into account that restrictive syndromes (thyroid disease and blow-out fractures) affect eye alignment differently than nerve or muscle dysfunctions (myesthenia gravis and cranial nerve dysfunction cause muscle palsy). In restrictive syndromes diplopia is caused by mechanical resistance to movement of the eye, and diplopia is most noticeable during attempted movements opposite the field of action of the involved muscle or muscles. With nerve dysfunctions, the deviation increases on attempted gaze into the field of action of the muscle. Recent paretic involvements are characterized by the following:

1. A larger secondary than primary deviation, and
2. A sudden onset of symptoms such as diplopia, blurring, and head tilt or turn.

The diagnostic field of action of each extraocular muscle is shown in Table 10.2. To properly diagnose noncomitancy, the examiner must evaluate the deviation in the primary position, in each of the six positions of gaze, and with each eye fixating. Evaluation is done monocularly and binocularly to allow determination of the affected muscles. Some tests that can be used for evaluation are the alternate cover test, the Hess-Lancaster screen, and the Maddox rod. A shortcut method to isolate a single cyclovertical muscle in recent noncomitancy is the Parks (1958) three-step method, which consists of various measurements of ocular alignment. It is not appropriate for lateral muscle palsies or when more than one muscle is affected. Determining which eye has the hyper component in primary position, in which field of gaze the hyper component increases, and, finally,

Table 10.2   Extraocular muscles and their fields of action

Right Eye			Left Eye	
Gaze Direction	*Muscle*		*Gaze Direction*	*Muscle*
R	RLR		L	LLR
L	RMR		R	LMR
L, down	RSO		R, down	LSO
L, up	RLO		R, up	LLO
R, up	RSR		L, up	LSR
R, down	RLR		L, down	LLR
Rotational separation	LLO		RIO	Rotational separation
Vertical separation	{ LSR RIO		RSR LIO }	Vertical separation
Patient's left	{ LLR RMR	Primary position	RLR LMR }	Patient's right
Vertical separation	{ LIR RSO		RIR LSO }	Vertical separation
Rotational separation	LSO		RSO	Rotational separation

whether the hyper increases on right or left head tilt allows differentiation of the affected muscle (Table 10.3).

Two tests are especially helpful for evaluating noncomitancy and subsequently monitoring therapy progress (Cohen and Soden, 1981). Using an arc perimeter or tangent screen, measure the following:

1. *Monocular field*: how far the patient can foveally fixate (follow) a target as it moves along the perimeter surface. This is measured in degrees.
2. *Binocular field*: to what extent the patient can bifoveally fixate (follow) a target along the perimeter surface before diplopia or suppression occurs, also measured in degrees. Anaglyphic or Polaroid techniques

Table 10.3   Three-step method for determining cyclovertical muscle

Paretic Muscle	*Hyper Eye in Primary Position*	*Hyper Greater on Gaze*	*Hyper Greater on Head Tilt*
LIO	R	R	R
RIR	R	R	L
RSO	R	L	R
LSR	R	L	L
RSR	L	R	R
LSO	L	R	L
LIR	L	L	R
RIO	L	L	L

help diplopia awareness. Frequently there is an area of suppression or confusion before diplopia is noticed. Figure 10.2 shows possible diplopia fields for a right lateral rectus paresis.

During and after optometric rehabilitation, these tests can be used to monitor therapy by checking whether the monocular fixation field has expanded. The extent of the binocular field before diplopia awareness also should increase. This allows objective assessment of therapy progress.

Pupillary and visual field studies should be done when diagnosing any noncomitancy (see Chapter 11 for more complete description). When pupillary function is affected, tumors or aneurysms are suspected. Etiologic factors are not determined in every noncomitancy, however.

REHABILITATION OF OCULOMOTOR DYSFUNCTIONS

In geriatrics it has long been recognized that the object of treatment is to restore function maximally based on the normal for the age of the patient and the condition present. This may seem obvious to the experienced clinician; however, attempts to restore function beyond normals for the age, visual condition, and individual patient will only result in frustration for both practitioner and patient. This may explain the reluctance of many optometrists to engage in the rehabilitation of visual dysfunctions of aged patients.

After an accurate history and diagnosis have been obtained, lens management, prism management, or both are used to improve binocularity maximally. Decisions about lens prescription types (bifocals, single vision reading, and so on) generally are made based on a case history of working conditions rather than any possible subsequent binocular therapy. The patient is reevaluated after 2 weeks to 1 month. If the patient still shows evidence of decreased binocular function (for example, macular suppression, decreased amplitude of fusion, fixation disparity, or decreased stereopsis) and symptoms persist, vision therapy is indicated if the patient can be properly motivated. Home vision therapy is generally sufficient for the rehabilitation of elderly patients' binocular dysfunctions, especially exodeviations. Occasionally, the management of esodeviations will need to incorporate office-based therapy.

Comitant Deviations

Binocular rehabilitation attempts to develop efficient, comfortable, well-sustained binocular vision using prisms, lenses, vision therapy, or a combination of these techniques. Motor and peripheral sensory fusion are generally already present. The rehabilitative therapies discussed in this chapter will be limited to lateral deviations. Although vertical heterophorias can be treated with vision therapy techniques, the processes needed are somewhat more complicated. Furthermore, experience indicates that vision therapy techniques for vertical

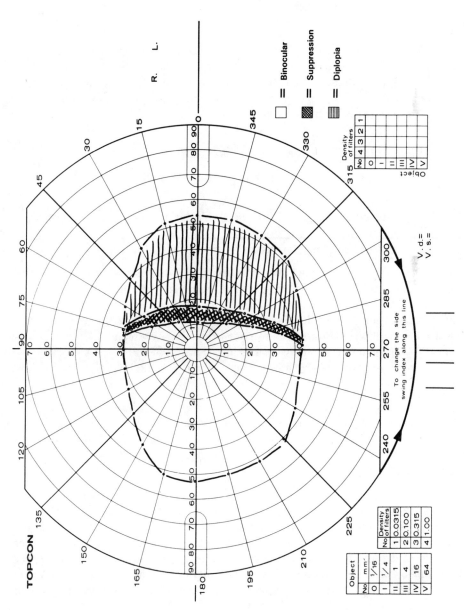

Figure 10.2. Possible diplopia fields for right lateral rectus paresis.

deviations are usually less successful in reducing symptoms of aged patients than vertical prism prescriptions.

Vision therapy is designed to maximally enhance stereopsis, version and saccadic ability, and vergence ranges. It is indicated at any age — even into the 90s — when symptoms exist and binocular findings are abnormal. When there are age-related decreases in monocular skills (pursuit and saccadic ability), a short period of monocular training may be needed (1 week to 2 weeks at most). Rehabilitation for the aged proceeds faster when binocular therapy accompanies monocular therapy and is emphasized exclusively after monocular skills are essentially equal.

Occasionally, elderly patients have problems with even very small heterophorias. Central suppression, reduced vergence ranges, poor version and saccadic ability, and reduced stereopsis influence the extent of these problems. Rehabilitative therapy using appropriate lens and prism corrections is done when these "general skills" problems exist.

Rehabilitative Management of Exophoria

The overall goals in the rehabilitation of exophoria in the elderly patient follow:

1. Sustained compensation for the exodeviation using increased convergence ability.
2. Comfortable binocular vision for needed visual tasks.

Refractive management is usually less successful than vision therapy management for exophoria. Obviously, overminusing is inappropriate for presbyopic patients, and base-in prism can actually increase the exodeviation because of prism adaptation (Carter, 1965; Henson and North, 1980). Vision therapy is generally sufficient without modification of the refractive correction. However, base-in prism can be useful when vision therapy is not possible.

The following are vision therapy goals for the elderly patient with exophoria:

1. Increase voluntary fusional convergence maximally (break points).
2. Enhance jump vergences (recovery points).
3. Establish central and foveal sensory fusion in free space at the ortho position.
4. Enhance stereopsis.
5. Develop reflex vergences.

The following lists give typical rehabilitative vision therapy procedures for symptomatic near and distance exophoria. Procedures are listed in the order usually prescribed for home therapy, and all procedures are not necessary for every patient. Aged patients with symptomatic exophoria at distance and near are managed using rehabilitative vision therapy techniques from all four lists. Therapy for both distance and near exophoria is grouped into two parts: vergence training and antisuppression/stereopsis training. Home therapy is prescribed from each category, and the level of difficulty is increased with improved binocular responses.

Vergence Training for Near Exophoria:

1. *Pencil push-ups.* A detailed target is moved from arm's length closer until fusion is lost. This technique is sometimes combined with lights, anaglyphs, or both for antisuppression training.
2. *Colored circles (Mast/Keystone).* These provide a flat fusion convergence demand and can be modified for antisuppression training simultaneously.
3. *Aperture-rule trainer.* Using a single aperture, positive fusional vergence training is done using antisuppression and stereoscopic targets. This is often combined with a distance target for jump vergence training.
4. *Eccentric circles.* Using these circles with stereopsis demand, fusion training is done by crossing the eyes to develop convergence ability. This technique can be combined with two targets for jump vergence training.
5. *Near point chiastopic fusion.* This develops convergent fusion using two ordinary objects (often with antisuppression cues) such as coins, thumbs, buttons, and so on.
6. *Anaglyphic reading.* Using a Polaroid or anaglyphic grid of bars and spaces, combined with appropriate glasses, antisuppression training is done. This technique can be combined with lenses or prisms for simultaneous vergence training (Gibson, 1955).
7. *Mirror stereoscope.* A Wheatstone-type stereoscope using two mirrors for dissociation and shaped in the form of a W, using various targets, can train vergence ranges of 40 Δ base in to 50 Δ base out.
8. *Brock's Posture Board.* With the use of anaglyphs and lights on a Plexiglas board, near antisuppression tests can be done. The technique can be combined with lenses and prisms.
9. *Three-eye mirror method.* A circle is drawn on a mirror. The patient converges and fuses his or her eyes to see one eye fused in the center and two eyes on the outside — all inside the circle. This technique can be combined with a letter on the mirror for jump vergence training.
10. *Combinations.* All these techniques can be combined to increase vergence demand, reduce suppression, and enhance stereopsis.

Antisuppression/Stereopsis Training for Near Exophoria:

1. *Polachrome Orthoptic Trainer.* Vectograms or tranaglyphs (Bernell Corporation, South Bend, IN) and appropriate spectacles are used in antisuppression and convergence therapy (Vodnoy, 1970).

2. *Pola-mirror push-ups.* The patient looks at his or her eyes in a mirror while wearing Polaroid glasses. Any "blacking out" of one lens (suppression) is noted (Griffin and Lee, 1970). The mirror is moved closer and farther away.
3. *Eccentric circles*
4. *Anaglyphic reading*
5. *Brock's Posture Board*
6. *Aperture-rule trainer*
7. *Orthofusor, base-out kit (Bausch & Lomb,* Rochester, NY). The Polaroid kit is used to improve positive fusional vergence and give antisuppression and stereoacuity training.
8. *Bar reading* (custom-made). A septum is placed between the reading task and the patient to dissociate one eye from the other. Suppression is noted when words are missing. This technique can be combined with lenses and prisms for vergence training.
9. *Combinations.* All these techniques can be combined to increase vergence demand, reduce suppression, and enhance stereopsis.

Vergence Training for Distance Exophoria:

1. *Voluntary convergence.* During the training of willful crossing of the eyes, visual stimuli sometimes are used. Patients are to become aware of the feeling in their eyes as they converge.
2. *Ductions and versions.* Some improvement of saccadic and version ability is often helpful. A swinging Marsden ball can train pursuit movements. Any two targets can be used for saccadic training.
3. *Pencil push-aways.* A detailed fixation target is held close and gradually moved farther away. Sometimes anaglyphs and a light are used.
4. *Hand-held Brewster's stereoscope.* This is a refracting stereoscope with a septum. Using any of the hundreds of stereograms available, vergence and antisuppression training are done. Vergence demand is varied by changing the target separation or fixation distance (tromboning).
5. *Prism demand flippers.* With the use of prisms in a lens holder, vergence demand is changed in discrete steps. This technique can be combined with antisuppression exercises (anaglyphs or Polaroid glasses) for powerful training of vergence and fusion ability.
6. *Chiastopic fusion at far.* Two pictures with suppression cues give a fusion demand. Near chiastopic fusion usually must be learned first.
7. *Risley prism for pursuit.* This variable prism, which can be used to increase vergence demand, may need to be combined with antisuppression exercises.
8. *Polachrome orthoptic trainer.* Vectograms or tranaglyphs (Bernell Corporation) and appropriate spectacles are used in antisuppression and convergence therapy (Vodnoy, 1970).

9. *Vis-a-vis walkaways.* Both examiner and patient wear Polaroid glasses. The patient is to tell of any blacking out of one of the examiner's eyes. This also can be done with a mirror by the patient alone (Griffin, 1976).
10. *Combinations.* All these techniques can be combined to increase vergence demand, reduce suppression, and enhance stereopsis.

Antisuppression Stereopsis Training for Distance Exophoria:

1. *Peripheral stereopsis.* With the use of large stereoscopic targets (Root rings or Brock's rings), stereopsis responses are elicited peripherally. The patient works to increase the distance from the test so that the test, as well as subsequent stereopsis demand, becomes more central.
2. *Television trainer.* An anaglyphic or Polaroid attachment for the television is available. When appropriate spectacles are worn, suppression is noted when part of the picture turns black. This technique can be combined with prisms or lenses for simultaneous vergence training.
3. *Brock string techniques.* A string is held from a distant target to the nose. The patient sees two strings crossing at the visual axes' crossing point. Beads can be put on the string to increase diplopia awareness, and anaglyphs can help eliminate suppression.
4. *Pola-mirror training with afterimages.* A mirror and Polaroid lenses are combined with afterimages. The goal is to see crossed afterimages and both eyes (no suppression).
5. *Pola-mirror training with two mirrors.* This is the same technique as in Item 4, but this one uses two mirrors so that fixation distances can be altered to increase or decrease vergence demand and fusion difficulty. It also can be combined with afterimages.
6. *Chiastopic fusion at far*
7. *Hand-held Brewster's stereoscope*
8. *Prism bar for saccadic vergences.* Prism bars increase vergence demand in discrete, rapid steps. They often are combined with antisuppression exercises. Prism bars can be custom made for each patient to give maximal training (Wick, 1974).
9. *Combinations.* All these techniques can be combined to increase vergence demand, reduce suppression, and enhance stereopsis. When home therapy is appropriate, detailed instruction sheets can help insure patient compliance. Figure 10.3 shows a typical instruction sheet for home therapy using push-up convergence. Other sheets can and should be prepared for each rehabilitative technique, and examples will be given throughout the chapter.

As with young patients, the primary therapeutic consideration in treating exophoria in the elderly is the patient's ability to compensate for the deviation (an ability that has large individual variations). Because of normal reductions in

These exercises will develop the coordination and focusing ability of your eyes when you are looking at near objects and when you look from far to near objects. You will know you are doing the exercise or exercises correctly when you can fuse the two sets of circles into one circle, with a smaller circle inside that stands out or falls away.

Exercise a total of _____ minutes each day. After you can accomplish Procedure 1, add one new procedure each week as you do the exercises. In the beginning you may experience some discomfort such as headaches and eyestrain, so you may have to limit the exercises to a few minutes. As your ability improves, your discomfort will disappear, and the exercise time can be increased. Remember that exercising 15 minutes daily is better than exercising 2 hours once a week! It would be best if you did this exercise at _____, _____, and _____ each day. Try to establish a routine so that you always do the exercises at the same time each day.

Procedure 1: Hold the two cards together with A's overlapping. Hold a pencil centered between the circles. Look at the top of the lead, and observe the circles on either side without looking directly at them. Slowly move the pencil toward your nose (always looking at the lead and keeping it centered) until you see *Four* large circles, or more than two. Continue moving your pencil. Observe the center large circles approaching each other until you see them overlap (superimpose). You then will see *Three* large circles with the center one under the pencil. The center large circle will have a smaller circle inside it that appears to be behind the large circle. If the center circle looks even with the large circle, you are not using one of your eyes (supression).

Note: If you find that only one eye is being used, then in order to use both eyes, do the following:
1. Blink your eyes rapidly.
2. Cover one eye, and then quickly remove the cover.

Next, try to clear the letters. While you continue to maintain the fused circles and depth (one circle behind the other), concentrate on holding the letters clear.

Correct Response: When Procedure 1 is done correctly, you should see three large circles. The center one should be *clear* and composed of two circles — one behind the other.

Note: This exercise also can be done with the *B's* overlapping. These are the correct responses:
1. When the *A's* overlap, the center circle should appear behind the larger circle.
2. When the *B's* overlap, the center circle should appear ahead of the larger circle.

If you cannot see the depth or see it as the reverse of the previous description, you are doing the exercise incorrectly and need to try again.

Procedure 2: Repeat Procedure 1, but without the aid of the pencil. When you can easily fuse the circle without the pencil, begin moving the cards apart. Keep moving them farther apart until the center circle blurs and then breaks into two. Repeat the exercise _____ times, trying to get the cards farther apart each time.

Procedure 3: Look to a detailed distant (more than 10 feet away) object, and make it clear. Then look to the cards and fuse the circles, making the center clear and single and noticing the depth. Repeat this until you can easily look from a distant object to the cards and fuse them when they are separated by 12 inches or more. No pencil is to be used in this exercise. Remember to clear the distant object, then look to the cards and fuse and clear the circles. Move the circles farther apart each time.

Procedure 4: Place the cards against a wall at a distance of about 5 to 6 feet. The cards should be 5 to 6 inches apart. Fuse them in the same manner you have been using for near. When you can fuse and clear the cards easily at this distance, begin moving them farther apart each time.

Procedure 5: When you can fuse the cards (at 5 to 6 feet away) when they are about 2 feet apart, being alternating your fixation from the fused cards at a distance to a detailed near object. Repeat this until you can easily look from the fused cards to the near object, making each clear before you look to the next one.

Procedure 6: Fuse the cards at a distance of 5 to 6 feet with the cards approximately 12 inches apart. Walk toward the cards (keeping them fused) as close as you can until they get blurry or split into two. Repeat this, trying to walk closer each time before the center circle breaks into two. Always try to maintain the correct response: The cards should be clear, and you should see the depth.

Figure 10.3. Patient Instructions: Home Vision Therapy — Free Fusion Rings (Convergence).

overall vergence ability in the elderly, the magnitude of the deviation is important to the final outcome. Rehabilitative vision therapy alone is generally sufficient for the treatment of exophoria. Frequently, a vertical and lateral heterophoria coexist, and it is occasionally difficult to decide whether it is necessary to correct the vertical phoria. When the vertical phoria is not corrected and initial lateral vergence training is unsuccessful, vertical prism correction frequently is needed to reduce symptoms and insure the success of lateral therapy.

Some older patients complete all the rehabilitative therapy techniques with little symptomatic relief. These patients require a decrease in overall convergence demand for comfortable, efficient binocularity. Vergence demand can be reduced with base-in prisms or extraocular muscle surgery when the deviation is large enough at all distances. After the deviation has been reduced with prism or surgery, some patients need further vision therapy to eliminate persistent conditions such as foveal suppression and fixation disparity or to develop fine stereopsis.

Rehabilitative Management of Esophoria

The overall goals in the rehabilitative management of esophoria are the following:

1. Enhance compensation of the esodeviation through increased divergence.
2. Provide comfortable binocular vision for needed visual tasks.

Prescription modification is more helpful for esodeviations than for exodeviations and may be successful in relieving symptoms without vision therapy or with minimized therapy time. Patients with a distance esophoria frequently are helped by base-out prism. Vision therapy then is done if needed to enhance sensory fusion and give the patient the most comfortable clear binocular vision possible.

The following are vision therapy goals in the management of esophoria:

1. Extend fusional convergence maximally.
2. Enhance awareness of stereopsis.
3. Exercise the present ability to achieve sensory fusion (especially peripheral fusion) in as many varied instruments as are available in office.
4. Increase fusional divergence (break points) by teaching "relaxation" of the eyes through mental effort.
5. Enhance jump vergence ability (recovery points).
6. Establish central and foveal sensory fusion at the angle of deviation by using instruments and then not using instruments.
7. Develop reflex vergences.

Rehabilitative therapy procedures for esophoria attempt to increase disparity (fusional) divergence involuntarily as a response to increased sensory fusion (stereopsis) demands. Sensory fusion is maintained by adding stereopsis to flat fusion skills. Fusional divergence is stimulated reflexly by increased demand. Because of the absence of accommodation (compensated by plus additions for clear vision at near), there are seldom symptomatic near esophorias.

The home rehabilitative therapy sequence for distance esophoria follows.

Vergence Training for Distance Esophoria:

1. *Ductions and versions.* Some improvement of saccadic and version ability is often helpful. A swinging Marsden ball can train pursuit movements. Any two targets can be used for saccadic training.

2. *Pencil pushaways*. A detailed fixation target is held close and gradually moved farther away. Sometimes anaglyphs and a light are used.
3. *Eccentric circles*. Using these circles with stereopsis demand, fusion training is done by turning the eyes out to develop divergence ability. This technique can combine with two targets for jump vergence training.
4. *Prism demand flippers*. Using prisms in a lens holder, vergence demand is changed in discrete steps. This technique can be combined with anti-suppression exercises (anaglyphs or Polaroid glasses) for powerful training of vergence and fusion ability.
5. *Brock string techniques*. A string is held from a distant target to the nose. The patient sees two strings crossing at the visual axes' crossing point. Beads can be put on the string to increase diplopia awareness, and anaglyphs can help to eliminate suppression.
6. *Combinations*. All of these techniques can be combined to increase vergence demand, reduce suppression, and enhance stereopsis.

Antisuppression Stereopsis Training for Distance Esophoria:

1. *Prism demand flippers*.
2. *Hole-in-hand game*. The patient looks through a tube with one eye while holding a hand in front of the other eye. The patient strives to see both the hand and an object in the field of view through the "tube-hole" in the hand.
3. *Hand-held Brewster's stereoscopes*. This is a refracting stereoscope with a septum. Using any of the hundreds of stereograms available, vergence and antisuppression training are done. Vergence demand is varied by changing the target separation or fixation distance (tromboning).
4. *Brock string techniques*
5. *Polachrome orthoptic trainers*. Vectograms or tranaglyphs (Bernell Corporation) and appropriate spectacles are used in antisuppression and convergence therapy (Vodnoy, 1970).
6. *Flannel board training*. Red, green, and yellow pieces are made to put on a piece of black flannel. Using anaglyphic glasses, antisuppression exercises can be done. This technique is often combined with lenses and prisms and distance anaglyphic targets.
7. *Worth dot lights*. Four lights — one red, two green, and one white — are arranged in a diamond pattern. They are used with anaglyphs and moved nearer and farther as a good antisuppression technique. This technique can be combined with lenses and prisms for simultaneous vergence training.
8. *Bagolini's striated lenses*. These lenses with fine striations cause a visible streak when the patient looks at a light. Any suppression is noted

when one line or part of a line disappears (Winter, 1971). This technique can be combined with lenses and prisms for vergence training.

9. *Combinations.* All of these techniques can be combined to increase vergence demand, reduce suppression, and enhance stereopsis. Figure 10.4 shows a typical home therapy instruction sheet for an esophoria rehabilitation technique.

Rehabilitative Management of Central Suppression and Fixation Disparity

When aged patients have reduced visual skills and binocular instabilities, fixation disparity, foveal and macular suppression, or both are frequently found. Goals in rehabilitation include the following:

1. Eliminate central suppression.
2. Establish bifoveal fixation.
3. Develop fine stereo-acuity.

These exercises will develop good binocular vision while your eyes are diverging (turning outward) as if looking at distant objects. You will know you are using both eyes correctly in each procedure when the pictures viewed are seen as one, they are seen clearly, parts of the targets seen by each eye alone are present simultaneously, and depth is seen in certain cards.

Exercise a total of _____ minutes each day, and increase the number of procedures in each session as you can do them. In the beginning you might experience discomfort such as headaches and eyestrain, so that you may have to limit the exercises to a few minutes. As your ability improves, your discomfort will disappear, and the exercise time can be increased. Remember that exercising 15 minutes daily is better than exercising 2 hours once a week! It would be best if you did this exercise at _____, _____, and _____ each day. Try to establish a routine so that you always do the exercises at the same time each day.

Procedure 1: Place the instrument on a table at a comfortable height, with light falling evenly on the target cards. The double-aperture slider is placed at the position marked 1 or 2 on the front rutler. The target cards should be placed at the 0 position on the back ruler. The AP1 and AP2 cards are the targets for the procedures. To see the targets through the double aperture, place the tip of your nose against the end of the front ruler. If you are wearing a bifocal, tip your head back slightly, and place your lower lip against the ruler. Concentrate and actively try to fuse the targets at all times. Do not be discouraged if you are unsuccessful at first. Repeated efforts at looking at the targets and attempting fusion will lead to success.

Look through the double aperture at card AP1 (later, follow the same procedure with AP2). Close your left eye, and your right eye will see only one box with a black cross. Close your right eye, and your left eye will see only one box with a black ball. The ball is seen only by the left eye, and the cross is seen only by the right eye. If necessary to achieve this, move the aperture slider toward or away from you. Your eyes are now in this position:

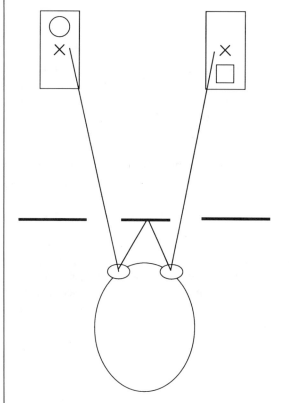

The right eye sees the target on the right side of the card.

The left eye sees the target on the left side of the card.

Look with both eyes, and make the two targets into one target.

Correct Response: When you have made the two targets into one (fusion), you will see this:

One box with the cross and ball are seen simultaneously.

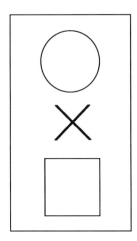

Note: If either the cross or the ball is seen alone, it means that although both your eyes are open, the visual information from one of your eyes is not being received (suppression). The result is that of closing one eye. One of your goals in this exercise is to become aware of the information from both eyes and unify it into one visual percept (sensory function). To do so, follow these steps:

1. Cover and uncover one eye, exposing both targets for brief periods while attempting fusion.
2. Blink your eyes rapidly, looking for fusion between blinks.

If you see two boxes instead of one, the visual information is being received, but your eyes are not aimed correctly. Your second goal is to diverge your eyes correctly so that sensory fusion can take place. To do so, look over the aperture slide across the room at a target. You should feel your eyes going outward. As you keep your eyes in an outward position, just notice the targets in the foreground. Now direct your attention to the targets. You should see them as one, and as you concentrate, the fused picture should clear. Repeat this procedure until you can maintain *one fused clear* target.

Figure 10.4. Patient Instructions: Home Vision Therapy—Double Aperture Rule Trainer.

Refractive management includes modification of the refractive correction using prism. Prescriptions are designed using forced vergence fixation disparity curves (see Figure 10.1). Prism is prescribed to reduce fixation disparity to zero (associated phoria) when steep curves are present. Prism is prescribed to center the flat portion more approximately on the y-axis (center of symmetry) when flat forced vergence fixation disparity curves are measured. Careful refractive management can reduce the need for rehabilitative therapy, enhance therapy success, or both.

Successful rehabilitative therapy of central suppression and fixation disparity requires targets that are small and detailed enough to necessitate bifoveal fixation and enhance central sensory fusion. Using stereoscopic targets rather than flat fusion targets will aid motor processes and thus maintain bifoveal fixation. The techniques used are "finishing-off" procedures for heterophorias with reduced visual skills. Whenever possible, targets should be chosen that have

1. binocular contours,
2. foveal-sized suppression targets, and
3. fine stereopsis stimulation.

Typical home rehabilitative therapy procedures for fixation disparity and central suppression follow.

Vergence Training for Central Suppression and Fixation Disparity:

1. *Polachrome orthoptic trainer.* Vectograms or tranaglyphs (Bernell Corporation) and appropriate spectacles are used in antisuppression and convergence therapy (Vodnoy, 1970).
2. *Biopter cards, E series.* These are targets with antisuppression cues for use in Brewster-type stereoscopes. They are combined with changeable vergence demand in the stereoscope (tromboning).
3. *Spache binocular reading.* These are targets with antisuppression cues for use in Brewster-type stereoscopes. They are combined with changeable vergence demand in the stereoscope (tromboning).
4. *MKM binocular reading cards.* These are targets with antisuppression cues for use in Brewster-type stereoscopes. They are combined with changeable vergence demand in the stereoscope (tromboning).
5. *Combinations.* All these techniques can be combined to increase vergence demand, reduce suppression, and enhance stereopsis.

Antisuppression/Stereopsis Training for Central Suppression and Fixation Disparity:

1. *Cheiroscopic tracing.* Using a cheiroscope, targets are traced, colored or filled in. Training can be enhanced by having the patient close his or her eyes and then reopen them, striving to see all lines and colors previously drawn.
2. *Projectopter.* Tranaglyphs or vectograms (Bernell Corporation) are projected on a screen for distance antisuppression and vergence training.
3. *Titmus stereo slides.* Slides are used to enhance stereopsis. Vergence ability is altered using prisms and lenses.
4. *American Optical vectographic adult slide.* A projected polarized slide is used to monitor fixation disparity and suppression as prisms and lenses change vergence demand.

5. *Mallet Distance and Near Fixation Disparity Test Unit.* These fixation disparity tests are used with Polaroid glasses. Lenses and prisms can be used to train vergence while reducing fixation disparity and suppression.
6. *Combinations.* All of these techniques can be combined to increase vergence demand, reduce suppression, and enhance stereopsis. A home therapy training sheet is shown in Figure 10.5 for a typical antisuppression training technique.

A different prism correction frequently is indicated for aged patients for distance and near. Bifocals can be prescribed with cement-on or press-on prism segments. It is often better to provide bifocals for occasional reading only. For prolonged reading, a single vision reading correction incorporating the proper near addition and indicated prism correction is frequently the best and most comfortable rehabilitation possible.

These exercises will develop simultaneous perception from your two eyes when you are looking at a distance. You will know you are using both eyes when you can see the television clearly through both parts of the therapy device. Remember, your task is to see the whole television picture throught both parts of the device at once.

Exercise a total of _____ minutes each day, and increase the number of procedures in each session as you can do them. In the beginning, one part of the television may be dark, or you may experience some discomfort; therefore, you may have to limit the exercise to a few minutes. As your ability improves, your discomfort will disappear, and the exercise time can be increased. Remember that exercising 15 minutes daily is better than exercising 2 hours once a week! It would be best if you did this exercise at _____, _____, and _____ each day. Try to establish a routine so that you always do the exercises at the same time each day.

Procedure 1: Attach the therapy device to the television set vertically with suction cups.

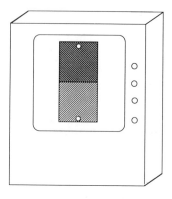

If the device is red and green, put the red part on top. It is very important that the device be vertical; otherwise, the therapy may be ineffective. Put on the special glasses provided by the doctor. If the glasses are red and green, put the red lens over your right eye. If the glasses are not red and green, be very careful to watch the television with your head straight upright. Turn on the television, sit _____ feet away from it, and watch it.

Correct Response: Looking at the television, you will see the television through both parts of the therapy device at the same time.

Note: During this exercise, if one part of the therapy device is black (cannot be seen through), the visual information from one of your eyes is not being received (suppression). The result is like closing one eye. If first one part of the device is black and then the other is black, it is similar to alternately closing one eye and then the other. The visual information is still being received only from one eye at a time. Your goal in these exercises is to become aware of the visual information from both eyes simultaneously.

If you find that only one eye is being used (suppression), do the following to use both eyes:

1. Blink your eyes rapidly, looking for the other eye's image between blinks.
2. Cover one eye; then quickly remove the cover.
3. Turn the room lights down or out.
4. Do any or all of the above in combination.

Ask yourself these questions, and be sure to tell your answers to the doctor evaluating your progress:

1. Does one part of the television therapy device ever go black? If so, when and how often?
2. Does the black part of the therapy device jump from top to bottom and back?
3. If both parts of the device are easy to see through, is the picture on the television clear or blurry?
4. Does this exercise get easier as I do it more often?

Procedure 2: Repeat Procedure 1 at a different distance (about _____ feet). Always try to maintain the correct response: clear, easy viewing through both parts of the therapy decvice at the same time.

Procedure 3: As Procedeure 2 becomes easy for you, move (closer) (farther) and continue trying to maintain the correct response.

Figure 10.5. Patient Instructions: Home Vision Therapy – Television Trainer.

Noncomitant Deviations

Management of the noncomitant deviation depends on whether it is of recent onset or is long-standing. Noncomitancy of recent onset requires accurate, immediate diagnosis and referral to the appropriate medial practitioner — usually an internist, ophthalmologist, neuroophthalmologist, or neurologist. The optometrist plays a significant role in diagnosing, directing the patient to the proper specialist, and judging the urgency of the situation. When the necessary medical care has been completed (and sometimes while it continues), functional aspects of the paretic noncomitant deviation are managed optometrically by fusion maintenance programs and ocular calisthenics to help prevent secondary contracture. These programs involve careful use of lenses, prisms, occlusion, and vision therapy.

When an extraocular muscle becomes paretic, its antagonist acts unopposed; an eye turn results from weakness of the paretic muscle and subsequent overreaction by the antagonist. Long-standing action by an unopposed muscle can lead to a slow contracture of that muscle. Contracture, which is thought to be caused by atrophy and hyalinization, frequently occurs over a long time course (months or years). When contracture occurs, even when the cause of the noncomitancy is muscle paresis, the paresis frequently lessens, the deviation becomes more equal, and a residual deviation remains. This is known as the "spread of comitancy." Rehabilitative intervention can help prevent and relieve the problems of noncomitancy (diplopia, spatial localization problems, and contracture).

When diplopia is a significant problem, prism and occlusion often can restore fusion or eliminate the diplopic image. Occlusion will always eliminate diplopia. However, this technique must be used cautiously, as spatial localization is impaired when an eye muscle is paretic. When critical or dangerous tasks are done (for example, driving, cooking, or dangerous work), the eye with the paretic muscle should be occluded.

Sector occlusion on a spectacle lens can help prevent diplopia when fusion exists in certain fields of gaze (Figure 10.6). Alternate occlusion can help give both eyes as much action into the paretic field of gaze as possible.

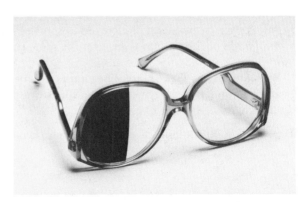

Figure 10.6. Spectacles with temporal occlusion.

Occlusion must be done in a manner consistent with attempts to prevent muscle contracture secondary to the paresis. Although it is doubtful whether any method of preventing secondary contracture is fully effective, preventive methods are important to try, and they can only help. The following optical techniques attempt to prevent contracture:

1. Conjugate prisms (bases in the same direction) may be worn. Both prisms are placed so that the eyes are forced to look in the direction of the field of the paretic muscle. This stimulates the paretic muscle and relaxes its antagonist.
2. A prism can be worn before the eye without the paretic muscle to force that eye into the field of gaze of the paretic muscle. This again attempts to relax the antagonist muscle and stimulate the paretic one.

Nonoptical methods of secondary contracture prevention are also possible. Medical techniques include anesthetic injection into the antagonist muscle, early recession surgery of the antagonist before contracture can develop, or both (O'Connor, 1943).

Optometric techniques for the prevention of secondary contracture are designed primarily to force the paretic eye toward the field of action of the affected muscle. Monocular therapy is designed for each eye while the other is occluded. The sound eye exercises in the field of action of the paretic muscle to relax the antagonist muscle and stimulate the paretic one. To exercise the eye with the paretic muscle, systematized programs requiring accurate fixations farther and farther into the field of action of the paretic muscle are used.

The following techniques can be used for monocular calisthenic therapy when there is a muscle paresis:

Sound Eye Fixing (gaze direction in field of action
of paretic muscle):

1. *Watching television or related activity.* This is done with the eyes directed in the field of action of the paretic muscle.
2. *Walking.* This is done with the eyes directed toward the field of action of the paretic muscle.
3. *Balancing exercises.* These are done with the eyes directed toward the field of action of the paretic muscle.
4. *Tracing exercises.* Targets are traced toward the field of action of the paretic muscle.
5. *Prism ductions: large prism changes.* Prism vergence is done in large steps toward the field of action of the paretic muscle. The patient tries to maintain fixation farther each time.

Paretic Eye Fixing (gaze direction toward action
of paretic muscle):

1. *Tracking a suspended moving ball.* The patient attempts to track a Marsden ball farther and farther into the field of action of the paretic muscle.

2. *Tracing exercises*
3. *Batting or ringing a moving, suspended ball.* The patient attempts to keep a circular ring around a swinging Marsden ball as it swings toward the field of action of the paretic muscle.
4. *Prism ductions: small prism changes.* Prism vergence is done in small steps toward the field of action of the paretic muscle. The patient tries to maintain fixation farther each time.
5. *Repeating Step 4 while walking.*
6. *Rotating pegboard.* The patient tries to put golf tees in a rotating perforated disk. Gradually the disk is moved toward the field of action of the paretic muscle.

Fusion should be maintained as much as possible in all cases of noncomitancy. Prism may be needed to restore fusion in the primary position. Sector prisms in Fresnel form can be used to give increasing fusion ability in the field of the paretic muscle. Prism power is determined empirically, and varying prism power can be used if noncomitancy is severe. Prism for fusion does not prevent secondary contracture.

Expansions of motor fusion ranges are indicated in practically all cases of muscle paresis. Motor fusion training is designed to give maximal fusion ability. Sensory fusion usually was present before noncomitancy developed, so this type of training may not be needed in all fields of gaze.

Vision therapy goals for patients with muscle paresis follow:

1. Maximally expand voluntary motor fusion ranges in the field of gaze *opposite* the paresis.
2. Develop reflex vergence in the primary position.
3. Expand fusional vergence training into the field of action of the paretic muscle.

Rehabilitative therapy is done in the manner indicated for the type of phoria present (see the section on therapy for comitant deviations). Therapy is similar for recent or long-standing noncomitant deviations. The progress of the therapy should be monitored according to the monocular field of view and binocular diplopia fields, which should increase as fusion and eye movement ability improve.

PROGNOSIS

Vision therapy is an effective procedure that can improve binocularity in presbyopic patients. These patients are able to learn therapy procedures easily and often carry them out more faithfully than do younger patients. Thus, the tradition of reserving vision therapy primarily for children or young adults is not justified. Problems such as blurred vision, tired eyes, or headaches after reading that are associated with binocular problems can be helped for most patients of any age.

To establish the prognosis for success of vision therapy in the elderly, Wick (1977) studied records of presbyopic subjects (n = 161) who had undergone vision therapy for convergence problems (n = 134) or general skills problems (n = 27). The age range was 45 to 89 years. Patients all had normal acuity for their age. After appropriate refractive management, vision therapy was prescribed as needed. When vision therapy was needed, exophoric patients generally were successful with 6 weeks of therapy, and esophoric patients were successful in 6 weeks to 8 weeks. Elderly patients generally carried out therapy procedures well, and home therapy was satisfactory for the majority. The conclusion of the study was that for binocular vision problems in the elderly that are treated with appropriate prism correction and vision therapy, symptoms are eliminated and test findings are restored to normal for the age and physical condition of the patient 92% (148 of 161) of the time. When the elimination of symptoms was the primary criterion, the success rate for therapy was 97% (156 of 161).

Approximately one-half of the patients who needed vision therapy remained asymptomatic after therapy was discontinued. In a 3-month follow-up to the study on vision therapy for patients with presbyopia, 47.8% (77 of 161) needed some additional therapy to remain asymptomatic. Generally, patients over age 70 years needed to continue with a maintenance therapy program (68.8%, or 22 of 32). These patients needed to continue minimal home therapy weekly or biweekly, with yearly examinations to assess visual function (Wick, 1977).

For elderly patients, just as for younger patients, exophoria responds better than esophoria to vision therapy alone. Vision therapy is generally the only necessary treatment for exodeviations. Esophoria, in contrast, often requires base-out prism management combined with vision therapy. Even when therapy causes symptoms to disappear, the magnitude of the heterophoria usually does not change. Patients more than 20 Δ exophoric and 15 Δ esophoric may have symptoms remaining after therapy. Extraocular muscle surgery can provide additional relief for selected cases.

Elderly patients who develop noncomitancy frequently have partial or complete recovery of paretic muscle function. The recovery of muscle function depends on the nerve innervation, the muscle involved, and the cause of the noncomitancy (Rucker, 1958; Rush and Younge, 1981). Overall rates of recovery of paretic muscle function based on the involved nerve are 48.3% for the third nerve, 53.5% for the fourth nerve, and 49.6% for the sixth nerve. When the cause of noncomitancy is vascular, the chance of muscle function recovery is approximately 70%. Usually recovery is within 3 months to 6 months. After that time, recovery of paretic muscle function is unlikely (Hugonnier and Hugonnier, 1969). When contracture does not occur or can be prevented by functional therapy and muscle function recovers, normal binocularity is restored.

The prognosis for comfortable binocular visual function in noncomitancy using the best medical management combined with appropriate optometric intervention (lenses, prisms, patching, and vision therapy) is probably 70 to 80%. Visual function may not be "normal," but the patient should be comfortable with minimal diplopia.

SENSORY ADAPTATION TRAINING
Monocularity

Elderly people frequently become monocular because of disease or accident. They often benefit from advice when adapting to this condition. For example, when monocularity comes suddenly, there is a loss of depth judgment, particularly for distances within arm's reach. Teaching the patient to touch a plate to the table or a teapot spout to the cup will reduce embarrassment and help prevent accidents. A description of monocular cues to depth — for example, size constancy, overlap, and perspective — and of proper head motion for increased parallax will help facilitate safer driving and parking.

Perceptual Rehabilitation

Declines in visual function with age can be attributed to a reduced ability to gather data (reduced saccades, version and vergence ability, visual acuity, and so on) as well as to a reduced ability to process the data gathered. Optometrists interested in the ability of children to process data gathered through vision and other senses have worked, through various types of visual/perceptual training, to increase abilities in this area.

Visual processing in the elderly significantly decreases when more complex processing tasks are attempted (Craik, 1977) because of an age-related slowing of the rate of information processing (Welford, 1964), different allocation of the resources that control visual function, or both (Hoyer and Plude, 1980). Perceptual function in the aged can be evaluated by the following techniques:

- Copy forms (adult variety) and an additional three-dimensional form.
- Motor free visual perception test.
- Reading test.
- Pegboard test.
- Jordan right-left test.
- Identification test using objects and pictures.

Optometric visual perceptual therapy is used to enhance attention span, form discrimination, and auditory and visual memory in children. Similar procedures can be used to improve visual perceptual function in the aged. A sequenced therapy program using sensory-motor interaction enhances basic visual perceptual skills for the aged, as well as for children.

Aphakic Rehabilitation

Patients with cataracts already have experienced visual function decrease and often are apprehensive about the prospects of life without sight. The optometrist can provide much assurance about the outcomes of surgery. Working closely with the ophthalmic surgeon will enable the optometrist to advise the patient about what to expect from aphakia or pseudophakia (see Chapter 11.) A careful explanation of the adaptation to, and correction options in, aphakia and the necessary spectacle correction (at least for near) in pseudophakia will help alleviate the fear and apprehension patients experience. Unfortunately, this necessary assurance sometimes is neglected in referrals back and forth between optometrist and surgeon.

Vision correction after surgery for cataracts presents some unique rehabilitative problems. First, visual acuity must be restored through the use of intraocular lens implants, contact lenses, or aphakic spectacle lenses, and each presents specific problems. Frequently, the patient must learn a new way of seeing because of that correction. Finally, convergence demand is increased by the surgery itself, especially for patients who do not have intraocular lens implants.

Aphakic spectacle lenses generally require the most comprehensive rehabilitative techniques. From a purely optical standpoint, an aphakic spectacle lens causes serious adaptive problems. The lenses magnify what is seen by over 25%, so objects appear larger and closer than they really are. Aphakic corrections significantly impair initial judgment of depth. The spherical aberration of high plus lenses causes pin-cushion distortion, that is, lines seem to curve inward, and movement of the eyes behind a fixed spectacle lens causes objects to swim.

The highly magnified central visual field of aphakic spectacle lenses overlap a portion of the peripheral field and produce a characteristic ring scotoma. The stronger a lens in plus power, the worse the problem is. At intermediate distances (10 to 2 feet), the scotoma causes problems that are not easily overcome. Objects, such as people and chairs, pop in and out of the blind area, and patients see things they cannot turn their eyes to look at, bump into objects, and have trouble negotiating their environment. Visual field limitations of aphakic spectacle lenses are best solved by contact lens correction.

Coordinating hand and eye movements also becomes difficult when aphakic spectacles are first worn, so coordination for near tasks frequently is impaired. Small wooden puzzles, building block figures, and jigsaw puzzles can be used to help patients redevelop the spatial judgment needed for daily tasks. Aphakic adaptation therapy sessions attempt to redevelop the depth judgment and head and eye movements necessary for accurate hand/eye coordination.

Convergence Requirements

Convergence requirements are altered by cataract surgery. Removal of the crystalline lens of the eye shifts the normal visual angle temporalward by 2° to 3° per eye. This shift causes an induced exophoria of 10 to 12 Δ for distance and near, which must be overcome by fusional (disparity) vergence reserves. Post-surgically induced exophoria combined with the usually receded near point of convergence in the aged can cause binocular problems that interfere with the aphakic patient's ability to read comfortably or for very long.

Convergence demands of binocular aphakic spectacle correction are affected by the following:

1. Phoria (pre-existing phoria combined with altered convergence demands that are caused by the change in the visual angle resulting from lens removal).
2. Interpupillary distance.
3. Spectacle lens vertex distance.
4. Correcting lens strength (both distance and bifocal additions).

Convergence requirements increase slightly with each diopter of distance lens power increase (provided the vertex adjustment, near additions, and interpupillary distance remain constant). This amounts to approximately 1 Δ of increased convergence demand for each diopter of distance correction. Increasing the bifocal addition causes dramatic increases in convergence demand.

Near work must be held closer to be clear, and the combined power of the distance lens and the bifocal increases vergence demand still more. Each diopter of increased bifocal addition power increases convergence demand about 12Δ. Each 2-mm increase in interpupillary distance increases convergence demands by about 1 Δ. Greater vertex distances increase convergence demand about 1 Δ per millimeter of increase.

Increased bifocal addition power is the most significant cause of increased vergence demand with aphakic spectacle correction. In general, prescribing the closest spectacle lens vertex distance and the weakest addition possible will minimize problems of increased convergence demand with initial aphakic correction. Aphakic patients who need strong (+ 14.00 to + 15.50 D) or very strong (greater than + 15.50 D) spectacle lens corrections with wide interpupillary distances have very large demands on near convergence and are best corrected with contact lenses, especially when strong (above + 2.50 D) near additions are needed.

Increased convergence demands with the spectacle correction of aphakia are treated with the rehabilitative therapy techniques previously described for near exophoria. These can be combined with puzzle tasks to enhance spatial awareness simultaneously. Rehabilitative therapy is generally successful in developing the convergence ability necessary for near tasks. Occasionally, prism segments or near reading corrections with base-in prisms are required for comfortable sustained near vision.

Difficulties in adapting to aphakic spectacle lenses are largely solved by contact lenses or pseudophakic correction. These corrections eliminate many of the size differences and spectacle lens distortions of aphakic spectacle lenses, thus causing significantly fewer adaptive problems. Increased convergence requirements after cataract surgery, however, are not eliminated by contact lens correction. Convergence therapy is still needed by many of these patients to obtain the best binocularity at near. Increased convergence requirements are reduced after intraocular lens implants, and convergence therapy is needed less frequently.

Intraocular Lens Implants

Intraocular lens implants are the management of choice after cataract surgery. This solves the problem of spectacle adaptation for cataract patients but can cause new problems when surgery initially is on only one eye: aniseikonia and anisometropia. The problem of aniseikonia also exists when contact lenses are used to correct monocular aphakia. Spectacle lens overcorrections, which are needed for clear vision at near, can be designed to minimize the problems of aniseikonia and anisometropia.

Aniseikonia and Anisometropia

Aniseikonia is a relative difference in the size, the shape, or both the size and shape of the ocular images. Clinically significant aniseikonia is aniseikonia that is greater than 0.75% associated with symptoms related to the use of the eyes (headaches, asthenopia, and spatial distortions) and that is not relieved by accurate refractive or motility correction (Bannon, 1965).

Intraocular lens implants and contact lenses to correct the refractive error after cataract surgery reduce aniseikonia to a minimum in unilateral aphakia. Aniseikonia usually is not considered in spectacle overcorrection of unilateral pseudophakic patients. Lens correction is always needed, even if just a near addition, for clear near vision. After a unilateral lens implant, there is an average ocular image size difference from 1.52 to 2.17% for various anterior chamber lenses (Choyce, 1961; Troutman, 1962). The image of the eye without the implant generally requires magnification. Contact lens correction of unilateral aphakia leaves approximately a 6% image size difference between the two eyes. This 2% to 6% image size difference causes symptoms for many patients.

The rehabilitation of aniseikonia after a unilateral lens implant or monocular contact lens correction of aphakia uses iseikonic lenses. Lens corrections are designed to equalize magnification as much as possible for the two eyes. Lenses are modified by making a thicker, steeper base curve lens for the eye requiring the magnification. If necessary, the opposite lens can be made thinner with a flatter base curve. Complete lens design techniques are available (Wick, 1973).

Increasing anisometropia during cataract development and after unilateral implants also can lead to binocular vision problems. This rapidly developed anisometropia causes prismatic differences in all fields of gaze, but it especially causes problems upon downgaze. Rehabilitation uses lens corrections for reading only or slab-off prism when bifocal lenses are used. The amount of slab-off prism to be prescribed can be measured using fixation disparity tests. In general, the amount measured by fixation disparity can be prescribed and is almost always less than the amount expected based on calculated prismatic differences between the two lenses. When contact lens corrections are used for unilateral aphakic correction, the contact lens is prescribed so that there is isometropic (equal) spectacle lens overcorrection. In this way, the problem of anisometropia and slab-off prism can be avoided with contact lens correction.

VISUAL-FIELD DEFECTS

Visual-field evaluations provide a functional assessment of the location, extent, and quality of the area of best vision (Bailey, 1978). The location, density, size, and number of scotomas are significant in determining the visual care of the patient (Jose and Ferraro, 1983). Recent field losses may be caused by life- or vision-threatening conditions, and patients with them should be referred to appropriate health-care practitioners.

When central visual-field defects affect visual acuity or patient fixation, the patient is best served by comprehensive low-vision evaluation. Some patients have binocular peripheral field loss. Careful analysis using the tangent screen, arc perimeter, and Amsler grid is indicated for optimal evaluation. When complex field loss (multiple scotomas, ring scotomas, peripheral islands of vision, and so on) is present, a low-vision evaluation should be done.

Partial monocular field loss is usually not a large problem, because the intact field of the other eye compensates adequately. However, occasionally when there is a high phoria, partial monocular field loss will cause fusion difficulty, and the patient will complain of transient diplopia or confusion. Vergence training and prism corrections are indicated for these patients to give the best possible fusion ability and minimize diplopia.

When binocular congruous field loss is present, techniques such as partial mirrors, mirrors, or prisms can increase the patient's awareness of objects located in the blind area. Bilateral conjugate prisms (with bases in the same direction) will enable the patient to become more aware of objects in the scotomatous area. Although prism does not expand the visual field, without it, the patient must make large head or eye movements toward the blind area to detect objects. Prism allows the use of small scanning eye movements to locate objects in the peripheral field. With the prism in place, the apparent position of objects is displaced toward the primary visual direction; objects are then easier for the patient to locate. Usually, visual acuity must be essentially normal for prism field enhancement; patients with reduced acuity need appropriate low-vision care.

A binocular mirror system also can be used for field defect rehabilitation (Goodlaw, 1982). Semitransparent mirrors with a 30% reflectant coating on the ocular surface are used to allow use of the remaining nasal fields, and temporal fields are seen by reflection. However, the two fields are seen simultaneously, and the mirror device is somewhat cumbersome. Generally, prisms are cosmetically superior and probably easier to adapt to.

Monocular mirrors can expand peripheral awareness by blocking out the seeing field of one eye and projecting a superimposed field of the lost area. The mirror allows the user to monitor major changes occurring in the blind field. Images seen in the mirror move rapidly with head movement and are reversed. The patient must learn to suppress the mirror image for many tasks and only use it when needed. Large eye movements, hand movements, or both are needed to look at an object in the blind field. The success rate with mirrors is not very high (Bailey, 1982) because of nausea or disorientation from the moving reversed mirror image.

Prism rehabilitation of visual field defects uses Fresnel prisms put on one sector of each spectacle lens. Prism power is chosen based on the lateral excursion of the patient's habitual eye movements. Larger eye movements allow prisms to be placed farther from the line of sight and lower powers to be used. Prism powers from 10 Δ to 30 Δ can be used, depending on the scanning area and the patient response. Initial prism power may have to be reduced as the patient's scanning ability improves.

Prisms are placed on the lenses where they will not interfere with primary gaze and normal eye movements. The patient should not be aware of the prisms during normal eye movements and should need only small scanning movements into the prisms to see objects in the blind field. Prisms usually are placed 1 mm or more away from the primary position of gaze (Jose and Smith, 1976; Weiss, 1972). They are placed on one lens at a time by occluding one eye and having the patient make eye movements into the blind field with the other eye while the prism is positioned. The leading edge of the prism is moved until the patient is just aware of the prism location. This procedure then is repeated for the other eye, and finally binocular adjustment is done so that both lines of sight simultaneously meet the prism edges. Generally, prisms must be used binocularly. When monocular prisms are used, patients may experience confusion when their gaze first encounters the prism and diplopia when looking further into the prism.

The necessity of using prisms is based on the location of the field loss. Right hemianopsias cause reading problems, because the patient has difficulty knowing where the next word is and often loses the line. Typoscopes, margin markers in books, and reading slits help the patient improve tracking ability. Occasionally, a patient is assisted by learning to read from right to left on an inverted book or by holding the book sideways and reading from the top down, thus avoiding reading into the scotomatous areas. Rehabilitative techniques will assist patients in learning these techniques when they are necessary.

Left hemianopsias cause fewer problems. Reading ability (right saccades) generally is not impaired, but patients tend to lose their place on returning to the next line. A marker (a finger or other object placed at the start of the next line) usually solves the problem. Superior field losses cause some problems. Because vertical (upward) scanning is difficult, base-up conjugate prism (with bases in the same direction) seems to be superior when prisms are required (Jose and Ferraro, 1983). Inferior field losses cause mobility problems and reading confusion when the patient tries to find the next line or scan a picture. Prism scanning aids are less successful than improving mobility with head movement, cane travel training, or both (Jose and Ferraro 1983).

Careful instruction and training can be valuable in the rehabilitation of visual-field defects. Patients must be told that scanning eye movements into the prisms may cause initial confusion and that objects, usually invisible, will appear suddenly in front of them. Images are displaced from their actual position by an amount that depends on the distance of the object seen.

Visual and perceptual rehabilitative therapy can improve judgment of object distance and location. The patient is seated, and objects are brought from the blind field into the seeing field at various distances and speeds (a swinging Marsden ball and ring work well). The patient is trained to judge correct responses by "ringing" the ball as it moves. As improvement is shown, the same and more complex tasks are repeated while the patient stands or walks. When mobility is substantially impaired, referral for mobility training can often greatly benefit the patient.

PATIENT EDUCATION, MONITORING, AND SELECTION

The availability of the most expert techniques and the finest instrumentation do not insure the success of therapy. The patient must be educated to understand alternative therapy (lenses or prisms, vision therapy, or both), along with the scope and magnitude of the problem. Unless the patient can be properly motivated and fully understands the need for, and the technique of, the treatment being used, management will not succeed. Literature describing lens corrections, vision therapy, heterophoria, stroke, and so on is valuable in explaining therapy and reinforcing patient cooperation. The following are psychologically sound techniques of greatly increasing patient cooperation with therapy:

1. It is best to work well within the patient's limitations in order to give a feeling of success at each session.
2. Emphasis on positive results is preferable to a detailed explanation of any dire results that could occur if the therapy is not completed.
3. Rehabilitative vision therapy, like any other health routine, must be done regularly. Help the patient set a time of day that insures the therapy's completion. Instructions to do therapy techniques 15 minutes each day at 9 in the morning, noon, and 6 in the evening are superior to simple instructions to do these techniques 45 minutes every day.
4. Written instructions often are helpful. A daily checklist showing results also can be used in more difficult cases. Routine instruction sheets can be prepared for the patient to reinforce a careful, friendly, personal explanation by the doctor. A typical home therapy instruction sheet is shown in Figure 10.7.

Monitoring rehabilitative therapy is simplified if the reasons for the therapy are kept in mind. It is important to question the patient about any decrease in symptoms, the amount of time spent in therapy, and the understanding of techniques. Therapy progress can be monitored objectively by repeating appropriate tests. Vergence ranges, the convergence near point, suppression tests, and forced vergence fixation disparity curves generally can be repeated as appropriate. As therapy progresses, vergence ranges expand, the near point of convergence improves, and suppression lessens. Forced vergence fixation disparity curves are especially helpful for monitoring near binocularity improvement of presbyopic patients. As binocularity improves, curves generally flatten; this indicates better compensation over a larger range of vergence changes.

Patients should be selected on an individual basis. Nearly all elderly patients can have some relief of symptoms related to faulty binocular vision when appropriate medical care is combined with subsequent optometric rehabilitative therapy as needed. Rehabilitative therapy consists of lenses and prisms combined with

PATIENT INSTRUCTIONS
Fixed Vectograms

The purpose of this therapy is to develop the coordination and focusing ability of your eyes. An additional benefit is a reduction in suppression which helps you use both eyes together so that you will obtain all the benefits of binocular vision. You will know that you are doing the techniques correctly when you can do the procedures quickly and easily without suppressing.

Perform therapy _____ minutes daily and increase the number of procedures in each session as you can do them. In the beginning you may experience discomfort, such as headaches, eyestrain, etc., and have to limit the therapy to a few minutes. As your ability improves, your discomfort will disappear and the therapy time can be increased. Remember that therapy 15 minutes daily is better than therapy two hours once a week. It would be best if you do this therapy at _____ each day. Try to establish a routine so that you always do the techniques at the same time each day.

There are many vectograms that can be used. Your doctor will give you the vectogram to use for your problem. An example of the types of techniques is discussed here. Ask your doctor if you have questions about how to use the vectograms you were given. Generally you should strive to observe all of the detail on the vectogram with no suppression or diplopia. Look from detail to detail spelling out the words or other tasks that require accurate attention and effort to keep the vectogram clear.

Procedure 1: View the vectogram through the polarizing glasses, which are designed to be used over your glasses if necessary. Do not remove or lift up the polarizing glasses when you refer to the instructions. Looking from picture to page provides additional therapy. Hold the vectograph so you are looking at it squarely with an evenly illuminated white surface behind it. Hold the picture about 20 inches from your eye. Study the picture carefully. The vectogram has a large number of fixation objects and you want to see them all single and clearly.

POSSIBLE TASKS: Consider the scene of the vectogram and let your eyes run around the course, always going slowly enough to see each part of it accurately. If there are letters, start with the letter *A* and jump quickly through the alphabet. Take a pointer and spell different words, touching each letter as you spell the word.

Procedure 2: Repeat the tasks of Procedure 1 except look up from the picture several times during each training period. The ability to look rapidly from the vectogram to distance and back again is important. Bring the vectogram in closer and repeat the procedure. You should be able to bring it in as close as 13 inches after practice.

Procedure 3: Prism alterations: Repeat the tasks of Procedure 1 using a special prism which you are to place in front of your _____ eye. First place the base in; next place the base out. Get a correct fusion response through the prism, then quickly remove it and regain the correct fusion response. Alternate the prism between base in and out, making sure that you never change the prism until the vectogram is single, clear, suppression-free, and seen with stereopsis.

Procedure 4: Lens alterations: Repeat the tasks of Procedure 1 using a special lens flippers, which you are to place in front of both eyes. Get a correct fusion response through the lenses, then quickly change them to the other power and regain the correct fusion response. Alternate the lenses between plus and minus, making sure that you never change them until the vectogram is single, clear, suppression-free, and seen with stereopsis.

Goal: To be able to view all the targets without diplopia, clearly, and comfortably at a close working distance.

Figure 10.7. Patient Instructions — Fixed Vectograms.

vision therapy to improve vergence ranges, eliminate suppression, reduce adverse adaptations after stroke, and improve motility in muscle weakness or restrictive syndromes.

When the patient is mentally capable of understanding instructions, therapy is generally successful in alleviating or reducing symptoms. As with all physical therapy, however, some patients are unwilling or unable to comply. These patients should be managed with lens or prism modification of the spectacle correction to give maximal symptom relief. Occasionally, patients have progressive problems that therapy can help only minimally. These patients need continued medical monitoring to be sure the condition is controlled maximally. Optometric rehabilitative therapy can be done concurrently to give the best possible relief of symptoms.

REFERENCES

1. Bailey, I.L. "Visual Field Measurement in Low Vision" *Optom. Monthly* 69 (1978): 697–701.
2. Bailey, I.L. "Mirrors for Visual Field Defects." *Optom. Monthly* 73 (1982): 202–206.
3. Bannon, R.E. *Clinical Manual on Aniseikonia.* Buffalo, N.Y.: American Optical Co., 1965.

4. Borish, I. *Clinical Refraction,* 3rd ed. Chicago: Professional Press, 1975.
5. Carter, D.B. "Fixation Disparity and Heterophoria Following Prolonged Wearing of Prism." *Am. J. Optom. Arch. Am. Acad. Optom.* 42 (1965): 144–152.
6. Choyce, D.P. "All-Acrylic Anterior Chamber Implants in Ophthalmic Surgery." *Lancet* 2 (July 22, 1961): 165–171.
7. Cohen, A.H., and R. Soden. "An Optometric Approach to the Rehabilitation of the Stroke Patient" *J. Am. Optom. Assoc.* 52 (1981): 795–800.
8. Cooper, J., and R. Duckman. "Convergence Insufficiency: Incidence, Diagnosis, and Treatment." *J. Am. Optom. Assoc.* 49 (1978): 673–680.
9. Craik, F.I.M. "Age Differences in Human Memory." In: J.E. Birren and K.W. Shaie (eds.). *Handbook of the Psychology of Aging.* New York: Van Nostrand, 1977.
10. Eskridge, J.B. "Flip Prism Test for Vertical Phoria" *Am. J. Optom. Arch. Am. Acad. Optom.* 38 (1961): 415–419.
11. Gibson, H. *Textbook of Orthoptics.* London: Hatton, 1955.
12. Goodlaw, E. "Rehabilitating a Patient with Bitemporal Hemianopia." *Am. J. Optom. Physiol. Opt.* 59 (1982): 677–679.
13. Griffin, J.R. *Binocular Anomalies: Procedures for Vision Therapy.* Chicago: Professional Press, 1976.
14. Griffin, J.R., and J.M. Lee. "The Polaroid Mirror Method." *Optom. Weekly* 61, no. 40 (1970): 29.
15. Hamasaki, D., J. Ong, E. Marg. "The Amplitude of Accommodation in Presbyopia." *Am. J. Optom. Arch. Am. Acad. Optom.* 33 (1956): 3–14.
16. Henson, D.B., and R. North. "Adaptation to Prism-induced Heterophoria." *Am. J. Optom. Physiol. Opt.* 57 (1980): 129–137.
17. Hirsch, M.J., M. Alpern, H.L. Schultz. "The Variation of Phoria with Age." *Am. J. Optom. Arch. Am. Acad. Optom.* 25 (1948): 535–541.
18. Hirsch, M.J., and L. Bing. "The Effect of Testing Method on Values Obtained for Phorias at Forty Centimeters." *Am. J. Optom. Arch. Am. Acad. Optom.* 25 (1948): 407–416.
19. Hofstetter, H.W. "A Comparison of Duane's and Donder's Tables of the Amplitude of Accommodation." *Am. J. Optom. Arch. Am. Acad. Optom.* 21 (1944): 345–363.
20. Hofstetter, H.W. "A Longitudinal Study of Amplitude Changes in Presbyopia." *Am. J. Optom. Arch. Am. Acad. Optom.* 42 (1965): 3–8.
21. Hoyer, W.J., and D.J. Plude. Attentional and Perceptual Processes in the Study of Cognitive Aging. In: L.W. Poon (ed.). *Aging in the 1980s: Psychological Issues.* Washington, D.C.: American Psychological Association, 1980.
22. Hugonnier, R., and S. Hugonnier. *Strabismus Heterophoria, Ocular Motor Paralysis.* Ed. and trans. Veronneau-Troutman. St. Louis: C.V. Mosby, 1969.
23. Jose, R.T., and J. Ferraro. "Functional Interpretation of the Visual Fields of Low Vision Patients." *J. Am. Optom. Assoc.* 54 (1983): 885–893.
24. Jose, R.T., and A.J. Smith. "Increasing Peripheral Field Awareness with Fresnel Prisms." *Opt. J. Rev. Optom.* 113 (1976): 33–37.
25. Maddox, E.E. *The Clinical Use of Prisms and the Decentering of Lenses.* Bristol, England: John Wright & Sons, 1893.
26. Morgan, M.W. "The Turville Infinity Binocular Balance Test." *Am. J. Optom. Arch. Am. Acad. Optom.* 26 (1949): 231–239.
27. Morgan, M.W. "Accommodative Changes in Presbyopia and Their Correction." In: M.J. Hirsch and R.E. Wick (eds.). *Vision of the Aging Patient.* Philadelphia: Chilton, 1960, pp. 83–112.
28. O'Connor, R. "Contracture in Ocular-Muscle Paralysis." *Am. J. Ophthalmol.* 26 (1943): 69.

29. Parks, M.M. "Isolated Cyclovertical Muscle Palsy." *Arch. Ophthalmol.* 60 (1958): 1027–1035.
30. Pitts, D.G. "The Effects of Aging on Selected Visual Functions: Dark Adaptation, Visual Acuity, Stereopsis, and Brightness Contrast" In: R. Sekuler, D. Kline, and K. Dismukes (eds.). *Aging and Human Visual Function.* New York: Alan R. Liss, 1982, pp. 131–159.
31. Rucker, C.W. "Paralysis of Third, Fourth, and Sixth Cranial Nerves." *Am. J. Ophthalmol.* 46 (1958): 787.
32. Rutstein, R.P., and J.B. Eskridge. "Studies in Vertical Fixation Disparity." *Am. J. Optom. Physiol. Opt.* 63 (1986): 639–644.
33. Rush, J.A., and B.R. Younge. "Paralysis of Cranial Nerves III, IV, and VI: Causes and Prognosis in 1,000 Cases." *Arch. Ophthalmol.* 99 (1981): 76–79.
34. Schor, C. "Analysis of Tonic and Accommodative Vergence Disorders of Binocular Vision." *Am. J. Optom. Physiol. Opt.* 60 (1983): 1–14.
35. Schor, C., and K.J. Ciuffreda. *Vergence Eye Movements: Basic Clinical Aspects.* Boston: Butterworths, 1983.
36. Schor, C., and V. Narayan. "Graphical Analysis of Prism Adaptation, Convergence Accommodation and Accommodative Vergence." *Am. J. Optom. Physiol. Opt.* 59 (1982): 774–784.
37. Sheedy, J.E. "Actual Measurement of Fixation Disparity and Its Use in Diagnosis and Treatment." *J. Am. Optom. Assoc.* 51 (1980): 1079–1084.
38. Sheedy, J.E., and J.J. Saladin. "Exophoria at Near in Presbyopia." *Am. J. Optom. Physiol. Opt.* 52 (1975): 474–481.
39. Sheedy, J.E., and J.J. Saladin. "Phoria, Vergence and Fixation Disparity in Oculomotor Problems." *Am. J. Optom. Physiol. Opt.* 54 (1977): 474–478.
40. Sun, F., L. Stark, A. Nguyen, J. Wong, V. Lakshminarayanan, and E. Mueller. "Changes in Accommodation with Age: Static and Dynamic." *Am. J. Optom. Physiol. Opt.* 65 (1988): 492–498.
41. Troutman, R.C. "Artiphakia and Aniseikonia." *Trans. Am. Ophthalmol. Soc.* 60 (1962): 590–658.
42. Vodnoy, B.E. *The Practice of Orthoptics and Related Topics,* 4th ed. South Bend, IN: Bernell Corp., 1970.
43. von Noorden, G.K. *Binocular Vision and Ocular Motility,* 4th ed. St. Louis: C.V. Mosby, 1990, p. 168.
44. Weiss, N.J. "An Application of Cemented Prisms with Severe Field Loss." *Am. J. Optom. Physiol. Opt.* 49 (1972): 261–264.
45. Welford, A.T. "Experimental Psychology in the Study of Aging." *Br. Med. Bull.* 20 (1964): 65–69.
46. Weymouth, F.W. "Effect of Age on Visual Acuity." In: M.J. Hirsch and R.E. Wick (eds.). *Vision of the Aging Patient.* Philadelphia: Chilton, 1960, pp. 37–62.
47. Wick, B. "Iseikonic Considerations for Today's Eyewear." *Am. J. Optom. Arch. Am. Acad. Optom.* 50 (1973): 952–967.
48. Wick, B. "A Fresnel Prism Bar for Home Visual Therapy." *Am. J. Optom. Arch. Am. Acad. Opt.* 51 (1974): 576–578.
49. Wick, B. "Vision Therapy for Presbyopes." *Am. J. Optom. Physiol. Opt.* 54 (1977): 244–247.
50. Wick, B. "Clinical Factors in Proximal Vergence." *Am. J. Optom. Physiol. Opt.* 62 (1985): 1–18.
51. Wick B., and R. London. "Vertical Fixation Disparity Correction Effect on the Horizontal Forced Vergence Fixation Disparity Curve." *Am. J. Optom. Physiol. Opt.* 64 (1987): 653–656.

52. Wick, R.E. Management of the Aging Patient in Optometric Practice. In: M.J. Hirsch and R.E. Wick (eds.). *Vision of the Aging Patient*. Philadelphia: Chilton, 1960, pp. 214–240.
53. Winter, J. "Striated Lenses and Filters in Strabismus." *Optom. Weekly* (June 10, 1971): 531–534.

Acknowledgment

My thanks to my father, Dr. Ralph E. Wick, for his help and support in all my writing and especially this chapter. He was free with his comments and suggestions, as usual.

11

Aphakia

Christina M. Sorenson

ETIOLOGIC FACTORS

Aphakia is the absence of the crystalline lens. The definition is broad and includes developmental abnormalities, trauma, surgical removal, and, in some cases, surgical removal of the cataractous crystalline lens and implantation of an intraocular lens (IOL). This chapter considers only the surgical removal of the crystalline lens without benefit of IOL implantation.

The development of the cataract is appropriately discussed in other sections of this book. All biologic systems are subject to myriad factors that accelerate senescence. These include oxidation, thermal effects (infrared radiation), photochemical effects (ultraviolet radiation), malnutrition, hormonal side effects, and errors in synthesis (Young, 1991). Both extrinsic and intrinsic forces act on the lens to produce molecular aggregation, oxidation, and insolubilization, accompanied by pigmentation, membrane fragmentation, and loss of enzymatic activity with predictable cataract development.

PATIENT SELECTION FOR SURGICAL APHAKIA

At present, surgical aphakia rarely is recommended because of the excellent results of microsurgical techniques and available technology. Absolute contraindications to IOL implantation include rubeosis irides and secondary glaucoma and chronic recurrent iritis (Stark et al., 1989). Occasionally, the patient's age may be a contraindication, but this may be slowly changing with the development of IOL materials and techniques (Heff et al., 1989). A few patients refuse to consider IOLs, and in some areas of the world these lenses are not available.

INCIDENCE OF SURGICAL APHAKIA

In the years before implantation, crystalline lens removal was the treatment for cataract development and the subsequent decreased visual acuity (Lazar, 1982). In 1950, Ridley (1951) began the first in a series of IOL implantations. In the years to follow, IOLs were placed into the anterior chamber (AC) of the eye.

The early patients of AC IOL placement often developed complications such as corneal decompensation and uveitis-glaucoma-hyphema syndrome (Rycroft, 1968; Apple et al., 1984). The AC placement of the IOL was improved upon, and now posterior chamber "in the bag" placement of IOLs is standard practice (Southwick and Olsen, 1984; Kraff et al., 1983). There are, however, still a number of patients who became aphakic before the development of IOLs.

Today, optometrists may encounter a few aphakic patients each year, and a decision must be made as to the best method of visual correction. Patients seek restoration of useful vision, and the goal must be visual rehabilitation. The correction options of the aphakic patient include spectacles, contact lenses, and/or several surgical procedures.

CORRECTION OPTIONS OF APHAKIA
Nonsurgical Correction of Aphakia
Spectacle Correction of Aphakia
The spectacle correction of aphakia has been discussed in texts and papers (Sloan and Garcia, 1979; Borish, 1983). The difficulties associated with aphakic spectacle correction are well known. Optically, difficulties arise from magnification, incorrect pantoscopic tilt, improper vertex distance, pincushion distortion, improper face form tilt, and ring scotoma with its "jack-in-the-box phenomenon" and restricted visual field. From a patient's view, difficulties with an aphakic spectacle correction may include altered depth perception, difficulty with hand-eye coordination, maintaining spectacles in precise adjustment for optimum acuity, binocularity, restricted visual field, and cosmesis (Borish, 1975; Kerr, 1981). Optical and fitting difficulties aside, the spectacle correction for the patient is usually relatively inexpensive and requires little or no follow-up compared with contact lenses and/or further surgery.

Patient selection for spectacle correction of aphakia may be based on patient personality, desires, and life-style. Because of the safety and efficacy of secondary IOL implantation, there may be an inclination for referral for surgical evaluation. However, many patients are frightened by surgery or are unable to undergo surgery because of concomitant illness(es). Some patients are unable to be compliant with postoperative follow-up and medications. Some patients may fall into one of the previously discussed, contraindicated categories of IOL implantation (Stark et al., 1989; Heff et al., 1989). Lastly, many aphakic contact lens successes may become contact lens failures for only a limited period of time.

The aphakic patient must adapt to an altered vision status. The aphakic spectacle correction may change magnification up to 25% to 35% (Guyton, 1979). This altered spatial perception may cause the patient to miss steps or reach for objects that are not located where they appear to be. The magnification of lens is a function of the vertex distance, lens thickness, and dioptric power (Borish, 1975). To minimize the magnification, the practitioner should be selective in the lens design and fitting technique. The dioptric power most often cannot be decreased without sacrificing visual acuity, even though a decrease in the power of the lens will minify magnification. Realistic options of shortened vertex distance, thinner lens and flatter base curve selection each decrease the total magnification of the spectacle prescription, allowing a "truer" spatial perception for the patient.

A roving ring scotoma (Figure 11.1) or the jack-in-the-box phenomenon is another common report by aphakics with spectacle correction (Welsh, 1967). Again, magnification and lens design can be altered to minimize this abberation. A decreased vertex distance, thin lens design, and flatter base curve all will aid in minimizing the magnification, thereby decreasing the jack-in-the-box phenomenon. Additionally, if the overall lens diameter can be increased, increasing asphericity by flattening the front curvature toward the edge of the lens will move the scotomatous area further peripherally, which decreases the edge prism power and thereby decreases the jack-in-the-box phenomenon. (It should be noted that this runs contrary to the MED Principle of Reiner [Reiner, 1982].)

Rotational eye movements will cause patients to experience a roving scotoma and increased prismatic effect (Fonda, 1981) whenever fixation takes place outside the optical centers. Many patients will adopt a central gaze with head movements rather than eye movements to reduce the roving scotoma and prismatic effect.

The refraction of the aphake can be achieved in several ways. Temporary cataract glasses or the "zero-error refracting glasses" are recommended by some experts (Reiner, 1982). Others prefer a trial frame refraction with exacting duplication directly to the spectacle correction (Midler, 1981). The use of Jannelli or Halberg clips (Figure 11.2) over selected frame (or the trial frame), keratometric readings, and retinoscopy provide the starting point for a manifest aphakic refraction. The manifest refraction is completed easily with the use of the trial lens set and a hand-held Jackson Cross Cylinder.

Convergence through a near addition may induce a base out effect created by the distance power. This can be corrected for by decentration of each segment 3.5 mm to 4.0 mm. A separate reading prescription might also be considered. The bifocal addition should be verified by a front vertex reading in a vertometer and

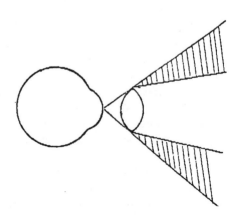

Figure 11.1 A schematic drawing of the "Jack-in-the-Box" phenomenon.

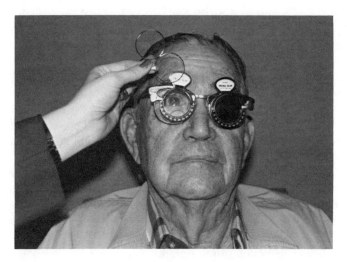

Figure 11.2 A temporary aphakic spectacle prescription is re-fined with the use of Halberg clips and over-refracting techniques.

not the back vertex power measurement, which is appropriate for the distance portion of the aphakic prescription (Malone et al., 1989).

In addition to specifying the power and the base curve, the measurement of vertex distance, including 1.0 mm lid thickness, and specification of desired pan-toscopic tilt (Reiner, 1982; Kerr, 1981) should be part of the prescription (Figure 11.3). The pupillary distance should be measured as exactly as possible to avoid

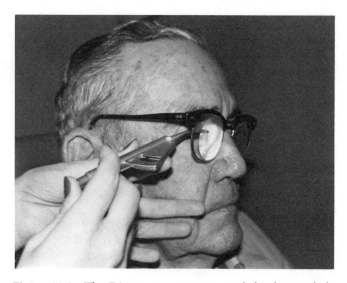

Figure 11.3 The Distometer measurement behind an aphakic spectacle correction.

induced prism. Instruments such as the Essilor Digital CRP are available for inter-pupillary distance (IPD) measurement, which, when used properly, make the IPD measurement repeatable and exacting monocularly and binocularly. The base curve may be omitted if an aspheric trade name lens is prescribed. The use of the lenticular design, where base curve specification is as flat as possible in the available plus lens blank, is advised only if prism correction is needed. An ultraviolet (UV) coating is desirable to protect the eye (Lerman, 1980; Miller, 1987; Newsome, 1985). A tint also may be recommended if there has been iris damage or an iridectomy performed. This may aid in glare reduction and greater patient comfort. (See Appendix A and Chapter 18.)

By use of the meticulous over-refraction technique, patients are well aware of the challenges that confront them at the time of dispensing. Close communication among the patient, the optician, and the doctor can alleviate patient adaptation difficulties.

Contact Lens Correction of the Aphake

Patients who are dissatisfied with an aphakic spectacle correction may be ideal contact lens candidates. Additionally, any monocular aphake will be an excellent candidate for a contact lens correction due to extreme anisometropia.

Practically, contact lenses (Guillon and Warland, 1980) perform as well as IOLs and are found to be optically "truer" than aphakic spectacles with regard to distorted field of view and magnification (Polse, 1981). Contact lenses and IOLs rotate with the eye and therefore avoid prismatic effects found with spectacle correction and eye rotation. Moreover, the contact lenses can be modified and updated, and their failure does not preclude the use of alternative methods of aphakic correction (Graham, 1988).

Contact lens fitting may begin as early as four weeks postoperatively in an uncomplicated cataract extraction without IOL implantation. The wound, cornea, and anterior chamber are inspected carefully. Signs of continued inflammation, chemosis, and poor wound apposition and injection indicate the need for further healing time. Stable manifest refraction and keratometric readings also aid to determine healing status.

Complications of contact lens wear are well known to every optometric practitioner. These include microbial keratitis, tight fit syndrome, striae/stromal edema, corneal erosion, neovascularization, blepharoconjunctivitis, punctate keratopathy, blepharitis, epithelial edema, giant papillary conjunctivitis, and epithelial microcysts. In the elderly aphakic patient, the practitioner also may note conjunctival bleb formation, loose or broken sutures, corneal dystrophies, iridectomy(ies), and meibomian gland dysfunction.

Successful contact lens correction includes proper fitting, material selection, compatible ocular condition, and, most importantly, patient compliance. It is imperative that patients understand the necessity of routine follow-up care, daily care of the lenses, and long-term sequelae of contact lens use.

Graham et al. (1988) have noted that patient age plays an important part in contact lens success. Daily wear contact lenses are found to be successful 89% of the time in the patient younger than 70 years of age, while the new daily wear contact lens patient of greater than 70 years of age shows a failure rate of 73% due to the inability to handle the contact lens. Koetting et al. (1988) noted great success in the aphakic extended-wear contact lens population, stating a success rate of 95%, with an average patient age of 61.8 years.

Normal corneal physiologic characteristics may be compromised with the aphakic contact lens because of the center thickness required and resultant hypoxia (Guillon and Morris, 1981). Development of the aspheric designs allows for the same central power with reduction of center thickness (Holden and Mertz, 1984). This allows for an improved transmission of oxygen and potentially less stress on corneal physiology with the contact lens in place.

Material for the aphakic contact lens includes polymethyl methacrylate (PMMA), various hydrogel materials, and various rigid gas-permeable (RGP) materials. In some cases, the PMMA material is not used because of the oxygen barrier. RGP materials generally fit larger to improve comfort and stability. These larger designs require a flatter fitting philosophy to maintain alignment across the posterior lens surface (Bridgewater, 1991). Additionally, UV-filtering properties have been added to some of the newest generation plastics to protect the retina from UV-A and UV-B electromagnetic radiation. UV light and blue light have been implicated in the development of macular changes and cataract development (Taylor et al., 1992).

The aphakic patient may be aided in the handling of the contact lenses through the use of a magnification mirror and/or a contact lens inserter. These, in conjunction with established finger placement, tactile clues, and lighting, all allow for improved contact lens insertion and removal.

Fitting contact lenses to a patient who is unhappy with the correction afforded with spectacles frequently results in restored spatial perception and mobility. Contact lens adaptation for the aphakic patient includes all the adaptation difficulties noted by any contact lens wearer. It may also include adaptation to differing insertion and removal techniques as the lid tissue changes in its tonicity with age.

Because of decreased corneal sensitivity, patients should be uncompromising in their wearing time and cleaning routines to avoid contact lens related ocular complications. (See Appendix B for information on aphakic contact lenses that are available in soft, rigid gas-permeable materials. Also see Chapter 9.)

Spectacle-Contact Lens Combination for the Aphake

The patient who enjoys the use of a contact lens correction but does not achieve full correction at distance and/or near will benefit from a combined contact lens–spectacle correction. A monocular aphake will note reduced diplopia, restored binocularity, and visual field with a contact lens–spectacle combination. This patient may note slight central suppression and reduced stereopsis resulting from residual anisometropia.

Techniques and instrumentation will be identical to that of an aphakic contact lens fit and a routine over-refraction. For the monocular aphake, a contact lens that overcorrects or undercorrects the patient to match the refractive error of the fellow phakic eye may be a method to achieve clear single binocular vision with the habitual spectacle prescription. (See Chapters 8 and 9.)

Surgical Correction of Aphakia
Secondary IOL Implantation for the Correction of Aphakia

IOLs implanted into the eye at a later date should be considered as a second surgical procedure to replace an extracted cataract. Secondary IOLs are often considered the treatment of choice in the rehabilitation of the aphakic patient (Wong et al., 1987; Swinger, 1987). Patients are evaluated on the basis of their general health and their ocular health. Evaluation of the AC angle, vitreous, and retina is performed routinely. Contraindications for secondary AC and/or posterior chamber (PC) IOL implantation may include a high risk of retinal detachment, chronic recurrent uveitis, and rubeosis irides. Relative contraindications may include glaucoma, cystoid macular edema, vitreous in the AC, and abnormal AC anatomy (Leatherburrow et al., 1988; Swinger, 1987). Corneal endothelial cell count/evaluation is commonly done when secondary procedures are considered. An eye with a relatively low cell count of less than 1,000 cells/mm^2 (Jaffe, 1981) may be a relative contraindication for the inexperienced surgeon (Maloney, 1988; Jaffe, 1981). However, with the use of viscoelastic substances, the risk of corneal decompensation through endothelial cell damage has been greatly reduced (Maloney, 1988). When it is contraindicated to perform a secondary IOL placement, the surgical procedure of epikeratophakia may be considered (Durrie et al., 1987). Patients should be counseled as with any intraocular surgical procedure and with the understanding that secondary procedures may carry a greater risk of complications (Hayward et al., 1990).

Secondary PC IOL implantation is performed when the posterior capsule is still intact. This technique is also used when the anatomy is such that a sulcus-fixated IOL will remain in place or when a PC location IOL can be safely sutured in place. A PC IOL is the procedure of choice so long as there are no contraindications (Lindstrom et al., 1982). Intraocular lenses are widely available, are accurate in refractive error correction, and have a relatively brief postoperative course.

Secondary AC IOL implantation is performed when the posterior capsule is absent or when the anatomy is such that a posterior placement is not possible. The anterior chamber is currently the most common location for secondary IOLs. Surgeons rely on their experience, expertise, and discretion to determine secondary IOL placement.

The power of the IOL is calculated with consideration of the keratometric readings, axial length, AC depth, and IOL placement. (Surgical technique and the patient's astigmatic regression curve may also play a role with the seasoned cataract surgeon.) Through the use of established formulas, such as the R.D. Binkhorst II shown in Table 11.1, the power of the anterior or posterior chamber IOL is calculated.

Table 11.1 An IOL calculation for posterior chamber placement and anterior chamber placement with a postoperative refractive aim of −0.75 diopters (R.D. Binkhorst II IOL calculation only)

	Primary	*Secondary*
Axial length	23.10	
AC depth	4.10	4.80
Keratometric value 1	45.00	
Keratometric value 2	45.87	
Postoperative refraction	−0.75	
Emmetropia Power	17.47	18.61

Primary		*Secondary*	
Refraction	*Implant*	*Refraction*	*Implant*
−1.95	20.00	−2.12	21.50
−1.17	19.00	−1.00	20.00
−0.78	18.50	−0.63	19.50
−0.40	18.00	−0.28	19.00
−0.03	17.50	0.08	18.50

IOLs were first implanted by Ridley in 1949. The lens was placed in the posterior chamber and made of glass. Through the years, the ideal location for IOL placement has led surgeons to place the lens in the PC, the AC, the iris plane with iris fixation, and in the iris fixated with posterior chamber support.

The PC is the location of choice following extracapsular cataract extraction with an intact capsular bag. Both the optic and the haptics of the IOL are behind the iris plane within the PC. The haptics support the IOL within the capsular bag or within the ciliary sulcus. Occasionally, the PC IOL haptics may make use of a transscleral suture to aid in haptic positioning if anatomy dictates.

AC placement following extracapsular or intracapsular cataract extraction with the haptics and the optic of the IOL within the AC of the eye is the most common in secondary IOL implantation. The haptics support the IOL in the angle of the AC.

Materials have also gone through a metamorphosis during the search for the ideal intraocular composition. Materials selected for IOLs are of high optical quality, are inert within a biological system, allow for long-term lens stabilization, and are easy to insert without induced inflammation. Polymethyl methacrylate, polypropylene, Perspex CQ and silicon are materials in use currently.

IOLs may be the ideal correction for aphakia as they reduce the aberrations and magnification found in other forms of correction. The successful use of the IOL lies not only in surgical skill but also in the determination of the postoperative refraction. The postoperative refractive aim is selected by the surgeon depending on patient needs. Binocularity and minimal anisometropia are most desirable. Many surgeons prefer to aim for a postoperative refractive error of low myopic amounts. This allows for near-task function by the patient, reduction of magnification induced by the IOL, and, in case of error of IOL calculation, may leave the patient myopic rather than hyperopic, which is often most tolerated by the patient.

IOL power calculation formulas are available for each style of IOL. The variables are the desired postoperative refractive aim, the keratometric readings, the axial length of the eye, and the postoperative AC depth of the eye.

The keratometric readings carry with them two sources of error: the calibration of the instrument and the index of refraction used by the instrument. These influences on the postoperative refraction have not been fully determined.

The axial length of the eye is determined by A-scan biometry. The A-scan must be aligned properly along the visual axis to obtain an accurate ultrasonic measurement. Global compression must also be avoided so as not to foreshorten the axial length.

The velocity of sound in each of the tissues is multiplied by the time it takes to pass through the tissue to yield the tissue thickness. The corneal thickness and velocity are often omitted from the equation for calculation of the axial length in determination of the intraocular lens power. One millimeter of error in the measurement of the axial length will result in an error of three diopters in the postoperative refraction. Solid A-scan probes allow for crisp echoes and accurate determination of the axial length in situ.

The postoperative AC depth makes use of an average value for each type of implant as influenced by the IOL thickness and the design of its haptics determine the expected positioning within the eye. Approximately 1 mm of error in AC depth will result in one diopter of error in the postoperative refraction. Expected postoperative recovery in secondary IOLs is approximately four to 12 weeks. Best visual acuity is usually achieved by six to nine weeks. Occasionally, there may be a loss of one to two lines of visual acuity with secondary IOL placement (Alper, 1989). Other possible complications include cystoid macular edema, retinal detachment, corneal decompensation, uveitis, glaucoma, pseudophakodenesis, and vitreous loss (Hayward et al., 1990). Generally, one can expect an improvement in visual functioning with secondary IOL implantation.

Future optometric care will continue to grow as co-management comes into greater usage. The optometrist may manage patients from one day postoperatively through their final refraction and continuing ocular health examinations.

Visual adaptation by patients is usually achieved within one to two weeks postoperatively. The postoperative spectacle prescription can be given as early as four weeks after the surgery. The update in the glasses aids patients in their acculturation to the changed spatial perception and acuity, both at distance and at near.

The following extraocular refractive procedures are now coming into greater use by the trained ophthalmic surgeon. The improvement of the technical difficulties with the newer procedures allows for this greater use. The determination of these procedures is still very selective because they are sometimes inaccurate and may demonstrate a decreased visual acuity with irregular astigmatism. It is interesting to note that the myopic procedures of keratomileusis and epikeratophakia at this time show greater accuracy in the postoperative refraction.

Hyperopic Keratomileusis

Hyperopic keratomileusis (HKM) is a method of reshaping the corneal surface to change its optical power. A disc of cornea is shaved off with a microtome, quickly frozen, and lathe-ground to a plus-shaped lenticule of predetermined power by subtracting tissue from the periphery of microkeratomed section. The reshaped corneal tissue then is returned to its original position within the patient's corneal stromal bed and sewn into place. Re-epithelialization takes place over this donor cryolathed lenticule. The steepened central corneal curvature and increased dioptric power brings the light rays into focus on the retina.

A non-freezing hypermetropic keratomileusis of Barraquer-Krumeich-Swinger (also known as planar lamellar refractive keratoplasty or PLRK) was first conceptualized in 1958 by Jose Barraquer (1980). The non-freeze technique is technically easier to learn, requires less instrumentation, and allows for greater survival of keratocytes with less damage to the donor cornea (Savala et al., 1988). The non-freezing method may allow for less variation in the expected postoperative result and a better quality of vision (Boyd et al., 1987; Savala, 1988). Conversely, the freezing technique requires a cryolathe, technical support of the instrumentation, technical expertise, and a freezing method. Freezing of the tissue causes a delay in healing.

Keratomileusis is often not done because secondary IOLs are a better option. The best aphakes for this procedure are between eight and 11 diopters of hypermetropia. If greater than 11 diopters hypermetropic, the patient will be left undercorrected; the refractive technique of choice is non-freeze epikeratophakia for this patient.

Rehabilitation for non-freeze keratomileusis is rapid. Epithelial defects are few, and graft clarity is often excellent. Optometric care can begin as early as one week postoperatively. Suture removal is commonly performed at three to four weeks postoperatively. Most patients can expect to achieve a greater visual potential within two months from their surgical date. A stable refraction is reached within one year postoperatively. Spectacles can be prescribed as early as two months postoperatively, with expected updates over the following months. Patient adaptation to a new visual world begins as soon as re-epithelization is completed.

Epikeratophakia

Epikeratophakia is another operation that involves the addition of tissue to modify corneal thickness and thereby the refractive power to alter the focusing of the light rays onto the retina. The corneal epithelium is removed, and an annular keratectomy is made. The donor predetermined plus-shaped lenticule is sewn to the prepared area of the patient's cornea. The epithelial cells of the patient will heal over this donor lenticule, leaving the newly shaped donor cornea and the patient's own epithelium and keratocytes. (See also Werblin-Kaufman-McDonald Epikeratophakia.)

Epikeratophakia can be done for patients in whom a primary or secondary IOL implantation is not feasible. This requires no entry into the eye and can be repeated, and it is reversible up to one year after the surgery (Swinger, 1987). This surgical technique is also feasible on corneas that are thinner than normal (<0.5 mm centrally), as the resultant cornea will be thicker with the addition of tissue. In thicker than normal corneas (>0.75 mm centrally), the postoperative recovery may not result in the achievement of the potential visual acuity (Boyd, 1987).

Patients with severe dry eye syndrome, extreme lagophthalmos, and severe blepharitis are not good candidates for epikeratophakia because these conditions may hinder re-epithelization over the donor tissue.

Tissue selection for epikeratophakia does not require fresh and viable cornea tissue (although viable tissue may be preferable); a centrally prepared disc can be transported and stored easily, safely, and for long periods of time (longer than tissue used for corneal transplantation) of up to two months (McDonald, 1987).

Expected postoperative recovery is on the order of months (Kaufman and McDonald, 1984). Scarring in the area of the annular keratectomy is expected. Optometric care of these patients often is started as soon as re-epithelization begins in one to two days. Sutures often are removed at three to four weeks postoperatively (Swinger, 1987). It is at this time also that patients will begin their adjustment to the change in their refractive error. Visual acuity continues to improve over time (McCartney, 1987) (Table 11.2).

Table 11.2   Surgical correction of aphakia — procedure comparison

Rehabilitation	Surgical Skill and Instrumentation	Preoperative Refractive Error	
Intraocular Secondary intraocular lens implantation			
Posterior chamber	Average	Most refractive errors	4 weeks
Anterior chamber	Average	Most refractive errors	4-8 weeks
Extraocular Lamellar refractive keratectomies			
Keratomileusis (HKM)	high	< +11.0 D	12 mos
Epikeratophakia (EPI)	>Average, training	Up to +30.0 D	4 mos

Experimental/Investigational Methods for the Surgical Correction of Aphakia

Intracorneal Implant/Corneal Inlay

Choyce polysulfone corneal inlay, or an intracorneal hydrogel implant, places a material optically and biochemically compatible with human corneal tissue into a pocket of the host cornea between the corneal epithelium and Bowman's layer. The refractive power is changed on the visual axis only. The inlay can be removed and exchanged through the original superior pocket incision.

This procedure is not yet approved by the Food and Drug Administration (FDA). It is performed in England and is found to be effective, but safe in only two-thirds of the patients; the remaining one-third developed corneal interface opacities and exudate around the inlay (Choyce et al., 1987). Fenestrated inlays have been done in animals with greater success and fewer side effects, and research is beginning in the use of the fenestrated corneal inlays in humans (McCarey, 1990; Oberlin et al., 1987). Theoretically, the correction with the use of the corneal inlay is −20.00 diopters to +20.00 diopters.

Photoablation for Corneal Refractive Surgery

The excimer UV laser, the carbon dioxide laser, the hydrogen fluoride laser, and variants of the YAG laser are all currently under investigation in corneal refractive surgery.

Laser light is used to excise tissue at a molecular level and reprofile the cornea. The reprofiling may be used to determine and create the lenticules with greater accuracy and with less loss of keratocytes, reducing difficulties with surface re-epithelization, thus allowing a shorter postoperative recovery. Additionally, the laser may be used in conjunction with any of the previously discussed techniques to reduce residual refractive errors.

Many methods are available to patients for the correction of aphakia. It is up to each optometrist as an eye-care practitioner to determine which of these methods will best allow each patient to achieve the fullest visual rehabilitation.

REFERENCES

1. Young, R. *Age Related Cataract*. New York: Oxford University Press, 1991, pp. 33–91.
2. Stark, W.J., A.C. Terry, A.E. Maumanee, (eds). *Intraocular Lenses: Changing Indications in Anterior Segment Surgery*. 1989, pp. 69–75.
3. Heff, L.K., P.S.F. Tseng, W. Yong. "Current Trends in the Correction of Aphakia: A Local Perspective." *Ann. Acad. Med. Singapore* 18, no. 2 (1989):172.
4. Lazar, P. "Recent Developments in Ophthalmology, Advances in Correction of the Optical Problems of the Postoperative Cataract Patient." *Arch. Dermatol.* 118(1982):526–527.
5. Ridley, H. "Intraocular Acrylic Lenses." *Trans. Ophthalmol. Soc. U. K.* 71 (1951):671–721.

6. Rycroft, P.V. "Acrylic Implants and Keratopathy." *Perspect. Ophthalmol.* 1 (1968):215–218.

7. Apple, D.J., N. Mamalis, K. Loftfield, et al. "Complication of Intraocular Lenses. A Historical and Histopathological Review." *Surv. Ophthalmol.* 29(1984):1–54.

8. Southwick, P.C. and R.J. Olsen. "Shearing Posterior Chamber Intraocular Lenses. Five Year Postoperative Results." *J. Am. Implant Soc.* 10(1984): 318–323.

9. Kraff, M.C., D.R. Sanders, H.L. Lieberman. "The Results of Posterior Chamber Lens Implantation." *J. Am. Implant Soc.* 9(1983):148–150.

10. Sloan, A.E. and G.E. Garcia. *Manual of Refraction,* 3rd ed. Boston: Little, Brown & Co., 1979, pp. 147–151.

11. Borish, I.M. "Aphakia, Perceptual and Refractive Problems of Spectacle Correction." *J. Am. Optom. Assoc.* 54, no.8 (1983):701–711.

12. Borish, I.M. *Clinical Refraction,* 3rd ed. Chicago: Professional Press, Inc., 1975, pp. 941–956.

13. Kerr, C. "Clinical Aspects of the Correction of Aphakic Spectacles." *Trans. Ophthalmol. Soc. U. K.* 101(1981):440.

14. Guyton, D.L. Aphakic Spectacle in Perspective. American Academy of Ophthalmology. Signet Optical Corporation. Baltimore: The Wilmer Ophthalmological Institute, The Johns Hopkins University School of Medicine, 1979 (videotape).

15. Welsh, R.C. "Defects of Vision through Aphakic Lenses." *Br. J. Ophthalmol.* Volume 51 (1967):306.

16. Reiner, G.L. "Aphakic and Pseudophakic Spectacle Management." *J. Am. Optom. Assoc.* 53, no. 4 (1982):296.

17. Fonda, G. "Spectacle Correction for Aphakia. The Prismatic Effect." *Surv. Ophthalmol.* 26, no. 3, (1981):154–156.

18. Midler, B. "The Aphakic Correction." *Can. J. Ophthalmol.* 15, (April 1981): 57–58.

19. Maloney, R.K., K.M. Miller, D.L. Guyton. "Aphakic Reading Adds. An Error in Traditional Teaching." *Ophthalmology* 96 (1989):1253–1256.

20. Lerman, S. *Radiant Energy and the Eye.* Boston: Macmillan, 1980.

21. Miller, D. (ed.). *Clinical Light Damage to the Eye.* Springer-Verlag, 1987.

22. Newsome, D. *Ultraviolet Effects on the Retina.* Presented at the FDA Ophthalmic Devices Panel Meeting, Washington, DC, May 13, 1985.

23. Guillon, M. and J. Warland. "Aniseikonia and Binocular Function in Unilateral Aphakes Wearing Contact Lenses. *J. Br. Contact Lens Assoc.* 1980; 3:36–38.

24. Polse, K.A. "Aphakia." In Mandell, R.B. (ed.). *Contact Lens Practice.* Springfield: Charles C. Thomas, 1981, Chapter 27.

25. Graham, C.M., J.K.G. Dart, N.W. Wilson-Holt, R.J. Buckley. "Prospects for Contact Lens Wear in Aphakia." *Eye.* 2 (1988):48–55.

26. Koetting, R.A., C.J. Metz, D.B. Seibel. "Clinical Impressions of Extended Wear Success Relative to Patient Age." *J. Am. Optom. Assoc.* no. 3, (1988):164–165.

27. Guillion, M. and J. Morris. "Corneal Response to a Provocative Test in Aphakic Patients." *J. Br. Contact Lens Assoc.* 4(1981):162–167.

28. Holden, B.A. and G.W. Mertz. "Critical Oxygen Levels to Avoid Corneal Edema for Daily and Extended Wear Contact Lenses." *Invest. Ophthalmol. Vis. Sci.* 25 (1984):1161–1167.

29. Bridgewater, B.A. "Fitting Philosophy of RGP Designs." Mesa, Arizona: Paragon Optical, 1991.

30. Taylor, H.R., S. West, B. Munoz, et al. "The Long-term Effects of Visible Light on the Eye." *Arch. Ophthalmol.* 110 (1992):99–104.

31. Wong, S.K., D.D. Kock, J.M. Emory. "Secondary Intraocular Lens Implantation." *J. Cataract Refract. Surg.* 13 (1987):17–20.

32. Swinger, C. "Cornea, Refractive Surgery and Contact Lens." *Trans. North Am. Acad. Ophthalmol.* New York: Raven Press, 1987.
33. Leatherbarrow, B., A. Trevett, A.B. Tullo. "Secondary Lens Implantation: Incidence, Indications and Complications." *Eye* 2 (1988):370–375.
34. Maloney, W.F. *Textbook of Phacoemulsification:* San Francisco: Lasenda Publishers, 1988.
35. Jaffe, N.S. Corneal Edema. In *Cataract Surgery and Its Complications,* 3rd ed. St. Louis: C.V. Mosby, Chapter 17.
36. Durrie, D.S., D.L. Jubrich, T.R. Deitz. "Secondary IOL Implantation vs. Epikeratophakia for the Treatment of Aphakia." *Am. J. Ophthalmol.* 103 (1987):384–391.
37. Hayward, J.M., B.A. Noble, N. George. "Secondary Intraocular Lens Implantation: Eight Year Experience." *Eye* 4 (1990):548–556.
38. Lindstrom, R.L., W.S. Harris, W.A. Lyle. "Secondary and Exchange Posterior Chamber Lens Implantation." *Am. Intraocul. Implant Soc. J.* 8 (1982):353–358.
39. Alper, J. *Ind. J. Ophthalmol.* 37, no. 2 (April–June 1989):54–57.
40. Barraquer, J.I. *Queratomileusis y Queratofaquia.* Bogota: Litografia Arco, 1980.
41. Savala E. Y., J. Krumeich, P. Binder. "Clinical Pathology of Non-freeze Lamellar Refractive Keratoplasty." *Cornea* 7, no. 3 (1988):223–230.
42. Boyd, B.F. *Refractive Surgery with the Masters. Highlights of Ophthalmology.* 1987, 24.
43. McDonald, M.B. Cornea, Refractive Surgery and Contact Lens. Trans New Orleans Am. Acad. Ophthalmology, 1987 (transcript).
44. Kaufman, H.E., M.B. McDonald. "Refractive Surgery for Aphakia and Myopia." *Trans. Ophthalmol. Soc. U. K.* 104 (1984):43–47.
45. McCartney, D.L. "Current Surgical Management of Aphakia." *Cataracts, Trans. North Am. Acad. Ophthalmol.* 2 (1987): 205–223.
46. Choyce, P. "Polysulfone Corneal Inlays. Personal Interview Between the Editor and Dr. Peter Choyce, M.D." *Refractive Surgery with the Masters. Highlights of Ophthalmology* 1987, pp 226.
47. McCarey, B.E. *Refraction and Corneal Surgery. Current Status of Refractive Surgery with Synthetic Intracorneal Lenses:* Barraquer lecture 6 (1990):40–46.
48. Oberlin, T.P., R.L. Peiffer, A.S. Patel. "Synthetic Keratophakia for the Correction of Aphakia." *Ophthalmology* 94, no. 8, (1987):926–934.

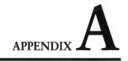

APPENDIX A

Ophthalmic Lenses

Aphakic lenses currently available, including spherical power range, cylindrical power range, bifocal style, center thickness, index of refraction, asphericity, can be found in the following publications:

- *Physicians Desk Reference for Ophthalmology*, Section Four, "Ophthalmic Lenses", Montvale, NJ: Medical Economics Data, Inc., updated annually.
- *Lenses, Frames Products Guide*, Newport Beach, CA, updated annually.

APPENDIX **B**

Aphakic Contact Lens Materials

Aphakic contact lenses available currently, including power range, base curve diameter, material, water percentage, center thickness trade name, manufacturer, DK/L can be found in the following publications:

- *Contact Lenses and Solutions Summary,* Publishers Contact Lens Spectrum, updated yearly.
- *American Journal of Optometry,* yearly review of contact lens materials.
- *Physicians' Desk Reference for Ophthalmology,* Section on Contact Lenses, Montvale, NJ: Medical Economics Data, Inc., updated annually.

SUGGESTED READINGS

1. "The Properties of Lenses Used for the Correction of Aphakia." J.K. Davis, D.L. Torgersen; *J. Am. Optom. Assoc.* 54, no. 8(1983):685–693.
2. "Aphakic and Pseudophakic Spectacle Management." G.L. Reiner, *J. Am. Optom. Assoc.* 53, no. 4(1982):296.
3. I.M. Borish. "Aphakia: Perceptual and Refractive Problems of Spectacle correction." *J. Am. Optom. Assoc.* 54, no. 8(1983):701–711.

12

Care of the Visually Impaired Elderly Patient

Alfred A. Rosenbloom, Jr.

Between 1970 and 1980, the U.S. population aged 60 and over grew by about 18% while the total population expanded by only 9%. According to the 1980 census information, life expectancy at birth is now over 73 years of age, and people living to age 65 can expect to live for an average of 16 more years (National Council of the Aging, 1982).

Today's greater life expectancy is accompanied by a higher incidence of ocular and degenerative disorders. According to Kirchner and Peterson (1979), nearly 25% of the elderly population, or over 6 million U.S. citizens, have some form of visual impairment. In making a statistical projection to the year 2000, a study by Kirchner concluded that the 1977 National Council for Health Statistics (NCHS) survey population of severely visually impaired individuals over age 65 will double (Kirchner, 1985). The vast majority of these individuals can be helped with a comprehensive low-vision care program and appropriately prescribed low-vision aids.

There are also demographic and psychosocial dimensions to the burgeoning population of elderly people. Women and nonwhites have the highest incidence of severe visual disabilities. Furthermore, approximately two-thirds of visually impaired older people have at least one other impairment, such as orthopedic impediments, paralysis, or hearing loss. Older people in the United States are demanding that more attention be paid to the quality and comprehensiveness of their health care. Serving these needs is truly a continuing challenge.

This chapter considers four aspects of the problem: (1) contemporary aspects of low-vision and aging as frames of reference; (2) effective optometric care for the elderly; (3) essential clinical skills and understandings; (4) new directions in elderly patient care.

CONTEMPORARY ASPECTS OF LOW-VISION CARE
The Elderly in Western Society

In the future, health-care providers will serve a greatly increased number of people in the 70- to 90-year age range. Data show that approximately 21% of the

U.S. population is 55 or over, 15% is 60 or over, and 12% is 65 or over (45 million, 33 million, and 24 million people, respectively). The number of people over age 65 is growing at twice the rate of the general population. People in this age group represent one of every eight U.S. citizens and head one of every five households. Those over 75 are in the fastest growing group of all.

Contrary to popular opinion, the majority of older people in the United States live independent lives (Population Resource Center, 1981):

- Only 5% over age 65 are institutionalized.
- Nearly three-quarters aged 65 to 74 are home owners.
- In the 65 to 74 age group, 62.6% are living with a spouse; 24% live alone, and most of these are women.
- One-half of all women over 75 live alone.
- Two-thirds of all households are headed by people over age 55.

In other developed countries, the elderly population makes up an even larger proportion of the whole.

The incidence of visual impairment increases markedly among the elderly. Robbins' (1981) survey of patients examined at the Low Vision Clinic, Kooyong, Melbourne, Australia, indicated that patients aged 80 or more make up about 35% of the patient population. Within this group, those aged 80 to 89 years represent the modal group, a distribution that closely follows that reported by Sorsby (1972) for both the United Kingdom and for Wales. This finding has particular clinical relevance since in the aging U.S. population, two-thirds of the low-vision population are already over the age of 60.

Aging

Aging describes physiologic and related changes in a person's life from maturity to death, including adjustment to the total environment. It is a continuous and highly individualized process, especially in the area of health. Each person adjusts to old age differently.

The impact of vision loss is rarely felt in isolation from the other losses associated with growing older. No two people experience visual loss or the changing self-perceptions associated with aging in the same way. The impact of visual impairment, however, is felt more keenly because of other problems associated with aging (for example, physical and physiologic changes; economic limitations; loss of social independence; and altered roles in the family, work place, and community) (Weg, 1982).

The Jarvik (1975) longitudinal study of a random sample of elderly people suggests that those who engage in cognitive, emotive, and physical activities on a regular basis throughout adulthood age more successfully than those who are relatively inactive. Activities of later life, rather than those of earlier years, are related to successful aging.

The optometrist's role is to understand the effects of aging in dealing with vision rehabilitation. The optometrist seeks to help patients with impaired vision to live fulfilling and useful lives and enjoy self-sufficiency, emotional independence, and satisfactory social interactions. Too often the practitioner's goals are aimed at physical well-being; social and psychological aspects are not given the emphasis they deserve.

EFFECTIVE OPTOMETRIC CARE FOR THE ELDERLY

The optometrist should adhere to five key principles for geriatric patient care, regardless of the nature of the patient's disease, disability, or impairment:

1. Distinguish *aging* from *disease*.
2. See the patient as a *whole person*, focusing on health status, ability, psychosocial well-being, and socioeconomic needs.
3. Use a *team approach*; use support resources from the family; community services; health care and rehabilitation; social service counseling; and occupational therapy, including environmental support services.
4. Emphasize the *goals* of geriatric patient care. These include prevention, preservation, restoration, and maintenance leading to the enrichment of quality of life.
5. Improve the patient's *quality of life* by facilitating independence and goal-directed activity.

Effective optometric service involves the art and science of patient care. Patients have become discontented, critical, and hostile as the *art* of health care gradually becomes separated from the *science* of health care (Remen, 1980). Patients have also become increasingly disenchanted with a specialized, high technology, health-care system that frequently treats "health problems" rather than human needs (Grayson, et. al., 1977; McKay, 1980). To overlook these attitudes diminishes the doctor-patient relationship. The practitioner must view patients as individuals with special needs and abilities.

Because health problems in the elderly tend to be complex, effective communication between patient and health provider is essential. Indeed, older adults share with everyone the dual needs for self-importance and social acceptance. Physical limitations often cause older adults to feel isolated. Deficits in hearing and vision may interfere directly with communication. The optometrist should understand the psychological stress that often accompanies aging: loneliness, a sense of uselessness, and anxiety over increasing dependency and impending death.

The care of the elderly patient should be effective, humane, and tailored to the limitations and priorities of each individual. In addition to obtaining information essential to a correct diagnosis and treatment plan, the optometrist should assess the cognitive and psychological states of elderly patients, their ability to carry out activities of daily living, and their socioeconomic needs. See Chapter 2 for mini-mental and depression screening measures. The practitioner must be sensitive to the patient's psychological set; the patient's expressed and perceived needs; the collection of clinical data; and an agreed-upon plan of action paced to the individual's needs, understanding, and motivation.

Psychological and Functional Effects of Low Vision

Ocular and degenerative disorders tend to increase in incidence and severity among elderly persons. For a complete discussion of these changes, see Chapters 2 and 4.

Many "normal" aging changes are exacerbated for the low-vision patient (Lederer, 1982). To understand the visual performance characteristics of low-vision patients, it is necessary to differentiate between optical effects and neural effects (Lubinas, 1980). For example, a patient with an optically reduced visual loss resulting from irregularities in the refractive surfaces or media usually suffers from a degradation of the visual image. This deficit results from excessive intraocular scatter, which causes lower visual acuity and reduced contrast sensitivity. This patient has greater difficulty with resolution tasks, and as the angular extent of scatter broadens, resolution capacity and performance suffer.

In some patients visual acuity may remain unaffected, but contrast sensitivity of all objects within the visual field is diminished. Marron and Bailey (1982) showed that loss of contrast sensitivity and loss of visual field were approximately equally important contributions to impaired mobility because of decreased vision. They also showed that visual acuity was a relatively poor predictor of mobility performance. Research results by Cunningham and Johnston (1980) suggest that the detection of low-contrast objects (such as steps, pavement, and textures) is critical for pedestrian mobility. Jos Verbaken (personal correspondence, 1982), of the Department of Optometry, University of Melbourne, measured the contrast threshold for a luminous edge profile using a photographic plate technique in 349 consecutive clinic patients with normal acuity. The data showed that the edge contrast threshold is constant between the ages of 5 and 49 and declines steadily thereafter. For the 80 to 89 age group, the contrast threshold was twice as great as in the younger age group.

With increased intraocular scatter and absorption of light by the media, higher than normal luminance levels are necessary. If the individual's environment includes poorly designed light fittings, dimly lit passageways, shadows surrounding objects, and impairments such as disability glare, performance difficulties are increased.

Regardless of their causes, losses involving structures within the neural pathway are most commonly expressed as visual field defects. Central field losses typically affect low-vision patients with a reduction in visual acuity. These losses may be complicated by metamorphopsia, poor tolerance to variation in luminance, dependence on high luminance levels, lowered contrast sensitivity, and poor mobility despite an intact peripheral visual field. The size and extent of scotomas limit sensitivity of the retina, as only objects of sufficient size, illuminance, or contrast will be recognized within these areas. If these scotomas are numerous, the correct localization and subsequent evaluation of visual information may become so difficult that some patients, despite relatively good visual acuity, are unable to read with any efficiency even when using magnification. This effect may be likened to the crowding phenomenon, in which letters can be seen but not interpreted by some amblyopic patients.

Although not as common as central field losses, peripheral field losses are important within the low-vision population. Mobility and the ability to detect environmental hazards are hindered when poor dark adaptation makes patients dependent on high light levels. The fact that older people require higher levels of illumination to meet their visual needs is well established, but frequently overlooked. The role of the practitioner in the assessment of the response of older patients to illumination levels and the appropriate standards for domestic lighting are described by Lovie-Kitchin and Bowman (1985) and Merz (1982).

Psychological Set

In addition to physical conditions and aging changes, a patient's performance is influenced by the attitude of the practitioner. Sinick (1976) notes that professional personnel in service settings may fail to realize the presence of prejudice despite their commitment to a professional service role. In so doing, they may become condescending, overprotective, and insensitive to the basic needs of elderly people. Members of the rehabilitation team must confront their own attitudes toward visually impaired people to render the most effective services.

In caring for the elderly person, professionals must recognize that an elderly person's well-being is as important as that of younger individuals. A shortened life span is no basis for making compromises in the scope or quality of health care services.

A recent World Health Organization (1981) meeting noted that the identification of the elderly population as the most vulnerable group for visual impairment has important implications for health planning. A number of factors explain the reasons why the elderly may be relatively neglected in the provision of services:

1. A number of elderly patients cannot effectively communicate their needs and may be reluctant to seek professional help. Moreover, practitioners often assume that elderly patients are less readily rehabilitated than more youthful patients.
2. Elders often accept the gradual loss of vision and therefore fail to seek appropriate help.
3. Professionals may believe they are examining patients too late in the disease process to permit optimal treatment and prevent disability.

Barraga and Morris (1980) report that many elderly patients resist attempts at visual rehabilitation because they fear their inability to achieve visual expectations, fear becoming more independent and possibly losing the care and emotional support of family and friends, and lack a desire to invest extra time and effort. These authors also suggest that motivation may decline because patients do not understand that low-vision devices only enhance blurred or distorted visual images rather than restore vision. Elderly patients also often do not understand that visual performance may vary from day to day. Mehr (1974) notes: ". . . the patient must be ready and eager for help, *not* seeking restoration of his former vision without limitations. For the patient playing 'yes, but' or preferring dependency to increased visual abilities, a program of masterful inactivity is preferable to an expensive aid." In making a decision about an appropriate therapeutic plan for the low-vision patient, the optometrist must consider the psychosocial factors influencing the patient's readiness.

In addition, the visually impaired person may also face inadequacy in all daily activities, such as dressing, grooming, personal hygiene, eating, telling time, caring for clothes and personal effects — virtually every facet of daily life. He or she may need to relearn many routines. Social insecurities and communication difficulties are experienced; independence may be reduced, and self-esteem affected.

Thus, the cognitive and psychological states of elderly patients, their ability to perform daily activities, and their socioeconomic frameworks should be assessed clinically. The services available to assist patients in maintaining their independence should be established. To the extent that practitioners can develop understandings about, and sensitivities to, the realities of being and growing old, they will enhance the quality of the interpersonal relationships with their patients.

ESSENTIAL CLINICAL SKILLS AND UNDERSTANDINGS

Five aspects of providing optometric care for the aged visually impaired person include the case history interview, low-vision examination and functional assessment, therapeutic approaches (appropriate low-vision designs and accessory aids), low-vision patient management, and patient education and compliance.

Case History Interview

The success of the rehabilitation process depends on the quality and scope of the case history. The history for elderly patients should establish their specific needs and desires, their ability to adapt to new situations, their motivation to learn new visual habits, and their understanding of the uses and limitations of the visual aids. If an elderly patient lives with sighted family members, efforts may be directed toward finding aids that allow participation in normal family activities (for example, television, card paying, sewing, and games). If the patient lives alone, more attention may be focused on functional tasks, such as reading mail and identifying labels on medicine bottles and canned goods (Rosenbloom, 1982). Other important case history information includes ocular and health history, visual capabilities at distance and near, illumination requirements, life-style history, present and previous interests, independent travel abilities, education and reading interests, vocational and avocational activities and goals, and familiarity with rehabilitation services.

The patient should be the primary source of information in gathering the case history; if doubt arises as to accuracy, other sources such as family or friends should be consulted. To compile a complete case history, multiple sessions may be needed to minimize patient fatigue.

Key questions for the case history interview include the following:

- What is the duration of the visual impairment?
- What is the ophthalmologic diagnosis, treatment, and prognosis?
- What is the state of the patient's general health?
- What drugs or medications are being taken, and for what purposes?
- Do any other health or psychosocial factors impair the patient's life-style?
- What is the patient's present level of visual functioning?
- Are there preferred light levels? Is there sensitivity to glare?
- What are the patient's principal vocational, recreational, and daily living activities?
- Are orientation and mobility impaired? Can the patient travel independently and successfully in familiar and unfamiliar surroundings?
- What are the patient's primary visual needs and expectations?
- Is reading an important activity? If so, reading of what type and purpose?
- Are any low-vision devices or appliances being used?
- What is the patient's life-style? Is the patient living with others or alone?
- Are there psychological readiness and motivation for visual rehabilitation?

This information is useful not only for in-office questioning by the practitioner, but also in a pre-examination interview by telephone or by a low-vision assistant in the office.

Low-Vision Examination and Functional Assessment

Michaels (1985) notes that the clinical examination of the aging eye does not differ in essentials from that of any other eye, except that it takes more time, more tact, and more patience. "It takes more time because older people frequently have many nonspecific complaints, poorly expressed, and sequentially muddled. Some symptoms may go unreported because of memory loss, fear, or indifference. It takes more tact because, in the nature of things, some senescent diseases are not only chronic but often irreparable. It takes more patience because the aged eye often suffers multiple defects which must be sorted out." (See Chapter 7.)

Flexibility and readiness to alter standard procedures are necessary to secure the most accurate and reliable findings. The visual examination must be adapted to the special needs and requirements of the patient. Environmental setting, test distance (usually 10 feet or less), and surrounding illumination are important considerations. Use of the trial frame (including clips for overrefraction), trial lenses, and low-vision printed acuity test charts add accuracy, flexibility, and improved patient control. Bailey and Lovie-Kitchin (1976) note that the examiner may wish to predict how much change in working distance, dioptric power of an addition, or magnification is required to enable the patient to read a certain size print. They also recommend using a chart with unrelated words arranged in a logarithmic size progression.

Much of the examination procedure follows a conventional pattern: determination of visual acuities at far and at near; internal and external ocular health examination; retinoscopy; tonometry and slit-lamp biomicroscopy; binocular indirect ophthalmoscopy; ophthalmometry; determination of central and peripheral visual fields, including use of the Amsler grid; and distance and near point subjective testing with low-vision and accessory devices suited to the needs and capabilities of the patient.

Functional assessment requires a full understanding of the patient's needs and the complex interaction of factors that influence the perceptual response. These factors include the acuity level required for tasks at various working distances; luminance; figure-ground and contrast differences; and contour interaction relationships involving size and style of type, spacing, and print quality. It is important to realize that magnification alone may not improve function in terms of daily activities, orientation, and mobility in the environment. Visual performance is correlated poorly with visual acuity. Accurate refractive technique is of utmost importance, as is the prescription of proper light levels for the patient's various environments. The goal of the low-vision practitioner should be to improve function by whatever means to enhance quality of life for the patient.

When possible, previously acquired skills must be reactivated by the practitioner's continuing encouragement, guidance, patience, and empathy. Techniques for achieving accurate clinical findings and their evaluation are described in Chapter 7.

Therapeutic Approaches (Appropriate Low-Vision Designs and Accessory Devices)

Low-vision devices that are most valuable to elderly patients include hand and stand magnifiers, compact telescopic systems for spot checking, high plus reading additions in bifocal or single vision designs, microscopic types of reading lenses, closed-circuit television systems, and various nonoptical or accessory aids.

A decision on what type of device(s)to prescribe depends not only on the optometric evaluation derived from the case history and examination findings, but also on the evaluation and interpretation of the functional field of vision. According to Faye (1984), the visual field is the single most important factor affecting visual function. Faye identifies three types of field defects that can influence the practitioner's decision on therapeutic correction: no demonstrable field loss, functional field loss involving retinal disease marked by central or paracentral scotomas, and peripheral field loss.

No Demonstrable Field Loss

Typically, patients with no demonstrable field loss complain of blurred vision or an image poorly resolved centrally, haze, or a sensation of glare. The evaluation of visual performance depends on the type and size of test objects, contrast, illumination levels, pupil size, and figure-ground interaction.

Therapeutic approaches to a blurred or poorly resolved image include telescopic devices, which help some patients retain their ability to read street, bus, and directional signs and avoid obstructions in travel. For such short-term spotting tasks, hand-held monocular telescopes from 2.5 to $10\times$ are available.

Stand magnifiers often are used by patients with hand tremors, by those with aphakia where added magnification for reading is needed, and as a supplemental correction for the occasional reading of small print.

Most informational display signs can be identified with 20/70 vision under suitable illumination. Patients with diffusely blurred vision need telescopes with good light-gathering properties — often a prism monocular with the largest field. For reading, high addition spectacles, hand or stand magnifiers, or telemicroscopes should be prescribed according to near reading acuity.

Functional Field Loss Involving Retinal Disease Marked by Central or Paracentral Scotomas

Faye (1976) notes the common denominators of macular disease: visible pathology of ophthalmoscopy, central or paracentral field defects of varying density, decreased central acuity, and central scotoma. Peripheral field functions remain relatively normal. Visual complaints may vary from lack of clear vision, recognition of faces, and disappearance of parts of words to search difficulties in travel vision.

The specific design of the low-vision device depends on the patient's level of visual acuity, preference and adaptability, and requirements for daily living. In descending order of frequency, the aids commonly prescribed for elderly patients are single-vision or bifocal spectacles, hand and stand magnifiers (2 to $9\times$ power), hand-held and spectacle-mounted telescopes (2.5 to $8\times$), telemicroscopic units, and closed-circuit television. Stand magnifiers often are used by patients with hand tremors, by those with aphakia where added magnification combined with the bifocal power is needed for reading, and as a supplemental correction for the occasional reading of small print.

Peripheral Field Loss

The practitioner must also differentiate between overall contraction of the visual field and sector or hemianopic losses. The most potentially disabling form of functional vision impairment is peripheral field loss. Magnification may not help those with peripheral field loss. Indeed, many patients adopt techniques in traveling and reading that prove more effective than the use of low-vision aids.

Patients with irregular scotomatous patterns often have unpredictable near-vision responses. They may identify isolated letters more easily than words, and they may use eccentric viewing and angling of reading materials. An accurate assessment and interpretation of the central and peripheral visual fields should be performed before low-vision devices or a rehabilitation program is considered.

In prescribing low-vision devices, the practitioner must consider the relative advantages and limitations of various devices. High addition spectacles may be ineffective as low-vision devices because of the close distance they impose. Tele-microscopes alleviate the working distance difficulties, but the field of vision becomes small.

Low-powered hand and stand magnifiers can increase the working distance and allow the patient to adapt to a preferred image size. Patients with small central or paracentral fields may prefer closed-circuit television because of the flexible reading distance and the improved ease and speed in reading, as well as the illumination and contrast controls.

Accessory devices for mobility and orientation should be considered. Light control is especially important. For patients with sector or hemianopic field defects, trials should be conducted with prisms of varying power and position. Mirrors have been used with some success by patients with homonymous hemianopias. Prisms also can enhance mobility and scanning, but their success with the elderly tends to be limited. With elderly people, the success rate with all these techniques is relatively low and depends on patient motivation and adaptability. As a consequence, patients should participate in selecting the best compromise. Adaptive training by the orientation and mobility specialist is most desirable.

Accessory or Nonoptical Devices

Accessory or nonoptical devices take many forms. These include large-print materials, matte black cardboard reading slits (typoscopes) and amber acetate sheets to improve contrast, reading stands, adequate illumination, the use of fiber-tipped pens, and visors to control light intensity and glare. Talking Books should be recommended where there are limited or unsuccessful trials with optical devices; this is especially appropriate if reading is an important part of a patient's life-style. Other technological advances include text-to-speech synthesizers, large-print computers, and image intensifiers.

Accessory or nonoptical devices should be considered to reduce glare and heighten contrast and illumination. Patients can control outdoor glare by wearing hats with wide brims; visors that attach to the eyeglass frame; and absorptive lenses that reduce ultraviolet (UV) and infrared radiation as do NOIR and Corning photochromic lenses. Tinted lenses may lessen glare but may also reduce reading acuity.

Disability glare presents a special challenge in the diagnosis and management of the elderly patient. Jacobs and Saabin (1982) of the Department of Optometry, University of Melbourne, indicate that elderly patients with cortical cataracts are so sensitive to disability glare that many are housebound at night. Contrast threshold or contrast sensitivity functions of these patients can be essentially normal in low photopic luminance (about 30 footcandles), but thresholds for high and medium spatial frequency targets are drastically reduced in the presence of any bright glare source. Because these patients often have 20/20 acuity, their problems can be overlooked by the examiner who does not specifically ask about night vision or glare problems during the case history. These patients can be helped with advice on lighting design to reduce luminance levels and restore contrast. Also, clear antireflective coatings, side and sun shields, and a cardboard reading mask of the appropriate length and width (typoscope) to reduce glare from the surrounding field and improve contrast generally are recommended. Large-print materials, marking pens, heavily lined writing paper, and reading lamps and stands are a few of the many available aids.

Contrast and Color represent important environmental design considerations. Gradual yellowing of the lens occurs with age, and, as a result, blue light is absorbed and scattered selectively. Thus, blues become darker and less vivid, and there is a perceptual increase in warm tones. The degree of color bias that occurs with age is quite variable because lens changes vary considerably from individual to individual. Typically, during old age, there is a diminished ability to differentiate among similar light tones (pastel colors) or dark shades (blacks, brown, navy) (Hiatt, 1990). Almost any color can be made more visible by improving light intensity, by using full-spectrum light sources, and by using color in a highly contrasting mode. Generally, lighting should be placed on the side of the eye capable of best near vision; it should be direct, close, and adjustable so that the light can be angled to reduce reflected glare.

The optometrist needs to stress the appropriate use of color contrast as an important factor in managing the environment for older people. For instance, decorating homes or facilities for older people should provide color contrast between walls and floor. A knowledgeable use of color also can accent stairways and steps and demarcate other changes in terrain.

The use of nonoptical or accessory devices is especially important because contrast sensitivity is generally lessened in low-vision patients. Cullinin (1978) identified the importance and effects of poor lighting control: "Among those surveyed who had recently been seen at specialist's clinic, over 60% apparently saw worse at home than they did at the time of examination." Poor lighting in the home is virtually a universal problem.

A loan system for optical devices that allows a patient to become accustomed gradually to the effects of greater magnification is often desirable. This adaptive process requires reassessment, supervision, and counseling on a continuing basis as frustrations and new needs emerge.

Various patterns of reinforcement or encouragement are needed to keep the patient's enthusiasm and motivation high. Adaptive training should be flexible and emphasize the most effective use of residual vision. Home visits by the assistant or allied professional should be considered. Questions about patient compliance and problems of illumination and contrast in the home often can be resolved by on-site assessment. Since comprehensive low-vision care is time consuming, help from an understanding, experienced low-vision assistant is desirable. This frees the professional examiner for those procedures necessitating special skills and knowledge.

Low-Vision Patient Management

The management of adaptive problems in the low-vision patient requires more than the prescription of devices. Proper management frequently requires painstaking instruction and supervised training to create and sustain motivation for visual tasks along with the use of training materials and activities chosen according to the patient's interests.

Depending on the clinical setting and the needs of the patient, the practitioner should make appropriate referrals. In same cases multidisciplinary care is unnecessary; in others, however, services should be coordinated. Where the services of several specialists are required, one member of the team must take responsibility for identifying needs and coordinating services. Establishing constructive relationships with the health-care and social service agencies is essential. Because of changing social and family structures, elderly patients must often seek other support systems. Social service agencies, senior citizen support groups, and religious and service organizations are available in the community for health-care and social support (Jacobs, 1984). The practitioner should furnish the patient and the patient's family with a list of resources in the community that will provide needed services. Periodic follow-up increases the patient's compliance and success.

Orientation and mobility professionals often may focus their efforts upon the home environment but not to the exclusion of other environments significant to their patients. The role of these specialists is to teach how to "utilize the remaining senses in establishing position and relationship to all significant objects in the environment and the subsequent capacity to move independently" (Hill and Ponder, 1976). The ultimate goal of orientation and mobility training is to enable the individual to enter any environment and travel safely, efficiently, and independently, by using a combination of these two skills. Orientation and mobility professionals and rehabilitation teachers frequently work together in providing individualized and comprehensive rehabilitation programs. These programs are most effective when they prevent or defer admission of patients into long-term care facilities. Indeed, independent living training may offer a viable alternative to nursing home placement.

All professionals and paraprofessionals involved in the care of the elderly low-vision patient should assist in the process of rehabilitation, which can be thought of as a transition from dependence to independence, and finally to inter-dependence. This transition can be typified by some commonly encountered phrases. The statement, "Of course, I can't read; you will have to do it for me," typifies dependence. Independence can be expressed by, "I will try to read this myself," but this also can be a stubborn and self-defeating experience leading to, "This print is just too small. No, you can't help me — I didn't want to read it any-way." Ideally, independence should lead to the ultimate state of interdependence: "I can read this section, but these words are too difficult. Could you help me, please?" This state of rehabilitation recognizes abilities and limitations and gra-ciously requests and accepts assistance. This process requires time, and the patient will fluctuate between stages. The optometrist should seek an understanding of the patient's present state.

The optometrist must be able to look behind the traditional stereotypes and focus on the special needs of each individual. These needs include independence and individuality, physical health and mobility, self-respect, dignity, and privacy. Good health and mobility, in turn, depend on the satisfaction of diverse sub-sidiary needs such as adequate services to compensate for loss of vision and hear-ing; a proper nutritional standard; adequate dental care; the maintenance of personal and household standards of cleanliness; and quality, accessible health service (Brearley, 1978).

Patient Education and Compliance

In contrast to the traditional model of health care, low-vision rehabilitation should be oriented to the person rather than to the disease. Such an approach establishes an ongoing, personal relationship with the patient. For the elderly patient unaccustomed to, or overwhelmed by, the diversified maze of the health-care system, the optometrist can develop a trusting relationship of support and encouragement. At the same time that this humanistic approach to health care is rightly desirable for the general population, it is critical for the elderly and will greatly enhance the patient compliance essential for successful low-vision rehabilitation.

There are few studies of patient compliance in optometry and medicine that specifically concern the elderly. Libow and Sherman (1981) found that for elderly patients who had medication prescribed, 50% deviated from the prescribed regi-men, and 70% did not comprehend the regimen. Errors in medication and self-medication have accounted for 25% to 95% of the noncompliance problem (Gabriel et al., 1977). Compliance difficulties are increased for the elderly for a variety of reasons. Explanations are given too rapidly or poorly, and written instructions are lacking. Environmental hazards such as weather conditions, transportation, or fear of crime deter patients from keeping appointments. Patients have trouble receiving or retaining instructions because of visual and hearing problems, or from loss of short-term memory. They are sometimes unable to open child-resistant medication containers and are confused about regimens with multiple medications (Ernst, 1981).

In a study using experimental and control groups, Talkington (1978) found that four factors significantly increased patient compliance (from 53% to 73%):

1. Good rapport and communication between the patient and the health provider has been established.
2. Effective interaction whereby the patient's concerns were understood and expectations were met.
3. Patient understanding of the health problem, causes, treatment regimen, expected outcome of treatment, and the consequences of noncompliance is achieved.
4. Patient participation in planning the treatment regimen, including the identification, analysis, and solution of problems that might interfere with compliance.

Practitioner's Role in Counseling and Patient Education

Patient education has many facets. The practitioner must realize that every low-vision problem is unique, and that individual differences increase with age. A slowing of motor functioning is not equated automatically with decreased learning ability; when older people can pace their own learning, studies show no significant age-related differences in ability. Diversity, rather than homogeneity, is the norm.

The pratitioner must pace the instructions according to the learning ability of the patient. The response rate and reaction time of the elderly are slower, but not because of lack of motivation. Rushing the elderly patient may result in frustration and reduced motivation. Fear of failure, frustration, and confusion can be reduced by simplifying the environment and the tasks demanded of the elderly person. Presentation of material in both amount and content should be planned so that it reduces the patient's potential for failure and increases the opportunity for success.

The optometrist must explain the low-vision device(s) (their purpose, use, and limitations); the adaptive training program and its goals; environmental variables, especially lighting; and the importance of continuing follow-up. Informational reinforcement can consist of handouts, demonstrations, discussions, and audio-visual aids; handouts are especially useful as a continuing reminder. Vivian and Robertson (1980; cited in Glazer-Waldman, 1983) developed guidelines for patient education that consider word choice, sentence length, and typography to maximize patient comprehension. They also suggest testing the education materials on a sample population before putting them into general use.

To ensure patient participation, the practitioner must provide sufficient opportunity for practice, repetition, and feedback about performance. Adaptive training must emphasize positive reinforcement for correct responses or procedures and re-training for incorrect ones. Evaluation involves assessment of the patient's progress at periodic intervals. An elderly person's sense of security, control, and orientation to the environment can be heightened with a set schedule of appointments at similar times, as well as the use of methods such as telephone inquiries or letter questionnaires. In all cases, rehabilitative success depends on the practitioner's ability to work together with the patient to realize attainable goals.

NEW DIRECTIONS IN ELDERLY PATIENT CARE

Today, emerging findings from reliable clinical studies make research in low-vision care of the elderly an exciting field of inquiry. New technological developments and the broader approach to patient management through involvement of allied health professionals adds to the research mandate to expand the boundaries of knowledge about health, disease, and sensory impairment during old age. The ultimate goal is optimum care of visually impaired elderly persons. This can be achieved by a synthesis of information from studies of normal aging and studies of disease in the elderly, yielding a data base that allows quantification of, and differentiation between, the effects attributed to age and those attributed to disease.

The focus for the future must be toward *research* and *development*. There is a need for greater scope and depth in basic and applied research on aging. Relevant topics range from basic biologic knowledge to the design of better healthcare delivery systems, including diagnostic and therapeutic approaches to visual-perceptual problems of aging people.

Assessment of Visual Performance

There is a need for greater research into visual performance. Topics include perceptual problems and adaptations; focusing, landmark spotting, and pursuit fixations involving movements of head, eyes, and body; adaptation to changing environmental conditions; optimal light levels indoors and outdoors; color cues; and figure-ground relationships.

Research should continue in the various conditions that cause loss of vision to allow the development of new procedures for alleviating their effects.

Studies of aging people who maintain good vision in spite of debilitating disease also are needed. Such studies might identify factors that offer preventive approaches to selected ocular diseases.

New techniques in the assessment of visual performance are needed, with improved correlation between clinical measurements of visual function and visual skills related to a person's life-style. This entails new instruments capable of measuring visual functions to understand the visual processes involved in everyday living.

There needs to be a greater understanding of the activity levels and interests of the elderly and their implications to behavior patterns of those with impaired vision. Such knowledge would enable the low-vision team to set realistic goals for rehabilitation.

The process by which elderly patients relearn skills necessary for the successful use of residual vision is poorly understood; consequently, soundly based techniques must be developed for extensive readaptation. This may involve perceptual relearning, the use of eccentric fixation, and methods of expanding the functional field of view.

The outcome of these and related studies may result in the development of a battery of tests used by the practitioner to create a profile of visual function for each visually impaired patient. With the development of this test profile, a multidisciplinary approach would be necessary to consider the patient's overall ability to perform common visually related tasks in everyday life. These data could then be used to implement life-style improvements with the use of specific low-vision devices.

Therapeutic Approaches

New low-vision devices must be designed for wider application, versatility, and patient acceptance. The technical challenge is to optimize optical design parameters in order to combine magnification with distortion-free fields of view.

New accessory devices are required for varied levels of patient disabilities and handicaps. The refinement of these devices may involve microprocessor technology, speech synthesis and recognition, and artificial intelligence. Closed-circuit television or similar display systems should be highly portable and gain additional technical features as supporting technology develops. Efforts should continue toward integrating large-character displays with computer and word-processing systems.

Lighting techniques must be examined in relation to intensity, spectral characteristics, heat properties, contrast, and the type of luminaires in various environments. Further objective and subjective evaluation is necessary to determine optimal lighting according to a person's near visual acuity, working distance, ocular disease type, and reading position to enhance patient comfort and visual efficiency.

The Emerging Role of the Health Professional in the Delivery of Low-Vision Patient Care

Another major focus must be on the education and preparation of health professionals for the delivery of care to elderly visually impaired people. A needs assessment study should be undertaken to determine the number and types of professionals needed to adequately serve the growing population of older blind and visually impaired people. Because there is a positive correlation between knowledge and attitudes, professional educators should consider planning strategies to impart knowledge about the aging process and about the health-care and social problems of the elderly early in school curricula. Training in gerontology should be undertaken at both professional school and the postgraduate levels (Rosenbloom, 1982). A health-care professional who understands the social, psychological, and economic aspects of aging can prevent exacerbations of illness, achieve patient cooperation with treatment programs, and interact more effectively with patients and their families.

Various alternative models of low-vision care delivery should be developed. Such models should delineate the total needs of the patient. The integration of the practitioner into a team is a necessary part of this planning; the nature of the interaction will depend on the health-care delivery mode — be it clinic, private or group practice, hospital, or domiciliary patient care.

Pioneer and current rehabilitation programs for the elderly blind and visually impaired should be analyzed and their relative merits evaluated in terms of basic concepts, standards, and principles. Innovative approaches, such as mobile units to provide low-vision care for the rural elderly, represent another health-care delivery need of increasing significance.

Multidisciplinary teamwork is especially important when caring for elderly patients. Delegates at the World Health Organization (1981) conference in Copenhagen emphasized the value of developing one or more comprehensive multidisciplinary centers that encompass patient care, planning, interdisciplinary research, and personnel training. These centers would be responsible for ameliorating the disability (but not necessarily prevent the disease), as well as for diagnosis, treatment, and rehabilitation. They should be staffed by specialists in the basic clinical, social, and public health sciences, bioengineering, and other technical disciplines.

In agency service, a need exists for in-service training of new staff to ensure a comprehensive approach to patient care. The actions of the low-vision team must dovetail the programs of care to insure successful rehabilitation. Feedback from patients is needed to evaluate the quality and adequacy of the services offered, for the most important member of any team is the low-vision patient.

A delivery system should be developed that is economically viable; disseminates new information and techniques; trains appropriate personnel; and provides grass roots care, specialized assessment, and ongoing support structures. Vision care should be evaluated continually at both the patient and the clinic levels to ensure cost-effective and relevant service delivery. This assumes that goals and objectives have been considered carefully and are realistic, given the limits of resources in personnel and money. Finally, patient care within the community should avoid unnecessary duplication.

Professional services for the low-vision patient have progressed a long way in the past 35 years since the first low-vision clinic was opened in the United States, and they still have a long way to go. New research, advanced technology, and multidisciplinary expertise will enhance our ability to meet important human needs.

There is not only technical expertise in rendering effective low-vision rehabilitation but also a personal and humane component. Perhaps the practitioner's greatest service lies in encouraging the visually impaired older person to become independent in every way possible and to learn as quickly as is practical the new skills needed to be once again a contributing member of society. The extent to which this is possible depends significantly on the practitioner's ability to foster the patient's aspirations, self-confidence, and potential to realize attainable goals. It is a challenge worthy of our best efforts.

REFERENCES

1. Bailey, I., and J. Lovie-Kitchin. "New Design Principles for Visual Acuity Letter Charts." *Am. J. of Optom. Physiol. Opt.* 53 (1976): 740.
2. Barraga, N., and J. Morris. *Program to Develop Efficiency in Visual Functioning.* Louisville: American Printing House for the Blind, 1980.
3. Brearley, P. "Aging and Social Work." In: *The Social Challenge of Aging.* D. Hobman (ed.). London: Croom Helm, 1978, p. 180.
4. Cullinin, T. "Low Vision in Elderly People: Light for Low Vision." Proceedings of a Symposium. London: University College, April 1978.
5. Cunningham, P., and A. Johnston. "Edge Detection: A New Test of Visual Function." Paper presented at the ANZAAS Jubilee Conference, Adelaide, Australia, May 1980.
6. Ernst, N. (ed.). *Pharmaceutical Interventions and the Aged.* Dallas: University of Texas Health Science Center, 1981.
7. Faye, E. *Clinical Low Vision.* Boston: Little, Brown, 1976.
8. Faye, E. "The Effect of the Eye Condition on Functional Vision." In: *Clinical Low Vision,* 2nd ed., E. Faye (ed.). Boston: Little, Brown, 1984, pp. 172–189.
9. Gabriel, M., J. Gagnon, and C. Bryon. "Improving Patient Compliance through the Use of a Daily Drug Reminder Chart." *Am. J. Pub. Health* 67 (1977): 968.
10. Glazer-Waldman, H. "Patient Education." In: *The Aged Patient: A Sourcebook for the Allied Health Professional,* N. Ernst and H. Glazer-Waldman (eds.). Chicago: Year Book Medical, 1983, Chapter 14.
11. Grayson, M., C. Nugent, and S. Oken. "A Systematic and Comprehensive Approach to Teaching and Evaluating Interpersonal Skills." *J. Med. Educ.* 52 (1977): 906–913.
12. Hiatt, L.G., Environmental Factors in Rehabilitation. In: S.J. Brody and L.G. Pawlson (eds.). *Aging and Rehabilitation II.* New York: Springer Publishing, 1990, pp. 151–153.
13. Hill, E., and P. Ponder. *Orientation and Mobility Techniques: A Guide for the Practitioner.* New York: American Foundation for the Blind, 1976.
14. Jacobs, P. "The Older Visually Impaired Person: A Vital Link in the Family and the Community." *J. Vis. Impair. Blind.* 78, no. 4 (1984): 154–162.
15. Jarvik, L. "Thoughts on the Psychobiology of Aging." *Am. Psychol.* (May 1975): 578.
16. Kirchner, C., and R. Peterson. "The Latest Data on Visual Disability from NCHS." *J. Vis. Impair. Blind.* 73, no. 4 (1979): 151–153.
17. Kirchner, C., and R. Peterson. "The Latest Data on Visual Disability from NCHS." *J. Vis. Impair. Blind.* 74, no. 1 (1980): 42–44.
18. Kirchner, C. *Data on Blindness and Visual Impairment in the U.S.* New York: American Foundation for the Blind, 1985.
19. Lederer, J. "Geriatric Optometry." *Aust. J. Optom.* 65, no. 4 (1982): 141–143.
20. Libow, L., and F. Sherman. *The Core of Geriatric Medicine.* St. Louis: C.V. Mosby, 1981.
21. Lovie-Kitchin, J., and K. Bowman. *Senile Macular Degeneration: Management and Rehabilitation.* Stoneham, MA: Butterworth, 1985.

22. Lubinas, J. "Understanding the Low Vision Patient." *Aust. J. Optom.* 63, no. 5 (1980): 227–231.
23. Marron, A., and I. Bailey. "Visual Factors and Orientation-Mobility Performance." *Am. J. Optom. Physiol. Opt.* 59, no. 5 (1982): 413–426.
24. McKay, S. "Wholistic Health Care: Challenge to Health Providers." *J. Allied Health* 9 (1980): 194–201.
25. Mehr, E. "Psychological Factors in Low Vision Care." In: *A Guide to the Care of Low Vision Patients.* J. Newman (ed.). St. Louis: American Optometric Association, 1974, p. 49.
26. Merz, B. "Lighting in Homes: A Study of Quantity and Quality." *Lighting in Australia* 2, no. 4 (1982): 26–28.
27. Michaels, D. *Visual Optics and Refraction. A Clinical Approach,* 3rd Edition, St. Louis: C.V. Mosby, 1985, p. 418.
28. National Council on the Aging. *Aging in North America: Projection and Policies.* Washington, DC: National Council on the Aging, 1982.
29. Population Resource Center. *Technology Adaptation and the Aging.* New York: Population Resource Center, 1981.
30. Remen, N. *The Human Patient.* New York: Doubleday, 1980.
31. Robbins, H. "Low Vision Care for the Over 80s." *Aust. J. Optom.* 64, no. 6(1981): 243–251.
32. Rosenbloom, A. "Care of Elderly People with Low Vision." *J. Vis. Impair. Blind.* 76, no. 6 (1982): 209–212.
33. Rosenbloom, A. "Optometry and Gerontology." *Optom. Month.* 73, no. 3 (1982): 143–144.
34. Sinick, D. "Counseling Older Persons: Career Change and Retirement." *Vocational Guidance Quarterly* 25, no. 1 (1976): 18–24.
35. Sorsby, A. *The Incidence and Causes of Blindness in England and Wales 1963–1968.* Reports on Public Health and Medical Subjects no. 128. London: Her Majesty's Stationery Office, 1972.
36. Talkington, D. "Maximizing Patient Compliance by Shaping Attitudes of Self-Directed Health Care." *J. Fam. Pract.* 6 (1978): 591–595.
37. Verbaken, J. Personal correspondence, 1982.
38. Vivian, A., and E. Robertson. "Readability of Patient Education Materials." *Clin. Ther.* 3 (1980): 129–136.
39. Weg, R. "The Image and Reality of 'Old': Time for a Change." *J. Am. Optom. Assoc.* 53, no. 1 (1982): 26–27.
40. World Health Organization. *The Use of Residual Vision by Visually Disabled Persons: Report on a WHO Meeting.* Euro Reports and Studies No. 41. Geneva: WHO, 1981.

SUGGESTED READINGS

1. Atchley, R.C. *Aging: Continuity and Change.* Belmont, Calif.: Wadsworth Publishing, 1983.
2. Committee on Vision, National Research Council. *Work, Aging, and Vision – Report of a Conference.* Washington, DC: National Academy Press, 1987, p. 32.
3. Conrad, K.A., and R. Bressler. *Drug Therapy for the Elderly.* St. Louis: C.V. Mosby, 1982.
4. Covington, T.R., and J. Walker. *Current Geriatric Therapy.* Philadelphia: W.B. Saunders, 1984.
5. Ernst, N.S., and H.R. Glazer-Waldman. *The Aged Patient: A Sourcebook for the Allied Health Professional.* Chicago: Year Book Medical, 1983.

6. Genensky, S.M., S.H. Berry, T.H. Bikson, and T.K. Bikson. "Visual Environmental Adaptation Problems of the Partially Sighted: Final Report." HEW RSA Grant 14-P-57997, 1979. Santa Monica, Calif.: Center for Partially Sighted, Santa Monica Hospital Center, 1979.
7. Hobman, D. (ed.). "The Social Challenge of Aging." *Aging and Social Work.* London: Croom Helm, 1978, p. 181.
8. Lovie-Kitchin, J.K. Bowman, E. Farmer. Technical Note: "Domestic Lighting Requirements for the Elderly." *Aust. J. Optom.* 66 (1983): 93–97.
9. Kwitko, M.L. Environmental Modifications for the Elderly. In: M.L. Kwitko and F.J. Weinstock (eds.). *Geriatric Ophthalmology.* Orlando, FL: Grune and Stratton, 1985, pp. 404–410.
10. Mehr, E.B., and A.N. Freid. *Low Vision Care.* Chicago: Professional Press, 1975.
11. Morgan, M.W. *The Optics of Ophthalmic Lenses.* Chicago: Professional Press, 1978.
12. O'Hara-Devereaux, M., L.H. Andrus, and C.D. Scott, (eds.). *Eldercare: A Practical Guide to Clinical Geriatrics.* New York: Grune and Stratton, 1981.
13. Rosenbloom, A.A. "Low Vision." In: *Principles and Practice of Ophthalmology,* G. Peyman, D. Sanders, and M. Goldberg (eds.). Philadelphia: W.B. Saunders, 1980, pp. 241–277.
14. Rosenbloom, A. "Low Vision: The Next Decade." Guest Editorial *J. Vis. Impair. Blind.* 86, no. 1 (1992):5.
15. Ross, M.A. *Fitness for the Aging Adult with Visual Impairment: An Exercise and Resource Manual.* New York: American Foundation for the Blind, 1984.
16. Sekuler, R., D. Kline, and K. Dismukes. *Aging and Human Visual Function.* New York: Allan R. Liss, 1982.
17. Simonson, W. *Medications and the Elderly: A Guide for Promoting Proper Use.* Rockville, MD: Aspen Systems, 1984.
18. Sloan, L. *Reading Aids for the Partially Sighted.* Baltimore: Williams and Wilkins, 1977.
19. Steinberg, F.U. (ed.). *Care of the Geriatric Patient,* 6th ed. St. Louis: C.V. Mosby, 1983.
20. Weale, R.A. *The Aging Eye.* London: H.K. Lewis, 1963.
21. Weale, R.A. *A Biography of the Eye: Development, Growth, Age.* London: H.K. Lewis, 1982.

13

Introduction to Special Non-Invasive Tests for the Assessment of Vision in Elderly Patients

J. Randall Pitman
Suresh Viswanathan
Robert L. Yolton

The need for electrodiagnostic, angiographic, psychophysical, imaging, and other special testing procedures arises when conventional testing cannot provide adequate assessment of a patient's visual function. Special testing is particularly useful for elderly patients, in part because conventional testing of the visual system can be hampered by the presence of media opacities. Conventional evaluations of elderly patients also can be difficult if the patient is unable to respond reliably or give valid information when tested subjectively. Special testing can overcome problems such as these and can be very useful in confirming tentative diagnoses or quantitatively monitoring the progression of known diseases in the elderly.

To properly use special tests, ophthalmic practitioners must not only realize when these tests would be beneficial for their patients, but they also must be able to select the appropriate test or tests, and properly interpret the results. In addition, practitioners should be able to describe the general testing procedures to their patients in order to alleviate their fears and prepare them for the testing environment that might appear somewhat threatening.

Based on these considerations, this chapter presents to the optometrist a practical guide to special testing.[1] It is designed to answer pertinent questions without getting into the intimate details of how to conduct special tests (for example, where to place electrodes on the patient). Detailed information regarding these procedures can be found in the references cited throughout the chapter, as well as in general references such as Carr and Siegal (1990), Fishman and Sokol (1990), and Regan (1989).

---

1. In preparing this chapter, the authors have assumed that the optometrist does not have access to the often expensive equipment required to perform special tests, but that special testing can be obtained from laboratories or consultants in the area. In this way, special ophthalmic tests are analogous to blood and other laboratory tests that are available on order.

ORDERING THE APPROPRIATE TEST

Once it has been determined that conventional testing is inadequate or inappropriate for a patient, the selection of the special test (or tests) to be conducted should be made by first determining which aspect of the patient's visual system needs to be assessed. To aid in this process, Figure 13.1 presents a flow chart showing a logical sequence to follow when considering referral for special testing. As indicated, special tests fall into three categories: (1) objective tests of retinal function, (2) subjective and objective tests of visual pathway integrity, and (3) imaging techniques.

If a disease affecting retinal function is suspected, this can be confirmed, further defined, or monitored objectively by using electroretinography (ERG) or electro-oculography (EOG). The question then arises as to which of these tests is most appropriate; the answer, of course, depends on the nature of the patient's problem. Flash ERG evaluates the inner and outer layers of the retina; focal ERG evaluates small portions of the retina; and pattern ERG evaluates ganglion cell function. Ordering an EOG is appropriate if a defect in the integrity of the retinal pigment epithelium (RPE) is suspected, but it is important to note that a normal EOG also depends on the integrity of the receptors and inner retinal layers. If the patient has difficulty with steady fixation or has poor saccadic movement, ordering an EOG probably would be inappropriate because reliable results depend on these skills.

In cases when the patient's problems suggest the use of special testing procedures, but there is no specific reason to suspect that the problems are confined to the retina alone, one of the subjective tests that evaluates the integrity of the entire visual pathway can be used. If the patient has clear media and is responsive to subjective testing, the test of choice probably would be perimetry, dark adaptometry, or contrast sensitivity, depending on the symptoms. Perimetry is a powerful subjective test that can be used for assessing disease of neurologic origin. Dark adaptometry is called for in cases of night vision difficulties, and contrast sensitivity is in order for those mysterious complaints of 20/20 vision that just does not seem quite right to the patient. For elderly patients with opaque media who respond well to subjective testing, laser interferometry, the potential acuity meter (PAM), or the blue field entoptoscope (BFET) can be used to determine the patency of the macular portion of the visual pathway.

When the validity of the patient's verbal responses cannot be relied upon, the most commonly used test to assess the visual pathway from the macula, up to and including the primary visual cortex, is the visual-evoked response (VER), in which signals from the cortex are recorded and analyzed by a computer.

If it is suspected that the patient has a disease affecting the structural integrity of the visual system (or other aspects of the central nervous system), imaging studies can be ordered to help define the nature and extent of the disease. Techniques include ultrasonography, which can image parts of the visual system not shielded by bone; computed axial tomography (CAT), which can be used to detect metallic foreign bodies, hard tissue injuries, space-occupying lesions, or

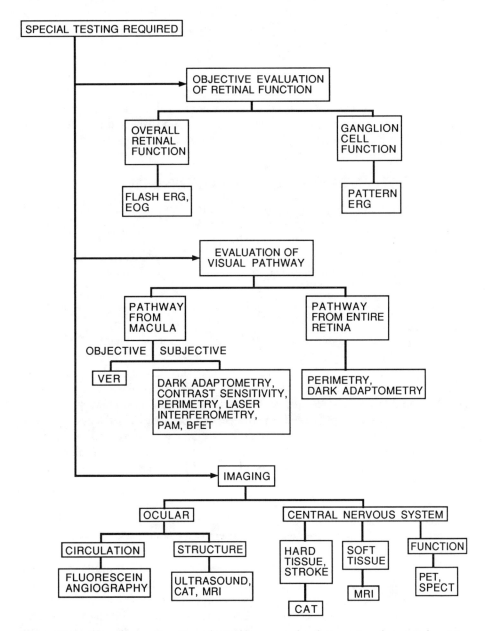

Figure 13.1 Flowchart suggesting a logical sequence for determining the special test (or tests) to order for a particular patient. The chart branches into retinal integrity, visual pathway, and imaging categories, with specific tests shown for each category.

hemorrhages; and magnetic resonance imaging (MRI), which is well suited for evaluating soft tissue injuries or degenerations. In the near future, other techniques such as positron emission tomography (PET) or single photon emission computed tomography (SPECT) will become more readily available for studying the metabolic function of selected brain structures.

Thus, many tests are available for the optometrist to use in evaluating a patient's visual system problems. The specific choice of a test (or tests) depends on at least three important factors: (1) the pattern of the patient's signs and symptoms, (2) the aspect or aspects of the visual system to be tested, and (3) the validity of the patient's subjective responses. By considering these factors, appropriate special tests can be ordered to determine the nature of a suspected disease, follow the course of a known disease, or rule out the presence of disease.

OBJECTIVE TESTS OF RETINAL FUNCTION

First to be considered are objective tests that give a specific indication of retinal function: electroretinography and electro-oculography. These tests are especially useful for patients with ocular opacities who are being considered for surgery, and, because they are objective, they can be used for those who cannot speak or otherwise communicate reliably.

Electroretinography

ERG is an electrodiagnostic test designed to measure the electrical potentials that arise from the retina in response to a flash of light (that is, flash ERG) or to a patterned stimulus (that is, pattern ERG) (Birch, 1989; Fishman and Sokol, 1990; Carr and Siegel, 1990). The flash ERG provides an objective indication of overall retinal function (Berson, 1987) or the function of a smaller area if a focused stimulus spot is presented. By using exceptionally bright flashes, the ERG can be used to assess the retina in elderly patients who have media opacities (Fuller et al., 1975). The pattern ERG can be used to assess ganglion cell function in glaucoma suspects or other patients who might have diseases that affect these cells (Rimmer and Katz, 1989).

Principles: Flash ERG

The flash ERG is a summed electrical response from cells across the entire retina. The ERG can be divided into a number of components, of which the a-wave and b-wave are the most commonly measured clinically (Figure 13.2). The a-wave is a small negative voltage (referenced to the cornea) primarily generated by retinal photoreceptors; the b-wave is a larger cornea-positive voltage generated by cells in the inner nuclear layer. Also seen with special recording configurations are oscillatory potentials that appear as small bumps riding on the b-wave (Fishman and Sokol, 1990). Ganglion cells and the optic nerve fiber layer do not appear to contribute to the flash ERG response (Gouras, 1970; Galloway, 1975).

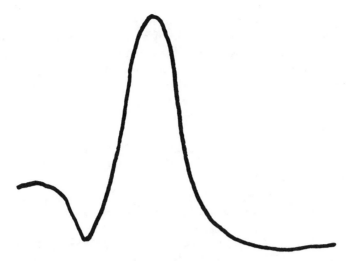

Figure 13.2 Schematic representation of the flash ERG waveform. The a-wave is the initial downward (negative) deflection in the trace, and the b-wave is the larger positive deflection.

Recording Methods

Recording electrophysiologic signals, such as those associated with the ERG, EOG, or VER, involves several basic procedures. These include (1) presenting a stimulus to the patient, (2) detecting an electrical response through surface contact electrodes, (3) amplifying and processing the electrical signal, and (4) displaying and/or recording the amplified signal.

In the case of the flash ERG, the patient usually is stimulated with diffuse strobe flashes presented in a Ganzfeld (a diffusing sphere into which the patient's head is partially placed; see Figure 13.3). Appropriate equipment can vary the duration, wavelength, and frequency of the light flashes presented in the Ganzfeld.

The patient's response is detected by a contact lens electrode, metallic fibers, or a foil strip (Fishman and Sokol, 1990) placed on the dilated and anesthetized eye. Signals from the ocular electrode and skin electrodes placed elsewhere on the body (typically near the lateral canthus and on an earlobe) are differentially amplified and displayed on an oscilloscope.

The ocular electrode is sometimes a problem for elderly patients, who may have fragile tissues. They may suffer a brief period of discomfort, including stinging, tearing, and injection following the procedure. However, these symptoms generally are minimal and usually last only a few hours.

Interpretation of Results

The ERG can be evaluated by comparing the amplitude and latency of the a-wave and b-wave components to expected values, to values from the other eye, or to both. Typical ERGs show b-wave amplitudes of roughly 0.5 mV, whereas a-wave amplitudes are about 25% of those for the b-wave. For the dark adapted eye, implicit times of the a-wave are typically about 20 ms, with the b-wave peaking at about 50 ms or less (Fishman and Sokol, 1990).

Abnormal ERG a- and b-wave responses can be caused by retinal disruptions such as large chorioretinal scars, detached retinas, vascular problems (Johnson et al., 1987; Johnson et al., 1988) and media opacities. A patient with cataracts, but with normal retinas, would be expected to have smaller than normal ERG amplitudes with corresponding long latencies (because of light absorbance and scatter by the lens). A patient with clear media and a retinopathy, such as a detachment, would have an ERG with reduced amplitude but normal latency (Gouras, 1970).

In patients with clear media, ERG a-wave amplitudes and latencies are not significantly correlated with age (Weleber, 1981), but several studies have indicated that b-wave amplitudes decrease with increasing age, especially after age 50 or 60 (Krill, 1972; Armington, 1974; Zollman et al., 1978; Weleber, 1981). This decrease is more evident when the intensity of the stimulus is increased (Weleber, 1981). In contrast, assuming that the ocular medium remains clear, ERG b-wave latency does not change with age (Weleber, 1981). However, as medium transparency decreases, stimulus intensity at the retina also decreases, causing a corresponding increase in latency and decrease in amplitude for all portions of the ERG wave-form.

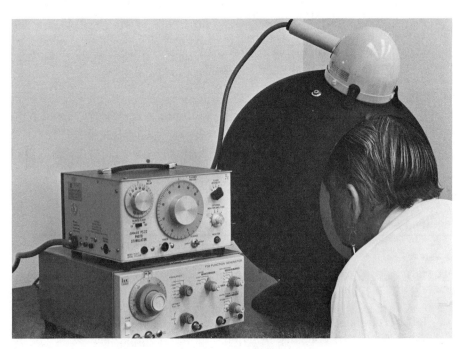

Figure 13.3 Patient presented with a uniformly diffused strobe-flash stimulus using a Ganzfeld dome during ERG recording.

In addition to changes in the a- and b-waves, changes in the ERG oscillatory potentials also can indicate abnormal retinal function. The oscillatory potentials have frequencies in the 100- to 160-Hz range, occur simultaneously with the b-wave, and probably are generated by cells in the middle or inner retinal layers. Loss of oscillatory potentials has been shown to indicate retinal ischemia, which might occur with the onset of diabetic retinopathy (Bresnick et al., 1984; Bresnick and Palta, 1987).

Because it has distinctive dark- and light-adapted responses, the ERG also can be used to differentiate rod versus cone degenerations. However, these more involved test procedures usually are not applicable to the elderly patient, since hereditary degenerations typically manifest themselves relatively early in life and are well documented by the time the patient reaches old age. For the interested reader, several reviews of ERG testing for receptor degenerations are available (Gouras, 1970; Weleber and Eisner, 1988; Carr and Siegel, 1990).

Bright-Flash ERG

For many elderly patients, the typical strobe stimulus (Grass Model PS22) must be replaced with an even brighter strobe to insure penetration of media opacities. Any response at all to this bright flash indicates a functional (but not necessarily perfect) retina. If the patient is contemplating surgical removal of cataracts or other media opacities, the presence or absence of the bright-flash ERG response can be used in making a prognosis for visual rehabilitation (Fuller et al., 1975).

As a word of caution, the standard, full-field ERG is a summed response from the whole retina, so the loss of a small but critical area, such as the fovea, usually would not be detected. Therefore, any predictions of postsurgical acuity based on full-field ERG data alone are tenuous. The value of the bright-flash ERG is that it gives a gross indication of retinal integrity. For a person virtually blind because of media opacities, some useful vision could be restored through surgery, even in the absence of a functioning macula. The bright-flash ERG, if recordable, gives reasonable hope for at least partial sight. A nonrecordable bright-flash ERG is not as conclusive. Again, because of the mass-response nature of the test, large portions of the retina may be damaged — thus producing no ERG — and yet the foveal region still may be functional. Because of these considerations, bright-flash ERGs should be followed up with other tests, such as bright-flash VER, laser interferometry, PAM, or BFET, that specifically assess central visual function.

Focal ERG

In distinction to the more commonly used full-field ERGs in which flashes are presented to the entire retina, focal ERGs have been used to demonstrate the response from a small portion of the retina. Focal ERGs use flash stimuli that are focused on small areas of the retina (for example, the macula) to isolate the response from these areas, but they produce much smaller signals than do full-field ERGs. For this reason, computer averaging usually is required to increase the amplitude of the ERG. Focal ERGs have shown some promise in evaluating the macula, but they are not yet readily available as referral tests.

Pattern ERG

It has been shown that ERG responses can be elicited by using a constant-luminance patterned stimulus such as a phase-reversing grating or a checkerboard (Rimmer and Katz, 1989). When these stimuli are used, the ERG is produced primarily by ganglion cells (which do not contribute significantly to the flash ERG). Pattern ERGs have been used to assess ganglion cell damage resulting from temporary occlusion of the central retinal artery, macular disease (Fish and Birch, 1989; Salzman et al., 1986), retrobulbar optic neuritis (Plant et al., 1986), glaucoma (Trick, 1987; Weinstein et al., 1988), and certain other diseases (Fiorentini et al., 1981). The objective nature of the pattern ERG can make it a powerful diagnostic tool for use with elderly patients, and when coupled with a laser-generated stimulus (see the section on laser interferometry), it can be used with patients who have almost opaque media.

The analysis of pattern ERGs is more complex than the analysis of flash ERGs, because computer averaging and processing of the pattern ERGs usually is required, and an electrode that does not interfere with the eye's optics (for example, a metallic fiber or foil as described in Fishman and Sokol, 1990) must be used. Thus, pattern ERG recording is typically available as a referral procedure only at teaching institutions and selected clinics. Additionally, it appears that pattern ERG amplitudes change with the age of the patient (Birch and Fish, 1988), so appropriate norms must be used when interpreting the results of this test.

Electro-oculography

Electro-oculography is another objective test of retinal integrity. It is particularly suited for testing the status of the pigment epithelium, but it evaluates certain other parts of the retina as well (Berson, 1987; Weleber and Eisner, 1988; Fishman and Sokol, 1990; Carr and Siegel, 1990). Like the ERG, it is a mass cell response, and, therefore, it generally does not allow fine discriminations to be made about the functional status of small retinal areas such as the macula. (Future applications of the EOG might allow these discriminations to be made, however. See Sunness and Massoff, 1986 for a presentation of techniques). It is less difficult to conduct an EOG than an ERG because a contact lens electrode is not needed. EOG testing does, however, require a reasonable degree of patient competence because targets must be fixated accurately (Doft et al., 1982).

Principles

In the resting (dark-adapted) state, there is normally about a 6-mV difference in electrical potential between the cornea (which is positive) and the back of the eye. This "standing potential" — which is produced largely by the pigment epithelial cells — varies with time in the dark, and a minimal value is reached 5 to 15 minutes after the lights are extinguished.

When the lights are turned on, the potential increases for about 5 to 15 minutes until a peak is reached. This increase is mediated by light striking the receptor cells and probably also involves activity of cells in the middle retinal layers (Carr and Siegel, 1990).

Methods
Following dilation of the irises, five skin electrodes are attached to the patient — one at each canthus and a reference electrode is placed at a remote location, usually the earlobe or mastoid. The patient is asked to alternate fixation between two target lights 30° apart. This produces an oscillating voltage at the electrodes, which is amplified and displayed on an oscilloscope or chart recorder. This voltage is recorded for about 15 minutes in the dark, then for 15 minutes in the light. Figure 13.4 shows a schematic representation of an EOG trace with the light peak and the dark trough indicated.

Interpretation of Results
The magnitude of the EOG depends on the state of the eye's light/dark adaptation. By dividing the maximum potential recorded during light adaptation (the light peak) by the minimum standing potential found during dark adaptation (the dark trough), a ratio called the Arden Index (AI) can be calculated. This value is commonly used as a clinical indicator of eye health.

Arden and Barrada (1962) found a significant negative correlation between age and the AI in normal subjects. For normal patients younger than 50 years old, Krill (1972) found that an AI less than 2.0 was abnormal; in patients older than 50 years old, a ratio of less than 1.85 was abnormal. Zollman et al. (1978) also reported decreases in the AI with age among their normal patients; the average index was 2.20 for patients aged 20 to 35 years, and 1.95 for patients aged 60 to 80 years.

An abnormal AI (lower than what is expected for the patient's age) indicates a widespread dysfunction of the retinal pigment epithelium or other retinal elements. This may be caused by a number of conditions, including malignant melanoma of the choroid (Staman et al., 1980; Jones et al., 1981), retinal detachment, acute disseminated choroiditis, vascular insufficiency, or hypertensive retinopathy (Arden and Barrada, 1962).

Occasionally, it is of interest to determine whether asymptomatic elderly family members are carriers of hereditary diseases. Electro-oculograms provide unique information regarding genetic traits for vitelliform macular dystrophy because patients who carry this trait (as well as those who manifest the disease) have abnormal EOGs (Berson, 1987).

As has been noted, the EOG is somewhat limited in its use because it requires the patient to make relatively accurate fixations. However, the EOG does provide an objective assessment of retinal integrity and can be critical for diagnosing certain pathologic characteristics — especially those involving the pigment epithelium.

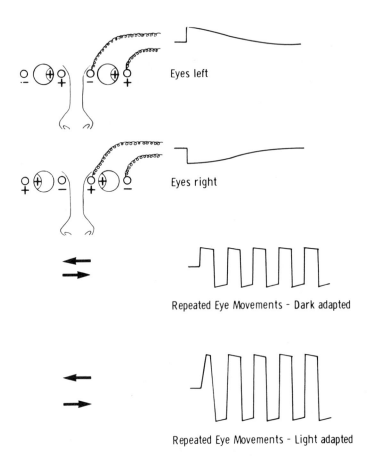

Eyes left

Eyes right

Repeated Eye Movements - Dark adapted

Repeated Eye Movements - Light adapted

Figure 13.4 Eye movements as indicated by the arrows produce an alternating voltage at the EOG electrodes. The amplitude of the voltage alternations is smaller in the dark (dark trough) and larger in the light (light peak). (Source: Reprinted with permission from Galloway, N.R. *Ophthalmic Electrodiagnosis.* Eastbourne, East Sussex, England: W.B. Saunders, 1975, p. 23.

TESTS OF VISUAL PATHWAY INTEGRITY

If a problem is suspected in the visual pathway, one of several objective and subjective tests can be ordered. The most commonly used objective test is the VER, which provides an indication primarily of macular pathway function up to, and including, the level of the visual cortex. In addition, laser interferometry, dark adaptometry, contrast sensitivity testing, perimetry, and use of devices such as the PAM and BFET allow subjective testing of important visual functions. Each of these tests, except the VER, requires that the patient can not only perceive a stimulus, but can also report what is seen.

Visual Evoked Response

The VER is an electrical potential generated primarily by neurons in the portion of the visual cortex representing the foveal region (Regan, 1972; Regan, 1989). Among the applications for VERs in elderly patients are: (1) detection of optic neuritis, (2) assessment of visual system patency, (3) preoperative prediction of postoperative visual acuity for patients with opaque media, (4) objective determination of visual acuity and refractive error, (5) objective color vision testing, and (6) objective visual field estimates (Sokol, 1976; Sherman, 1979; Regan, 1989; Fishman and Sokol, 1990; Carr and Siegel, 1990). VER recording is not invasive or painful, and requires only a minimal level of patient cooperation; this makes it possible to obtain recordings from nearly every type of patient.

Principles

Visual stimuli — either flashes of light or patterns — elicit cortical responses that can be detected through scalp electrodes placed over the occipital region of the brain. However, the VER itself is of such a small magnitude (about 5 μV), as compared with the normal electroencephalographic (EEG) "noise" (about 30 μV), that it must be specially processed before it can be analyzed. This is typically accomplished by using a computer that makes multiple measurements of the VER and then ensemble averages them. This produces a relative reduction in the amplitude of the EEG noise that accompanies the VER.

There are two major types of VER stimulus presentation systems in current use: transient systems in which a single, discrete change in the visual stimulus produces the response, and steady-state systems in which the VER is produced by a continuous change in stimulus luminance, pattern, and color.

The transient VER waveform has several components, most of which occur in about the first 200 ms after the stimulus (Figure 13.5). The most clinically useful of these components are the first and second significant negative deflections, usually labeled N-1 and N-2, and the first significant positive deflection, usually referred to as P-1. Two characteristics of these components — their implicit times (measured from stimulus presentation to peak response) and their amplitudes — are of diagnostic importance.

The steady-state VER is elicited by a continuously changing stimulus such as a phase-reversing checkerboard pattern. The continuous VER produced by such a stimulus is ensemble averaged to enhance the signal-to-noise ratio, and then further analyzed by using a fast Fourier Transform. The amplitude and implicit time (as determined from the phase angle of the VER) can be measured and used in a manner similar to corresponding data from transient stimulus presentations.

Methods

Typically, VER recording involves placement of one electrode on the scalp over the occipital pole and two more at other sites on the head or body. The patient is placed in a darkened room and presented with a visual stimulus, such as a bright light flash or phase-reversing checkerboard pattern. Following computer processing, VER records are displayed for analysis. The recording procedure can take 20 minutes to longer than an hour to complete, depending on the tests to be conducted.

Interpretation of Results

The VER implicit times are indicators of the time between stimulus presentation and the response of the cells in the visual cortex. Normal times depend somewhat on the stimulus being presented and usually decrease as intensity increases. Thus, each laboratory or clinic usually establishes its own norms for a population of patients who are presumably free from disease, and individual patient data are reported as deviations from these norms. An increase in the implicit time of VER components often is regarded as an indication of optic neuritis, which can be the result of a demyelinating disease such as multiple sclerosis (Asselman et al., 1975). However, because latencies normally increase with the

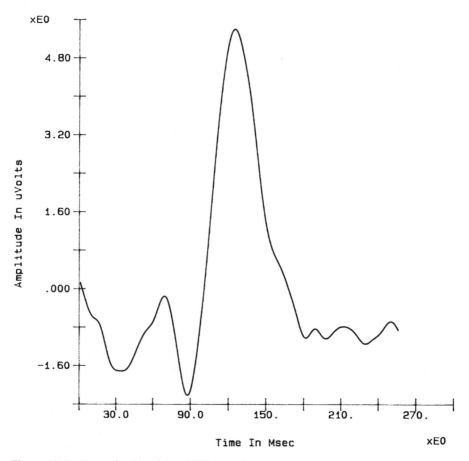

Figure 13.5 Example of transient VER waveform.

age of the patient (Celesia and Daly, 1977), evaluations of latencies should be made with respect to appropriate age norms.

Theoretically, VER amplitude data can be used for several purposes. Because VERs represent primarily foveal region activity, they are especially useful for testing the patency of central vision from the retina to the cortex (Vance and Jones, 1980). For elderly patients with media opacities, very bright or trans-scleral light flashes can be used to produce VERs (Rubin and Dawson, 1978; Thompson and Harding, 1978). A recordable bright-flash or trans-scleral VER can be a sign of potentially usable central vision, even in patients who have non-recordable bright-flash ERGs.

When patterned stimuli are used, maximum VER amplitudes are obtained when the patient's cortex "sees" the pattern most clearly. This makes it possible to determine the patient's refractive error by simply changing lenses until the VER amplitude is maximized. Conversely, acuity can be determined by reducing the size of the elements (checks) in a checkerboard until the pattern no longer produces a VER (that is, when the pattern cannot be differentiated from a uniform field). Contrast sensitivity functions also can be determined using evoked potential amplitudes. These functions can be especially useful for detecting and monitoring macular changes in the elderly.

Other applications of the VER include the assessment of hereditary or acquired color vision losses in which two-color checkerboards are presented (Kinney and McKay, 1974), as well as the assessment of large field losses in which stimuli are presented at various locations in the visual field (Cappin and Nissim, 1975; Wolfe, 1979). Neither of these procedures is totally successful with all patients, and data from VER field testing should be interpreted with particular caution if less than full-quadrant field losses are suspected (Regan and Milner, 1978).

In summary, whereas VER latency data are fairly reliable and have been shown to be sensitive indicators of optic neuritis (Asselman et al., 1975), VER amplitudes are quite variable and thus limit the usefulness of procedures that depend on these measurements (Van Brocklin et al., 1979). VER recording, however, is the best currently available objective means of determining the patency of the macular pathway from the retina to the visual cortex; as such, it can be a powerful diagnostic tool, especially for noncommunicative elderly patients.

Dark Adaptometry

Dark adaptometry is a subjective method for determining sensitivity to light as a function of time in the dark. Normal ranges have been established for the commonly used test equipment (Goldmann-Weekers Adaptometer made by Haag-Streit), and deviations from these norms can validate patient complaints of night vision difficulties.

Including the initial preadaptation phases, dark adaptometry usually takes at least 30 minutes and requires attentiveness on the part of the patient, as well as the ability to make timely responses. Some elderly patients may find the process

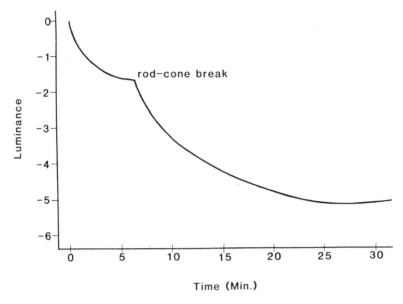

Figure 13.6 Dark adaptation curve showing the change in light sensitivity as a function of time in the dark for a normal person.

excessively fatiguing, and others may have difficulty concentrating on the test. These factors make it important for the optometrist to exercise reasonable care in the referral of patients for dark adaptometry. Older people should be advised to get adequate rest before the procedure to increase their alertness and endurance.

Principles

A curve showing the change in light sensitivity as a function of time for a normal person is shown in Figure 13.6. There are two parts of the dark adaptation curve: the upper arm corresponds to the action of the cone system, which is the dominant system for the first few minutes in the dark. (During this time, the rod system has not yet recovered enough sensitivity to match that of the cones.) As dark adaptation progresses, the cones become more sensitive until, after about 5 minutes, their sensitivity reaches a plateau. At this time, a transition (called the rod-cone break) takes place, after which the rods become more sensitive than the cones; overall sensitivity increases again until a final plateau is reached after approximately 20 to 30 minutes of dark adaptation.

Dark adaptometry data provide measurements of four important variables: (1) the time it takes for the rod-cone break to occur, (2) the cone threshold, (3) the rod threshold, and (4) the time to reach the final rod threshold. As aging occurs, the dark adaptation curve changes steadily, with the threshold for both rods and cones increasing. The time to the rod-cone break, however, remains constant (Pitts, 1982).

Note that the ordinate scale in Figure 13.6 is in log units of light intensity. Thus, it can be seen that a small change in the patient's threshold corresponds to a marked change in intensity of the test light. Gunkel and Gouras (1963) showed that an average increase in threshold of 0.5 log units occurs between the ages of 20 and 80 years (using a white stimulus). This means that a white threshold stimulus for an 80-year-old person is about three times as intense as it is for a 20-year-old individual.

The color of the stimulus can dramatically change the results of dark adaptometry, especially if the stimulus is at the blue end of the spectrum. For a violet stimulus, the change in the threshold of 1.8 log units between the ages of 20 and 80 years is apparently caused by changes in the aging lens (Gunkel and Gouras, 1963). Figure 13.7 shows the relationship between visual thresholds for various stimulus colors and age.

Methods

Dark adaptometry procedures vary slightly, depending on the clinic and the apparatus used; however, the basics are similar, especially if the standard equipment (a Goldmann-Weekers Adaptometer) is used. The patient is typically given a mydriatic and then adapted for a fixed amount of time to a light of a standard luminance (usually 5 minutes to a light of 1,400 to 2,100 apostilbs). The adaptation light then is extinguished, and the patient is asked to respond when the test light can first be seen. The test light is initially made too dim for the patient to see and then gradually increased in brightness until it can first be detected; this establishes the patient's threshold. The process is then repeated about every 30 seconds to 1.0 minute to follow the changes in threshold as a function of time in the dark. The procedure is continued until no further decreases in threshold are found (usually about 20 to 30 minutes).

Interpretation of Results

The elderly patient who complains of night vision difficulties may or may not be experiencing normal aging changes. Possible abnormal causes of night vision problems in the elderly include media opacities, vitamin A deficiencies, and other metabolic difficulties. Assuming that the ocular media are clear, dark adaptometry is a method by which normal age-related changes can be distinguished from abnormal changes that may require treatment. In addition, patients who show substantial, non-treatable decreases in sensitivity can be counseled to avoid night driving and other situations that require optimum performance in dim environments.

Contrast Sensitivity

A visual scene can be considered to be made up of a complex amalgam of light and dark bands. These bands, or gratings, can have different spatial frequencies (the number of bands or cycles per degree of visual angle), contrasts (the ratio of the brightness of the light and dark bands), and orientations in space (Nadler et al., 1990). Tests of Snellen acuity evaluate only sensitivity to high spatial frequencies, but most visual scenes contain low and mid-range spatial frequencies as well as high frequencies.

Loss of contrast sensitivity in the middle and low-frequency ranges can be bewildering to the patient, as well as to the examiner. Visual acuity can be corrected to 20/20, but the patient might still complain that things just don't look right. Before dismissing this complaint as unimportant or "psychological," con-

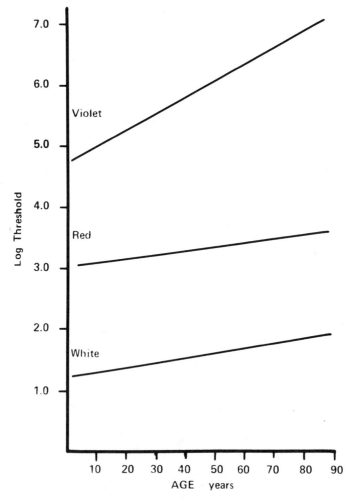

Figure 13.7 Relationship between age and the absolute thresholds for violet, red, and white test lights. Note that as age increases, so does the threshold — especially for the violet stimulus. (Source: Adapted with permission from Gunkel, R.D., and P. Gouras. "Changes in Scotopic Visual Thresholds with Age." *Arch. Ophthalmol.* 69 (1963): 5.

trast sensitivity testing should be ordered, especially since abnormal contrast sensitivity curves can result from corneal disease, glaucoma, optic neuritis, cataracts, diabetes, macular pathologies, amblyopia, and other abnormalities (Sjostrand and Frisen, 1977; Arden, 1978; Arden and Gucukoglu, 1978; Arden and Jacobson, 1978; Arundale, 1978; Weatherhead, 1980, Lund and Lennerstrand, 1981; Kupersmith et al., 1989; Miller and Sanghvi, 1990; Nadler, 1990; Cavallerano and Aiello, 1990; Arden, 1990; Storch and Bodis-Wollner, 1990).

Contrast sensitivity testing can be especially valuable for estimating the degree of visual impairment experienced by cataract patients. The loss of mid-spatial frequency sensitivity can make everyday tasks difficult, even with reasonably good Snellen acuity. The ability to estimate real-life impairment can be enhanced by subjecting cataract patients to a glare source during contrast sensitivity or Snellen acuity testing (Miller and Nadler, 1990; Prager, 1990; Nadler, 1990).

Contrast sensitivity testing can take less than 30 minutes using photographic plates (Arden, 1978), electronically generated stimuli, or poster style plates (Ginsburg and Tedesco, 1986), but testing with any of these devices requires a cooperative and responsive patient. To avoid this problem, the VER can be used to indicate a response to the grating (Prager, 1990).

Of special importance when dealing with elderly patients is the fact that contrast sensitivity changes with age (Derefelt et al., 1979; Owsley et al., 1983; Morrison and McGrath, 1985; Owsley et al., 1985). Once again, appropriate norms must be used to evaluate data from these patients.

Methods
The contrast sensitivity function is obtained by presenting the patient with a series of grating patterns having different spatial frequencies. For each spatial frequency, the contrast in a series of patterns decreases until the patient can no longer detect the grating; this determines the threshold for that spatial frequency. Thresholds can be graphed, as Figure 13.8 shows, to form a contrast sensitivity function.

Contrast sensitivity thresholds can be made more meaningful to ophthalmic practitioners if they are used to produce a Visuogram (analogous to an audiogram). In a Visuogram (Figure 13.9), the patient's response at each frequency is compared with the population norm (Bodis-Wollner, 1980).

Interpretation of Results
As indicated above, Snellen visual acuity is an indicator of high spatial frequency sensitivity; consequently, a loss in this part of the spatial frequency spectrum corresponds to a loss of visual acuity. Less easy to understand are the consequences of low- or mid-frequency losses. Patients having such losses describe the sensation as being like looking through a fog or looking at a "washed out" visual scene. Figure 13.10 is an attempt to visualize a high-frequency loss (a) and a low-frequency loss (c), as compared with normal frequency sensitivity (b). The scene, as a normal person would see it, contains low, medium, and high spa-

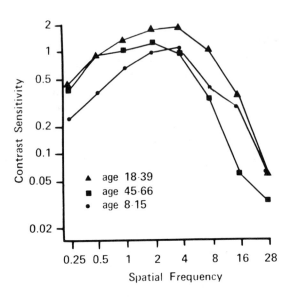

Figure 13.8 Normal contrast sensitivity functions from persons of different ages. Note the age-related changes. (Source: Adapted with permission from Arundale, K. "An Investigation into the Variation of Human Contrast Sensitivity with Age and Pathology." *Br. J. Ophthalmol.* 62 (1987): 214.

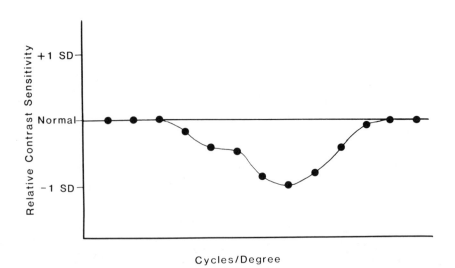

Figure 13.9 Contrast sensitivity data represented as a Visuogram in which the patient's data are expressed as deviations from normal values. Y-axis coordinates represent plus and minus one standard deviation (SD) from the population norm. Plus indicates above-normal and minus indicates below-normal (reduced) contrast sensitivity. The patient whose data are shown has a selective loss of mid-range spatial frequency contrast sensitivity.

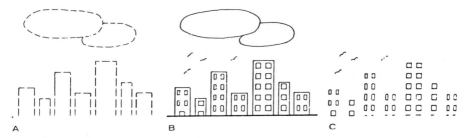

Figure 13.10 Schematic representation showing the effects that high- and low-spatial frequency sensitivity losses would have on a city scene. (A) shows a loss of high-frequency sensitivity: fine details such as birds and windows are missing, and the buildings and clouds are seen as gross shapes without sharp edges (indicated by dashed lines). (B) shows the scene as it would be seen by a normal person. The birds, windows, and building edges represent high-spatial frequencies. The general outlines of the buildings and clouds represent low frequencies. (C) shows the scene as it would appear to a person with a loss of ability to perceive low-spatial frequencies. Details are preserved, but gross shape information is lost. Source: Courtesy of Jurgen Meyer-Arendt, M.D., Ph.D.

tial frequencies. High-frequency loss results in a loss of detail vision. Low-frequency loss is more difficult to explain; fine details stand out, but the general shapes of large objects are lost.

Early investigations of contrast sensitivity showed little or no change with age (Arden, 1978; Arden and Jacobson, 1978), but more recent investigations indicate that normal variations do occur with age (Arundale, 1978; Derefeldt et al., 1979; Sekuler and Hutman, 1980; Sekuler et al., 1982; Skalka, 1980; Owsley et al., 1983; Owsley et al., 1985). These reports indicate a lessening of contrast sensitivity with increasing age; however, the amount of change and the frequencies at which it occurs vary with the investigator, the apparatus used, and the testing conditions.

In summary, contrast sensitivity testing can be a very useful clinical tool. It can help practitioners to understand the basis of patients' complaints, especially if 20/20 patients have difficulty in describing their problems and yet insist that "something just is not quite right with my eyes." For these patients, contrast sensitivity testing may reveal a mid- or low-spatial frequency loss, but the cause of that loss would need further exploration.

Perimetry

Perimetric assessment of visual fields is often an important diagnostic procedure, especially for elderly patients whose conditions suggest glaucoma, strokes, or central nervous system (CNS) lesions. Field testing equipment ranges from the simple use of the examiner's fingers in confrontation testing to the use of complex computer-assisted devices.

Methods

Perimetry can be divided into several categories based on the portion of the visual field being tested and the nature of the test stimulus. Bowl type perimeters are commonly used to test the entire field; the central 30° can be tested with a tangent screen; and the macular region can be explored further with the Amsler grid. Testing with the Amsler grid is especially important for elderly patients, because it can reveal metamorphopsia, which can be an early sign of age-related macular degeneration. Detection of this problem is especially important, since some types can be successfully treated with laser photocoagulation (Macular Photocoagulation Study Group, 1982).

Based on the nature of the stimulus presented to the patient, field testing also can be divided into kinetic and static perimetry. Kinetic perimetry uses a moving stimulus of a constant size, color, and luminance. By determining the boundaries of the visual field in which a particular target can be seen, an isopter can be plotted. By using different target sizes or colors, several isopters can be plotted, and a contour map of the island of vision can be created (Harrington, 1981). Tangent screens and Goldmann perimeters use the kinetic principle.

Static perimetry, in contrast, uses stationary targets. Multiple points in the visual field are selected, and lights at these points are simply turned on and off (Anderson, 1991). Static perimetry is generally considered to be more reliable than kinetic perimetry (Harrington, 1981). Another advantage of static perimetry is that retinal edema can be detected at an early stage by measuring and comparing visual fields obtained under mesopic and photopic conditions; kinetic perimetry is not as sensitive an indicator of these subtle retinal changes (Greve et al. 1976).

There are many automated perimeters now on the market which use the static perimetry principle (Schlindler and McCrary, 1981). Although their features vary somewhat, most use a computer to select the location and brightness of points to be presented and to record patient's responses. Because of the computerized nature of these perimeters, their presentations can be customized to meet the needs of individual patients. This is especially valuable for the elderly who might need a much slower testing pace and shorter sessions as compared to younger patients (Goodlaw 1981).

Most automated perimeters are able to present screening tests in which the ability of a patient to simply detect a spot is assessed, or they can determine the degree of vision loss at any point by finding the brightness threshold for detection of that point. Many of the perimeters also allow selection of test strategies designed to detect losses associated with glaucoma, tumors, or other specific problems.

Typically automated perimeters present their results using gray scale figures and/or give numeric values corresponding to the degree of field depression at different points. Some also provide a statistical analysis of the patient's field to determine how far it deviates from normal (Haley, 1987).

With the use of computerized devices, perimetry is becoming a technician's task in many practices. However, to completely define the defects uncovered by computerized perimeters using standard screening strategies, the visual field must be analyzed using custom strategies with the automated perimeters, or manually using Goldmann perimetry, a tangent screen, or an Amsler grid.

Interpretation of Results

The normal visual field shrinks with age, apparently in a continuous process starting in youth and proceeding on through senescence (Drance et al., 1967; Johnson et al., 1989; Haas et al., 1985). Until about age 50, the visual field size decreases slowly; after age 60 years, however, shrinkage becomes much more apparent, particularly in the temporal fields (Wolf and Nadroski, 1971). The changes may be the result of yellowing of the lens, changes in positions of the upper lids and/or the globe, neuroretinal decay, or artifacts that are the results of delays in reaction time (Drance et al., 1967). Normal aging changes must be considered when evaluating perimetry data from elderly patients. In addition, consideration should be given to the transparency (or lack of transparency) of the patient's ocular media (Guthauser and Flammer, 1988).

To aid in making the subtle distinction between cataractous visual field changes and those caused by other pathologic conditions such as glaucoma, Radius (1978) determined threshold isopters for five standard test stimuli in 148 eyes with varying degrees of cataractous lens changes. By correlating visual acuity with standard isopters (obtained with the Goldmann perimeter), Radius constructed a series of expected visual fields for patients with cataracts. By using these norms, it may be possible to detect subtle field changes that are caused by complicating pathologic characteristics in elderly patients with cataracts.

Laser Interferometry

Ophthalmic laser interferometry uses low-power, coherent light beams (lasers) to produce visible interference patterns directly on the retina (Green, 1981). Because this process is relatively independent of the optics of the eye, it is possible to produce interference patterns with fine or gross detail, even in eyes with media opacities or large refractive errors. Thus, interferometry provides a subjective means for determining the visual acuity that a patient could achieve if such problems could be eliminated. The process is not harmful (light power levels do not exceed normal daylight levels) and is especially useful for elderly patients when there is a question regarding whether they would benefit from cataract surgery. Totally accurate fixation is not required because the pattern covers a relatively large retinal area, and the patient would be expected to view the stimulus with the part of the retina providing maximum acuity. However, for the test to be conducted properly, the patient must be able to signal what is being seen reliably (unless interferometry is coupled with an objective assessment technique such as the VER; see Arden and Sheorey, 1977).

Principles
Interference patterns occur when two coherent beams of light interact. In simple terms, the two beams can be thought of as alternately reinforcing (producing bright bands) and canceling each other (producing dark bands). If the ocular media are clear and homogenous, the bands thus formed are very uniform. As opacities are introduced, disruption of the pattern occurs; however, it is still possible to produce perceptible interference bands through formidably dense media. Presumably, there are enough minute spaces in such media to allow sufficient unscattered light to enter the eye to produce the patterns (Green, 1970).

Methods
Commercial laser interferometers are available as slit-lamp attachments (Richter and Sherman, 1979). Prior to testing, the patient generally is given a mydriatic to allow more light to enter the eye. Interference bands then are produced on the retina and made progressively closer together (finer) until any further reduction makes individual bands indistinguishable. This provides a measure of the best visual acuity for the patient.

The procedure may be complicated somewhat by extraneous patterns that are introduced by the presence of media opacities. These extraneous patterns sometimes can confuse elderly patients, making it necessary to help them understand which patterns they should attend to. To assure that the patient is indeed responding to the correct stimulus, an indication of the orientation of the interference bands can be solicited. Band orientation is varied randomly by the examiner throughout the test, and failure of the patient to indicate the proper orientation is analogous to missing a letter in Snellen acuity testing.

Interpretation of Results
Studies show that in normal populations, there is a high correlation between visual acuities obtained with laser interferometry and Snellen acuities (Green and Cohen, 1971). Likewise, in a study of 150 patients (163 eyes) with cataracts complicated by retinal disease, preoperative predictions of visual acuity agreed very well with postoperative acuities in 140 eyes (86%). Of the remaining 23 eyes, 21 had better postoperative acuity than expected, and two had unexpectedly low acuities, apparently because of pathologic changes that occurred between preoperative and postoperative testing (Cohen, 1976).

Laser interferometry testing is especially recommended for patients with opacities and suspected macular changes, which together can result in moderately reduced visual acuity (about 20/80). For these patients, laser interferometry is valuable because it can differentiate between acuity losses that are caused by media opacities and losses that are the result of retinal degeneration.

Potential Acuity Meter

The PAM uses a Maxwellian view optical system to image a miniature Snellen acuity chart onto the patient's retina by projecting it through a relatively clear portion of the media. The PAM is commonly used to test visual acuity subjectively in patients with mild to moderate media opacities. For many cataract patients, it gives a prediction accurate to within two lines of postoperative Snellen acuity (Guyton, 1987). It is also useful for preoperative assessment of the retina, especially in cases of known or suspected posterior pole disease.

Methods

The potential acuity meter is mounted on a slit lamp so that its output beam can be moved by using the slit lamp's controls. The patient's refractive error is compensated by adjusting the PAM, and the light beam from the instrument is moved around on the cornea until it enters the eye through an area of less dense opacification, or a clear area in the media. The patient is asked to report when the chart is visible and then to read any letters that can be seen. Using this procedure, a subjective estimate of acuity can be obtained. Finding a clear area in the media often requires a considerable amount of searching, and this can be frustrating and tiring for some elderly patients.

Interpretation of Results

The PAM generally produces reliable results. Postoperative visual acuity predictions with a 95% accuracy have been reported by Minkowski et al. (1984) for cataract patients, and similar results also have been found by Christenbury and McPherson (1985). Not all reports of acuity predictions made with the PAM have been this good, however. Falsely low acuity predictions have been found mainly in patients with very dense media opacities (Guyton, 1987), and falsely good predictions have been reported by Faulkner (1983). These falsely good predictions occurred in cases of cystoid macular edema, serous detachment of the macula, recurrent surgically reattached retina, geographic atrophy of the macular pigment epithelium, and macular hole or cyst. The PAM predictions of acuity were better, however, than predictions made for these patients with a laser interferometer (Faulkner, 1983).

Blue Field Entoptoscope

The BFET is a very simple device used to subjectively assess macular function in patients with opaque media. It allows prediction of postoperative vision for cataract patients preoperatively, and may be one of the best tests available for this purpose with patients who have moderately dense media opacities. For patients with extremely dense opacities, however, this test can be less effective.

The test is based on the blue field entoptic phenomenon, which allows the patient to visualize white blood cells as they flow through the foveal and parafoveal capillaries (Duke-Elder, 1962). The cells appear to be rapidly moving white specks as seen against the bright blue field projected by the instrument. The phenomenon is based on the fact that white blood cells transmit blue light to a greater extent than do other blood components, and the transmitted light stimulates underlying photoreceptors (Loebl and Riva, 1978).

Methods
The patient views a 500-watt tungsten lamp through a 430-nm band-pass filter. The intensity of the blue light is increased in steps until the patient reports seeing "flying corpuscles" or "specks." The patient also is asked to approximate the total number of corpuscles seen, and how they are distributed in the field. The test does not require the patient to wear any form of refractive correction, and takes only a few minutes per eye.

Interpretation of Results
Normal patients report that about 25 to 40 corpuscles are seen at any one time (Minkowski and Guyton, 1984). In addition, the corpuscles must be distributed uniformly in the field (Loebl and Riva, 1978). If few or no corpuscles are seen, the blood flow to the foveal and parafoveal region could be compromised, and/or the retina in this area might be damaged. Both possibilities suggest poor postoperative acuities for cataract patients. With the criterion of 15 or more corpuscles visible at any time, Sinclair et al. (1979) predicted 20/40 or better postoperative visual acuity with 91% accuracy for a population of cataract patients.

Use of the BFET can produce results that are of significant value in counseling patients on the probable results of surgical treatment of media problems such as vitreal bleeds, corneal opacities, or cataracts. The accuracy of this test, its simplicity, and the relatively low cost of the BFET make this test of considerable value, especially for elderly patients who have trouble responding to more complex stimuli or demanding procedures.

IMAGING TECHNIQUES
Fluorescein Angiography

Fluorescein angiography is a special photographic technique that can be used to evaluate the vascular integrity of the choroid and retina (Behrendt, 1981; Zimmerman and Russell, 1986). Referral for angiography has been suggested for patients with ischemia, diabetic retinopathy, histoplasmosis, suspected malignancies, macular degeneration, disc edema, reduced visual acuity of unknown etiology, any area of retinal edema where the cause is not apparent, or other retinal abnormalities (Alexander et al., 1979). These conditions are important, not only because of their vision-threatening consequences, but because they can indicate that similar problems are occurring in other parts of the brain.

Principles and Methods

Fluorescein angiography involves taking a rapid sequence of photographs starting after the injection of dye into the patient's hand or arm vein. As the fluorescein passes through the fundus vasculature, it is excited by flashes of blue light (485 to 500 nm), which cause it to emit green-yellow light (525 to 530 nm). Filters in the fundus camera select for this green-yellow light, and photographs of the fluorescing vasculature against a dark background are produced. Several such photographs are taken each second, allowing the examiner to observe the progressive filling and draining of the choroidal and retinal vessels.

The testing process is contraindicated for patients who have had previous allergic or adverse reactions to fluorescein (about 0.6%, according to Stein and Parker, 1971) and for those who are unable to achieve a minimum degree of fixation during photography. Also, the photographs require a series of reasonably bright flashes delivered through the dilated pupil, and this can be somewhat uncomfortable for many patients.

Interpretation of Results

Several features of the vascular system can be studied in angiography photographs. Disruptions of the normal laminar blood flow in the vessels (especially the veins) can be detected; this turbulence often signals partial obstructions. The photographs also can show that some areas receive more fluorescein than normal or hold the dye after it has been cleared from the rest of the retina. This suggests edema, neovascularization, hemorrhage, or decreased retinal pigmentation. Other areas may receive less fluorescein than normal, suggesting ischemia or occlusion.

There is a negative correlation between age and the rate of filling for the retinal, optic disc, and peripapillary choroid vessels. Elderly patients typically have a slow filling rate (Schwartz and Kern, 1980), which can be mistaken as hypofluorescence if appropriate age-adjusted norms are not used. Such norms are developed most often by individual clinics and typically are based on experience rather than on published standards.

Ocular Ultrasonography

Ocular ultrasonography provides an objective assessment of the gross structural integrity of the globe and orbit (Smith et al., 1986; Dallow, 1986). Its chief advantage over optical techniques is that it can "see" beyond media opacities and give an indication of intraocular status. Among the pathologic features that ophthalmic ultrasonography can detect and help to differentially diagnose are vitreous and subretinal hemorrhages, vitreal membranes, retinal and choroidal detachments, foreign bodies, malignant melanomas, metastatic carcinomas, hemangiomas, senile macular choroidal degeneration, and a number of other orbital and/or ocular conditions (Hodes, 1976; Coleman, 1977; Hassani and Bard, 1977; Coleman et al., 1977; Coleman and Abramson, 1981; Coleman and Dallow, 1981b; Tani et al., 1980).

Elderly patients may express concern about possible side effects associated with the use of ultrasound. Although extremely intense ultrasound is potentially hazardous, average diagnostic power levels are several orders of magnitude below the levels that produce pain or tissue damage. There is no evidence of damage caused by power levels used in diagnostic ultrasonography, but cumulative effects of ultrasound have not yet been investigated thoroughly (Posakony, 1969; Coleman et al., 1977).

Principles

Ultrasound is high-frequency sound above the range of human hearing (above 20 kHz). When ultrasound waves cross a boundary between two heterogeneous tissues, some of the waves are reflected. The time it takes for this echo to return to a detector is recorded; knowing the velocity of sound in the particular ocular medium involved makes it possible to calculate the distance to the reflecting boundary.

Two scanning techniques — A-scan and B-scan — are commonly used and yield different types of information (Coleman and Dallow, 1981a). A-scan ultrasonography provides a linear representation of the eye; that is, it shows the location of tissue boundaries that would be encountered if a linear object — for example, a needle — was pierced through the eye. Typically this information is displayed as a series of peaks on an oscilloscope time (distance) line trace. Interpretation of these peaks can allow fine discriminations between tissue types to be made and can provide distance measurements between intraocular structures.

B-scan ultrasonography provides a two-dimensional view of the eye analogous to a histologic cross-section. It gives a picture-like representation of the eye and is very useful for detecting hemorrhages, tumors, and detachments. A combination of A-scan and B-scan often is used to make precise differential diagnoses of suspected pathologies.

Methods

Several types of transducers have been developed for use with ultrasound. Since ultrasound does not propagate well in air, one type makes direct skin contact through the closed eyelid, and the other is applied directly to the eye and uses water as a contact medium. The more elaborate ultrasonography instruments can make equally spaced B-scans across the eye to provide a comprehensive series of cross-sections. These usually are displayed on a cathode-ray tube and may be computer enhanced and photographed for permanent records.

Interpretation of Results

Interpretation of ultrasonography data largely involves detecting abnormal structures in the eye or orbit or determining that normal structures are displaced from their appropriate locations. Using B-scan, structures can be viewed in relation to the rest of the eye; tumors, foreign bodies, and blood clots can readily be located. By comparing data between the eyes, or to norms (which are often clinical impressions based on experience), tissue displacements also can be detected. Such displacements can indicate the presence of tumors, hemorrhages, or detachments.

A-scan often is used in making precise determinations of intraocular distances. Beyond detecting abnormal displacements of tissue, these distances (for example, from the cornea to the retina) have value in predicting the required power of an intraocular replacement lens.

Because of its noninvasive nature, ultrasonography can be used by various health-care professionals. With computer enhancement and imaging procedures, this test can provide valuable information about orbital and ocular structures.

Computed Axial Tomography

Perhaps the most commonly used technique for imaging structures in the brain has been the conventional x-ray. Using this procedure, x-rays are emitted from a stationary source, pass through the head, and expose a single photographic plate. More recently, however, systems have been developed in which the x-ray detector and/or source rotate around the patient to produce a cross sectional image. The image requires a computer for its analysis, hence the name "computed axial tomography" (CAT) (Grove, 1982; Galton, 1985; Marg, 1988; Tower and Oshinskie, 1989). CAT scans allow the imaging of the orbit and visual pathway either as flat sections or as three-dimensional reconstructions (Herman, 1980). Primary reasons for ordering CAT scans include detection of metallic foreign bodies or tumors; assessment of hard tissue injuries, for example, orbital fractures; and detection of vascular problems associated with strokes (Haik et al., 1986a; Haik et al., 1986b; Leib et al., 1986; Tower and Oshinskie, 1989).

Methods

The equipment used for CAT scans is quite large and formidable appearing. The scanner itself resembles a large doughnut into which the patient is placed. The most difficult part of the procedure is often the injection of an iodine-based contrast medium used to aid in visualizing blood vessels. Some patients react to the medium with symptoms including nausea, headache, or edema (Tower and Oshinskie, 1989). In extreme cases, reactions can involve bradycardia, cardiac arrest, or even death.

Following injection of contrast medium, the patient is advanced on a movable table into the center of the scanner, and the scans are made. To make multiple scans, the patient can be advanced further into the unit. The process takes several minutes per scan, and some patients experience claustrophobia in the scanner.

Although the images produced with the CAT system are extremely good, care should be taken in ordering CAT scans because of the risks associated with the ionizing radiation to which the patient is exposed, and the possibility of an allergic reaction to the contrast medium. As with any procedure, the risk-benefit ratio for CAT scans must be carefully considered for each patient.

Interpretation of Results

Typically, the results of a CAT scan are interpreted by a radiologist. Calcification and erosion of structures, intracranial masses, fractures of the orbit, muscle entrapment, results of cerebral vascular accidents, tumors involving the visual system, (for example, pituitary tumors), and other problems can be detected, assessed, and followed with CAT scans (Tower and Oshinskie, 1989). The high degree of image precision produced by CAT scans has greatly advanced the clinical management of problems such as these.

Magnetic Resonance Imaging

Like CAT, magnetic resonance imaging (MRI) (originally called nuclear magnetic resonance imaging) involves the production of detailed cross-sectional or three-dimensional images of various body structures (Galton, 1985; Tower and Oshinskie, 1989). Unlike CAT, however, no ionizing radiation is used. Instead, the combination of a magnetic field and radio waves force hydrogen atoms to emit signals that are detected by the MRI equipment. Because most of the hydrogen in the body exists in the form of water, MRIs actually show the concentration of water in various tissues. Because these concentrations vary, different tissues can be seen as separate from each other.

Major applications for MRI include assessment of soft tissue changes, tumors, and the effects of demyelinating diseases (for example, multiple sclerosis). MRI is not typically used to assess the effects of hard tissue damage or strokes. Because of the very strong magnetic fields used in MRI, the major contraindication to the technique is the presence of any metallic foreign object in the body (Tower and Oshinskie, 1989).

Principles and Methods

The MRI system consists of a large doughnut-shaped electromagnet that creates a magnetic field around the patient's body. The appearance of the equipment is quite similar to that of a CAT scanner. To produce an image, a strong magnetic field is used to align the polar atoms (for example, hydrogen) in the body, and a radio-frequency pulse is used to briefly disturb the alignment. This disturbance causes the atoms to emit radio-frequency signals that are detected by the MRI equipment.

To image a large structure such as the brain, the patient is placed inside the MRI unit, but special surface coils can be placed near the body to receive signals from smaller areas such as the eye (Saint-Louis et al., 1986; Galton 1985). In some applications, contrast medium is injected to help visualize structures, but often no medium is needed for MRI (Tower and Oshinskie, 1989). This fact, along with the high quality of images produced and the lack of ionizing radiation produced by the MRI equipment, makes this technique appropriate for imaging many ocular and related structures.

Typically, MRI takes about 40 minutes to complete, depending on the part of the body to be imaged. The MRI equipment makes a loud hammering noise in operation, and this, along with the feelings of claustrophobia associated with being in the doughnut, can be disturbing for some patients.

Interpretation of Results
Like CAT scans, MRIs are typically interpreted by a radiologist. MRIs of the orbital contents allow excellent visualization of muscles, masses, and tumors (Saint-Louis and Haik, 1986; Saint-Louis et al., 1986). MRIs of the brain are extremely useful for detecting the plaques associated with the neuronal degeneration caused by multiple sclerosis, and MRI is often used to help make the definitive diagnosis in this disease. In older patients, MRI can help to determine the cause of hearing loss, vertigo, progressive neural degeneration, and many other problems (Tower and Oshinskie, 1989).

Positron Emission Tomography and Single Photon Emission Computed Tomography

Positron and single photon emission tomography techniques are rapidly evolving methods used to produce images of metabolically active organs and tissues (Galton, 1985; Marg, 1988). These scans are used to demonstrate the metabolic level in brain nuclei such as those associated with processing sensory information (Marg, 1988). Specific applications include the study of multiple sclerosis, Parkinson's disease, schizophrenia, and Alzheimer's disease (Galton, 1985).

Methods
To conduct a PET scan, substances such as oxygen or glucose are converted to radioactive isotopes in a cyclotron and injected into, or inhaled by, the patient. These isotopes are then carried to metabolically active tissues where they decay by emitting positrons that interact with nearby electrons to produce radiation. SPECT scans are conducted in a similar manner, but radioactive xenon gas is typically inhaled or injected. The xenon is carried across the blood-brain barrier to active tissues in which it emits radiation as it decays.

Interpretation of Results
PET or SPECT equipment detects the radiation produced by the decaying isotopes and produces an image based on the amount of radiation coming from different tissues; metabolically active tissues will take up more of the isotope and therefore will be imaged against a background of less active tissue. The resolution of PET and SPECT scan images is not yet as good as it is for MRI or CAT images, but there is great promise for combining the excellent resolution of MRI or CAT with the ability of PET or SPECT to assess the functional status of different brain nuclei (Levin, 1989).

CONCLUSIONS

Special testing procedures offer the optometrist an opportunity to gain diagnostic insight beyond that afforded by conventional techniques. Difficulties that are encountered frequently among elderly patients, such as media opacities and communication difficulties, often can be overcome by ordering appropriate special tests.

To select appropriate tests for elderly patients, the patients' particular needs must be considered carefully. Subjective tests such as perimetry, contrast sensitivity, dark adaptometry, and those involving the use of the PAM and BFET depend on the ability of the patient to respond in a timely and reliable fashion. Certain objective tests also have special requirements; electro-oculography, for example, requires adequate fixation ability and relatively reliable eye movements. If there is some doubt as to the appropriateness of a particular test, consultation should be made with the laboratory or technician that will be performing the test.

Interpretation of the test results is perhaps the most critical area. The visual systems of elderly patients have undergone natural aging changes, and this makes it necessary to compare test results with population norms specific for the patients' ages.

Changes in test results can be expected with aging, but the actual values that should be considered normal for a particular age group often depend on the specific clinic in which the test is performed. This is particularly true with electro-diagnostic testing. Each clinic tends to have its own particular testing routine and apparatus, and small differences can affect test values significantly. Therefore, the doctor should consult with the particular clinic and inquire about the age norms that have been established in that clinic. If the clinic has no norms for elderly patients, data must be interpreted with caution.

With the appropriate use of special non-invasive tests, optometrists can monitor and manage patients more effectively, offer counseling regarding contemplated surgery for media opacity removal, and provide elderly patients, who have special needs, with more extensive assessment of their visual health and function.

REFERENCES

1. Alexander, A., J. Sherman, D. Horn. "Fundus Fluorescein Angiography: A Summary of Theoretical Concepts and Clinical Applications." *J. Am. Optom. Assoc.* 50, no. 1 (1979): 53–63.
2. Anderson, D.R. *Automated Static Perimetry.* St. Louis: C.V. Mosby, 1991.
3. Arden, G.B. New Methods of Diagnosis of Retinal Neural Damage Associated with Primary Open-Angle Glaucoma. In: Nadler, M.P., Miller, D., Nadler, D.J. (eds.). *Glare and Contrast Sensitivity for Clinicians.* New York: Springer-Verlag, 1990, pp. 76–84.
4. Arden, G.B. "The Importance of Measuring Contrast Sensitivity in Cases of Visual Disturbance." *Br. J. Ophthalmol.* 62 (1978): 198–209.
5. Arden, G.B., and Barrada, A. "Analysis of the Electro-oculogram of a Series of Normal Subjects." *Br. J. Ophthalmol.* 46 (1962): 468–482.

6. Arden, G.B., A. Barrada, J.H. Kelsey. "New Clinical Test of Retinal Function Based Upon the Standing Potential of the Eye." *Br. J. Ophthalmol.* 42 (1976): 449–467.
7. Arden, G.B., and A.G. Gucukoglu. "Grating Test of Contrast Sensitivity in Patients with Retrobulbar Neuritis." *Arch. Ophthalmol.* 96 (1978): 1626–1629.
8. Arden, G.B., J.J. Jacobson. "A Simple Grating Test for Contrast Sensitivity: Preliminary Results Indicate Value in Screening for Glaucoma." *Invest. Ophthalmol.* 17, no. 1 (1978): 23–32.
9. Arden, G.G., and U.B. Sheorey. "The Assessment of Visual Function in Patients with Opacities: A New Evoked Potential Method Using a Laser Interferometer." In: Desmedt, J.E. (ed.). *Visual Evoked Potentials in Man: New Developments.* Oxford: Clarendon Press, 1977.
10. Armington, J.C. *The Electroretinogram.* New York: Academic Press, 1974.
11. Arundale, K. "An Investigation into the Variation of Human Contrast Sensitivity with Age and Pathology." *Br. J. Ophthalmol.* 62 (1978): 213–215.
12. Asselman, P., D.W. Chadwick, C.D. Marsden. "Visual Evoked Responses in the Diagnosis and Management of Patients Suspected of Multiple Sclerosis." *Brain* 98 (1975): 261–282.
13. Behrendt, T. Fluorescein Angiography. In: Duane, T.D. (ed.). *Clinical Ophthalmology, vol. 3.* New York: Harper & Row, 1981, Chapter 4.
14. Berson, E.L. Electrical Phenomena in the Retina. In: Moses, R.A., Hart, W.M. Jr, (eds.). *Adler's Physiology of the Eye: Clinical Application.* St. Louis: C.V. Mosby, (1987), 8: 506–567.
15. Birch, D.G. "Clinical Electroretinography." *Ophthalmol. Clin. North Am.* 2 (1989): 469–497.
16. Birch, D.G., and G.E. Fish. "Focal Cone Electroretinograms: Aging and Macular Disease." *Doc. Ophthalmol.* 69 (1988): 211–220.
17. Bodis-Wollner, I. Detection of Visual Defects Using the Contrast Sensitivity Function. In: Sokol, S., (ed.). *Electrophysiology and Psychophysics: Their Use in Ophthalmic Diagnosis.* Boston: Little Brown, 1980.
18. Bresnick, G.H., K. Korth, A. Groo, et al. "Electroretinographic Oscillatory Potentials Predict Progression of Diabetic Retinopathy." *Arch. Ophthalmol.* 102 (1984): 1307–1311.
19. Bresnick, G.H., M. Palta. "Oscillatory Potential Amplitudes: Relation to Severity of Diabetic Retinopathy." *Arch. Ophthalmol.* 105 (1987): 929–933.
20. Cappin, J.M., S. Nissim. "Visual Evoked Responses in the Assessment of Field Defects in Glaucoma." *Arch. Ophthalmol.* 93 (1975): 9–18.
21. Carr, R.E., and I.M. Siegel. *Electrodiagnostic Testing of the Visual System: A Clinical Guide.* Philadelphia: F.A. Davis, 1990.
22. Cavallerano, J.D., and L.M. Aiello. Diabetes Mellitus and Visual Function. In: Nadler, M.P., Miller, D., Nadler, D.J. (eds.). *Glare and Contrast Sensitivity for Clinicians.* New York: Springer-Verlag, (1990), pp. 66–75.
23. Celesia, G.G., and R.R. Daly. "Effects of Aging on Visual Evoked Responses." *Arch. Neurol.* 34 (1977): 403–407.
24. Christenbury, J.D., and S.D. McPherson. "Potential Acuity Meter for Predicting Postoperative Visual Acuity in Cataract Patients." *Am. J. Ophthalmol.* 92 (1985): 746.
25. Cohen, M.M. "Laser Interferometry: Evaluation of Potential Visual Acuity in the Presence of Cataracts." *Ann. Ophthalmol.* 8, no. 7 (1976): 845–849.
26. Coleman, D.J. Ultrasonic Evaluation of the Vitreous. In: Freeman, H.M., Hirose T., Schepens C.L. (eds.). *Vitreous Surgery and Advances in Fundus Diagnosis and Treatment.* New York: Appleton-Century-Crofts, 1977.

27. Coleman, D.J., and D.H. Abramson. Ocular Ultrasonography. In: Duane, T.D. (ed.). *Clinical Ophthalmology*, vol. 2. New York: Harper & Row, 1981, chapter 26.
28. Coleman, D.J., and R.L. Dallow. Introduction to Ophthalmic Ultrasonography. In: Duane, T.D. (ed.). *Clinical Ophthalmology*, vol. 2. New York: Harper & Row, 1981a, chapter 26.
29. Coleman, D.J., and R.L. Dallow. Orbital Ultrasonography. In: Duane, T.D. (ed.). *Clinical Ophthalmology*, vol. 2. New York: Harper & Row, 1981b, chapter 26.
30. Coleman, D.J., E.L. Lizzi, R.L. Jack. *Ultrasonography of the Eye and Orbit.* Philadelphia: Lea and Febiger, 1977.
31. Dallow, R.L. "Ultrasonography of the Orbit." In: Haik, B.G. (ed.). Advanced Imaging Techniques in Ophthalmology. *Int. Ophthalmol. Clin.* 26, no. 3 (1986): 51–76.
32. Derefeldt, G., G. Lennerstrand, B. Lundh. "Age Variations in Normal Human Contrast Sensitivity." *Acta Ophthalmol.* 57 (1979): 679.
33. Doft, B.H., S.A. Burns, A. Elsner. "The Inverse Electro-oculogram." *Brit. J. Ophthalmol.* 62 (1982): 379–381.
34. Drance, S.M., V. Berry, A. Hughes. "Studies on the Effects of Age on the Central and Peripheral Isopters of the Visual Field in Normal Subjects." *Am. J. Ophthalmol.* 63, no. 6 (1967): 1667–1672.
35. Duke-Elder, S. *System of Ophthalmology.* St. Louis: C.V. Mosby, 1962, p. 445.
36. Faulkner, W. "Laser Interferometric Prediction of Postoperative Visual Acuity in Patients with Cataracts." *Am. J. Ophthalmol.* 95 (1983): 626.
37. Fiorentini, A., L. Maffei, M. Pirchio, D. Spinelli, V. Porciatti. "The ERG in Response to Alternating Gratings in Patients with Diseases of Peripheral Visual Pathway." *Invest. Ophthalmol.* 21, no. 3 (1981): 490–493.
38. Fish, G.E., and D.G. Birch. "The Focal Electroretinogram in the Clinical Assessment of Macular Disease." *Ophthalmology* 96 (1989): 109–114.
39. Fishman, G.A., and S. Sokol. *Electrophysiological Testing in Disorders of the Retina, Optic Nerve and Visual Pathway.* San Francisco: American Academy of Ophthalmology, 1990.
40. Fuller, D.G., R.W. Knighton, R. Machemer. "Bright-flash Electroretinography for the Evaluation of Eyes with Opaque Vitreous." *Am. J. Ophthalmol.* 80, no. 2 (1975): 214–223.
41. Galloway, N.R. *Ophthalmic Electrodiagnosis.* Philadelphia: W.B. Saunders, 1975.
42. Galton, L. CAT Scans. In: Galton, L. (ed.). *Med Tech: The layperson's guide to today's medical miracles.* New York: Harper and Row, 1985, pp. 111–115.
43. Galton, L. NMR. In: Galton, L. (ed.). *Med Tech: The layperson's guide to today's medical miracles.* New York: Harper and Row, 1985, pp. 286–289.
44. Galton, L. PET. In: Galton, L. (ed.). *Med Tech: The layperson's guide to today's medical miracles.* New York: Harper and Row, 1985, pp. 303–306.
45. Ginsburg, A.P., and J. Tedesco. "Evaluation of Functional Vision of Cataract and YAG Posterior Capsulotomy Patients Using the Vistech Contrast Sensitivity Chart." *Invest. Ophthalmol.* 27, no. 3 (1986): 107.
46. Goodlaw, E.I. "Assessing Field Defects of the Low-Vision Patient." *Am. J. Optom. Physiol. Opt.* 58, no. 6 (1981): 486–490.
47. Gouras, P. "Electroretinography: Some Basic Principles." *Invest. Ophthalmol.* 9, no. 8 (1970): 557–569.
48. Green, D.G. "Testing the Vision of Cataract Patients by Means of Laser-Generated Interference Fringes." *Science* 168 (1970): 1240–1242.
49. Green, D.G. Laser Devices in Measuring Visual Acuity. In: Duane, T.D. (ed.). *Clinical Ophthalmology*, vol. 1. New York: Harper & Row, 1981, chapter 66.

50. Green, D.G., and M.M. Cohen. "Laser Interferometry in the Evaluation of Potential Macular Function in the Presence of Opacities in the Ocular Media." *Trans. Am. Acad. Ophthalmol. Otolaryngol.* 75, no. 1 (1971): 629–637.
51. Greve, E., P. Bos, D. Bakker. "Photopic and Mesopic Central Static Perimetry in Maculopathies and Central Neuropathies." *Docu. Ophthalmol. Proc.* 14 (1976): 253–257.
52. Grove, A.S., Jr. "Computed Tomography in Ophthalmology." *Int. Ophthalmol. Clin.* 22, no. 4 (1986): 1–5.
53. Gunkel, R.D., and P. Gouras. "Changes in Scotopic Visual Thresholds with Age." *Arch. Ophthalmol.* 69 (1963): 4–9.
54. Guthauser, U., and J. Flammer. "Quantifying Visual Field Damage Caused by Cataract." *Am. J. Ophthalmol.* 106 (1988): 480–484.
55. Guyton, D.L. Preoperative Visual Acuity Evaluation. In: Smolin, G, Friedlaender, M, (eds.). *Int. Ophthalmol. Clin.* 27 (1987): 140–147.
56. Haik, B.G., L.A. St-Louis, M.E. Smith. "Computed Tomography in Ocular Disease." In: Haik, B.G. (ed.). Advanced Imaging Techniques in Ophthalmology. *Int. Ophthalmol. Clin.* 26, no. 3 (1986): 77–102.
57. Haik, B.G., L.A. St-Louis, M.E. Smith. "Computed Tomography of Extraocular Muscle Abnormalities." In: Haik, B.G., (ed.). Advanced Imaging Techniques in Ophthalmology. *Int. Ophthalmol. Clin.* 26, no. 3 (1986): 123–150.
58. Haley, M.J. (ed.). *The Field Analyzer Primer.* San Leandro: Allergan Humphrey, 1987, p. 2.
59. Harrington, D.O. *The Visual Fields: A Textbook and Atlas of Clinical Perimetry.* St. Louis: C.V. Mosby, 1981.
60. Haas, A., J. Flammer, U. Schneider. "Influence of Age on Visual Fields of Normal Subjects." *Am. J. Ophthalmol.* 101 (1985): 199–203.
61. Hassani, S.N., and R. Bard. "Evaluating the Eye Through Ultrasonography." *Geriatrics* 32, no. 10 (1977): 94–95, 99–101.
62. Herman, G.T. *Image Reconstruction from Projections.* New York: Academic Press, 1980.
63. Hodes, B.L. "Eye Disorders: Using Ultrasound in Ophthalmologic Diagnosis." *Postgrad. Med.* 59, no. 4 (1976): 197–203.
64. Johnson, C.A., A.J. Adams, R.A. Lewis. "Evidence of a Neural Basis of Age-Related Visual Field Loss in Normal Observers." *Invest. Ophthalmol.* 30, no. 9 (1989): 2056–2064.
65. Johnson, M.A., S. Marcus, M.J. Elman. "ERG Sensitivity Loss in Venous Stasis Retinopathy." *Invest. Ophthalmol.* 28 (1987): 319. Abstract.
66. Johnson, M.A., S. Marcus, M.J. Elman, et al. "Neovascularization in Central Retinal Vein Occlusion: Electroretinographic Findings." *Arch. Ophthalmol.* 106 (1988): 348–352.
67. Jones, R.M., R. Klein, G. DeVenecia, F.L. Myers. "Abnormal Electro-oculograms from Eyes with a Malignant Melanoma of the Choroid." *Invest. Ophthalmol.* 20, no. 20 (1981): 276–279.
68. Kinney, J.S., and C.L. McKay. "Test of Color-Defective Vision Using the Visual Evoked Response." *J. Opt. Soc. Am.* 64, no. 9 (1974): 1244–1250.
69. Krill, A.E. *Hereditary Retinal and Choroidal Diseases.* New York: Harper & Row, 1972.
70. Kupersmith, M.J., K. Holopigian, W.H. Seiple. Contrast Sensitivity Testing. In: Wall, M. and Sadun A.A. (eds.). *New Methods of Sensory Vision Testing.* New York: Springer-Verlag, 1989, pp. 53–67.
71. Leib, M.L. Computed Tomography of the Orbit. In: Haik, B.G. (ed.). Advanced Imaging Techniques in Ophthalmology. *Int. Ophthalmol. Clin.* 26, no. 3 (1986): 103–122.

72. Levin, D.N. "MRI and PET Data Merge in 3-D Images of Brain." *Diagnostic Imaging* 11 (1989): 150–157.
73. Loebl, M., and C.E. Riva. "Macular Circulation and the Flying Corpuscles Phenomenon." *Ophthalmology* 85 (1978): 911–917.
75. Lundh, B.L., and G. Lennerstrand. "Eccentric Contrast Sensitivity Loss in Glaucoma." *Acta Ophthalmol.* 59 (1981): 21–23.
76. Macular Photocoagulation Study Group. "Argon Laser Photocoagulation for Senile Macular Degeneration: Results of a Randomized Clinical Trial." *Arch. Ophthalmol.* 100 (1982): 912–918.
77. Marg, E. "Imaging Visual Function of the Human Brain." *Am. J. Optom. Physiol. Opt.* 65, no. 10 (1988): 828–851.
78. Miller, D., and M.P. Nadler. Light Scattering: Its Relationship to Glare and Contrast in Patients and Normal Subjects. In: Nadler, M.P., Miller, D., Nadler, D.J. (eds.). *Glare and Contrast Sensitivity for Clinicians.* New York: Springer-Verlag, 1990, pp. 24–32.
79. Miller, D., and S. Sanghvi. Contrast Sensitivity and Glare Testing in Corneal Disease. In: Nadler, M.P., Miller, D., Nadler, D.J. (eds.). *Glare and Contrast Sensitivity for Clinicians.* New York: Springer-Verlag, 1990, pp. 45–52.
80. Minkowski, J.S., and D.L. Guyton. "New Methods of Predicting Visual Acuity after Cataract Surgery." *Ann. Ophthalmol.* 16 (1984): 511–516.
81. Morrison, J.D., and C. McGrath. "Assessment of the Optical Contributions to the Age Related Deterioration in Vision." *Q. J. Exp. Physiol.* 70 (1985): 249.
82. Nadler, J.D. Glare and Contrast Sensitivity in Cataracts and Pseudophakia. In: Nadler, M.P., Miller, D., Nadler, D.J. (eds.). *Glare and Contrast Sensitivity for Clinicians.* New York: Springer-Verlag, 1990, pp. 53–65.
83. Owsley, C., R. Sekuler, D. Siemsen. "Contrast Sensitivity Throughout Adulthood." *Vis. Res.* 23, no. 7 (1983): 689.
84. Owsley, C., T. Gardner, R. Sekuler, et al. "Role of Crystalline Lens in the Spatial Vision Loss of Elderly." *Invest. Ophthalmol.* 26 (1985): 1165.
85. Pitts, D.G. "Dark Adaptation and Aging." *J. Am. Optom. Assoc.* 53, no. 1 (1982): 37–41.
86. Plant, G., R. Hess, S. Thomas. "The Pattern Evoked Electroretionogram in Optic Neuritis: A Combined Psychophysical and Electrophysiological Study." *Brain* 109 (1986): 469–490.
87. Posakony, G.J. Ultrasonic Transducers and Acoustic Waves. In : Gitters, K.A. (ed.). *Ophthalmic Ultrasound: An International Symposium.* St. Louis: C.V. Mosby, 1969.
88. Prager, T.C. Essential Factors in Testing for Glare. In: Nadler, M.P., Miller, D., Nadler, D.J. (eds.). *Glare and Contrast Sensitivity for Clinicians.* New York: Springer-Verlag, 1990, pp. 33–44.
89. Radius, R.L. "Perimetry in Cataract Patients." *Arch. Ophthalmol.* 96 (1978): 1574–1579.
90. Regan, D. *Evoked Potentials in Psychology. Sensory Physiology and Clinical Medicine.* London: Chapman and Hall, 1972.
91. Regan, D. *Human Brain Electrophysiology.* New York: Elsevier, 1989.
92. Regan, D., and B.A. Milner. "Objective Perimetry by Evoked Potential Recording: Limitations." *Electroencephalog. Clin. Neurophysiol.* 44 (1978): 393–397.
93. Richter, S.J., and J. Sherman. "Electro-oculography, Dark Adaptometry, and Laser Interferometry." *J. Am. Optom. Assoc.* 50, no 1 (1979): 101–104.
94. Rimmer, S., and B. Katz. "The Pattern Electroretinogram: Technical Aspects and Clinical Significance." *J. Clin. Neurophysiol.* 6 (1989): 85–99.
95. Rubin, M.L. and W.W. Dawson. "The Transscleral VER: Prediction of Postoperative Acuity." *Invest. Ophthalmol.* 17, no. 1 (1978): 71–77.

96. Ryan, S., and G.B. Arden. "Electrophysiological Discrimination between Retinal and Optic Nerve Disorders." *Doc. Ophthalmol.* 68 (1988): 247–255.
97. Saint-Louis, L.A., and B.G. Haik. Magnetic Resonance Imaging of the Globe. In: Haik, B.G. (ed.). "Advanced Imaging Techniques in Ophthalmology." *Int. Ophthalmol. Clin.* 26, no. 3 (1986): 151–168.
98. Saint-Louis, L.A., B.G. Haik, J.L. Amster. Magnetic Resonance Imaging of the Orbit and Optic Pathways. In: Haik, B.G. (ed.). "Advanced Imaging Techniques in Ophthalmology." *Int. Ophthalmol. Clin.* 26, no. 3 (1986): 169–186.
99. Salzman, J., W. Seiple, R. Carr, et al. "Electrophysiologic Assessment of Aphakic Cystoid Macular Oedema." *Br. J. Ophthalmol.* 70 (1986): 819–824.
100. Schindler, S., and J.A. McCrary. "Automated Perimetry in Neurophthalmologic Practice." *Ann. Ophthalmol.* 13, no. 6 (1981): 691–697.
101. Schwartz, B., and J. Kern. "Age, Increased Ocular and Blood Pressures, and Retinal and Disc Fluorescein Angiogram." *Arch. Ophthalmol.* 98 (1980): 1980–1986.
102. Sekuler, R., and L.P. Hutman. "Spatial Vision and Aging; Contrast Sensitivity." *J. Gerontol.* 35, no. 5 (1980): 692–699.
103. Sekuler, R., C. Owsley, L. Hutman. "Assessing Spatial Vision of Older People." *Am. J. Optom. Physiol. Opt.* 1982; 59(12): 961–968.
104. Sherman, J. "Visual Evoked Potential (VEP): Basic Concepts and Clinical Applications." *J. Am. Optom. Assoc.* 50, no. 1 (1979): 19–30.
105. Sinclair, S.H., M. Loebl, C.E. Riva. "Blue field entopic phenomena in cataract patients." *Arch. Ophthalmol.* 97 (1979): 1092–1095.
106. Sjostrand, J., and L. Frisen. "Contrast Sensitivity in Macular Disease: A Preliminary Report." *Acta Ophthalmol.* 55 (1977): 507–512.
107. Skalka, H.W. "Effect of Age on Arden Grating Acuity." *Br. J. Ophthalmol.* 64 (1980): 21–23.
108. Smith, M.E., D.J. Coleman, B.G. Haik. Ultrasonography of the Eye. In: Haik, B.G. (ed.). "Advanced Imaging Techniques in Ophthalmology." *Int. Ophthalmol. Clin.* 26, no. 3 (1986): 25–50.
109. Sokol, S. "Visually Evoked Potentials: Theory, Techniques and Clinical Applications." *Surv. Ophthalmol.* 21, no. 1 (1976): 18–44.
110. Staman, J.A., C.R. Fitzgerald, W.W. Dawson, M.C. Barris, I. Hood. "The EOG and Choroidal Malignant Melanomas." *Doc. Ophthalmol.* 49 (1980): 201–209.
111. Stein, M.R., and C.W. Parker. "Reactions Following Intravenous Fluorescein." *Am. J. Ophthalmol.* 75, no. 5 (1979): 861–868.
112. Storch, R.L., and I.B. Wollner. Overview of Contrast Sensitivity and Neuro-ophthalmic Disease. In: Nadler, M.P., Miller, D., Nadler, D.J. (eds.). *Glare and Contrast Sensitivity for Clinicians.* New York: Springer-Verlag, 1990, pp. 85–112.
113. Sunness, J.S., and R.W. Massof. "Focal Electro-oculogram in Age-related Macular Degeneration." *Am. J. Optom. Physiol. Opt.* 63 (1986): 7–11.
114. Tani, P.M., H. Buettner, D.M. Robertson. "Massive Vitreous Hemorrhage and Senile Macular Choroidal Degeneration." *Am. J. Ophthalmol.* 90 (1980): 525–533.
115. Thompson, C.R.S., and G.F.A. Harding. "The Visual Evoked Potential in Patients with Cataracts." *Doc. Ophthalmol. Proc.* 15 (1978): 193–201.
116. Tower, H., and L.J. Oshinskie. "An Introduction to Computed Tomography and Magnetic Resonance Imaging of the Head and Visual Pathways." *J. Am. Optom. Assoc.* 60, no. 8 (1989): 619–628.
117. Trick, G. "Pattern Reversal Retinal Potentials in Ocular Hypertensives at High and Low Risk of Developing Glaucoma." *Doc. Ophthalmol.* 65 (1987): 79–85.

118. Van Brocklin, M.D., R.R. Hirons, W.H. Langfield, R.L. Yolton. "The Visual Evoked Response: Reliability Revisited." *J. Am. Optom. Assoc.* 50, no. 1 (1979): 1371–1379.
119. Vance, J.R., and R. Jones. "Central Visual Field Contributions to the Visual-Evoked Response." *Am. J. Optom. Physiol. Opt.* 57, no. 4 (1980): 197–204.
120. Weatherhead, R.G. "Use of Arden Grating Test for Screening." *Br. J. Ophthalmol.* 64 (1980): 591–596.
121. Weinstein, G.W., G.B. Arden, R.A. Hitchings, et al. "The Pattern Electroretinogram (PERG) in Ocular Hypertension and Glaucoma." *Arch. Ophthalmol.* 106 (1988): 923–928.
122. Weleber, R.G. "The Effect of Age on Human Cone and Rod Ganzfeld Electroretinograms." *Invest. Ophthalmol.* 20, no. 3 (1981): 392–399.
123. Weleber, R.G., and A. Eisner. Retinal Function and Physiological Studies. In: Newsome, D.A. (ed.). *Retinal Dystrophies and Degenerations.* New York: Raven Press, 1988, pp. 21–69.
124. Wolf, E., and A.S. Nadroski. "Extent of the Visual Field: Changes with Age and Oxygen Tension." *Arch. Ophthalmol.* 86 (1971): 637–642.
125. Wolfe, P. "Utilizing the Visual Evoked Response (VER) for Visual Fields When Subjective Responses Are Not Attainable." *J. Am. Optom. Assoc.* 50, no. 1 (1979): 117–118.
126. Zimmermann, R.D., and E.J. Russell. Angiography in the Evaluation of Visual Disturbances. In: Haik, B.G. (ed.). "Advanced Imaging Techniques in Ophthalmology." *Int. Ophthalmol. Clin.* 26, no. 3 (1986): 187–214.
127. Zollman, R., L. Cary, S. Dippel, R.L. Yolton. "The Effects of Patient Age on Electroretinogram and Electro-oculogram Signals." *Rev. Optom.* 115, no. 1 (1978): 46–48.

14

The Delivery of Vision Care in Non-Traditional Settings

Gary L. Mancil

Optometric care traditionally has been provided in the private-practice setting with the optometrist's role in institutional and other out-of-office settings a recent development. This is largely due to the fact that patients typically seek non-emergency, primary care in individual, private, office settings. Older adults are well served in these settings. With current demographic trends of maintained independence continued over a longer number of years, the elderly population is generally able to continue with well-established, life-long, health-care-seeking patterns. Recent trends toward the development of Health Maintenance Organizations (HMOs), as well as the growing indigent population who must seek health care in publicly operated clinics means that private offices are no longer the only alternative for non-emergency, primary health care. Nevertheless, private-practice settings remain the major site for the provision of primary care.

This is also the most prevalent mode of practice for optometrists, and older adults who are physically fit to travel to such a setting for vision care should be encouraged to do so. While on-site services often are reserved for those who are truly unable to travel to receive care elsewhere, the growing mobile service delivery system in the United States (encompasing everything from health care to car repair) suggests that the convenience factor appeals to other segments of the population. For instance, relatively independent older adults residing in retirement communities may prefer to receive vision care on-site rather than travel to an office. In the future, this new service delivery trend may expand the applications of this discussion to a larger number of settings.

A growing number of older adults, however, are unable to continue receiving vision care in the private-practice setting. This change comes with the onset of fraility, most often seen in the so-called "old-old" population of older adults (those aged 85 years and older). With advancing age, patients are more likely to experience a variety of health problems (see Chapter 2), which may result in their experiencing a loss of independence and restrictions in their mobility. Approximately 10% of those over age 65 years become institutionalized at some point in their life. Approximately 80% of those over age 75 are likely to become dependent on others to a significant degree through some degree of visual disability alone (Fozard et al., 1977). This larger number of frail older adults who remain in the community but require significant assistance is growing much faster than the nursing home population.

Loss of independence is most often the result of age-related physical or mental health disorders such as atherosclerotic vascular disease (including cerebral vascular accident and congestive heart disease), adult onset diabetes mellitus, congestive obstructive pulmonary disease, age-related dementias (including Alzheimers' disease and Parkinson's disease), and degenerative joint disease (see Chapter 2). Three conditions—diseases of the heart, malignant neoplasms, and cerebrovascular diseases—are the major contributors to immobility and disability among older persons (Blake, 1981). For many of these patients, transportation to a doctor's office is lacking or available only through assistance from family, friends, community resources (which are infrequently found) or through considerable personal expense.

With decreasing personal independence, older adults are likely to be forced into new living arrangements, and the variety of settings in which they may choose to reside are sometimes described as the "housing continuum." For example, older adults could theoretically move along this continuum through various options ranging from a fully independent private home (sometimes receiving support from community resources) to a situation of total dependency. Along the continuum, they might use a non-independent private residence (incorporating regular assistive services such as homemaker/chore assistance and supportive medical services), a group home, congregate care or supported living arrangement (using full-time caretakers), or a so-called "life care" or "continuing care" community (combining independent living arrangements with the availability of extensive medical and supportive services). Adult day care/day hospital services provide a form of respite care (see below) for an older person's usual caregiver or short-term rehabilitation. Hospice care provides for the needs of dying patients and their families. Respite care provides temporary support to relieve stress of caring for frail elderly persons. Older adults recovering from an acute illness who are discharged from the hospital but are not well enough to return to the community may enter a convalescent hospital. In this instance, the treatment goal is to facilitate the expected return to the community. With the onset of greater dependency, a nursing home providing skilled and intermediate care may provide the greatest degree of supportive living.

OPTOMETRIC CONSIDERATIONS IN IMPLEMENTING VISION CARE PROGRAMS IN NON-TRADITIONAL SETTINGS

The initial steps in establishing a vision-care program as an outreach of an existing private practice concern an analysis of the practice itself. As providing care "on-site" necessitates the doctor and/or staff being away from the office, this must be an appropriate decision for the practice. A closely related issue that needs to be considered is that of expected reimbursement to the practice through the new program. As many patients encountered in so-called, non-traditional settings may be expected to rely on Medicare and/or Medicaid as their insurance (see Chapter 1), issues of accepting assignment and level of reimbursement often are predetermined by the insurance carrier. By obtaining information from the carrier in advance of implementing any new program, as well as evaluating the availability of practice time to devote to this activity, better decisions regarding the frequency and length of time the doctor is able to devote to out-of-office care can be made. Based on this analysis, practices adding an associate or experiencing reduced growth may be expected to benefit to the greatest degree from establishing new programs for outreach.

A second decision to be made is which opportunities for providing care in non-traditional settings are preferred. Settings geographically convenient to the doctor's practice should be considered first because of decreased travel time. Additional questions to consider in the process of making this decision are, how many potential patients may be accessed in a particular setting; what, if any, existing arrangements for vision care are in place; and what, if any, prior personal contacts and references are present to facilitate beginning a new program.

The question of whether a contractual agreement is to be established between the optometrist and the out-of-office setting should be determined in advance. Various options include serving on an "on-call," case-by-case basis, scheduling regular visits during which a predetermined, minimal number of voluntary patients are seen, and establishing a contract through which all existing and future patients will be examined on a regular basis with additional services provided as needed (including urgent or emergent services). Furthermore, the issue of exclusivity of the optometrist's services and recommendations regarding primary referral sources can be specified at this time.

Key Staff Interactions

The decisions of how to initiate contact and who to approach on the staff of an out-of-office setting are critical in that the initial impression made and reception given have the potential to set the tone of the entire vision-care program. A letter of introduction should be prepared and copies sent to the key administrator and other key staff identified (for example, nursing director and social worker). The optometrist's interest in serving the patients' visual needs, his or her qualifications and expertise in the area, and the intention to follow-up the introductory letter with a phone call requesting an appointment should all be stated. Whenever possible, the letter should be addressed to specific individuals rather than simply to unnamed positions or titles, and the follow-up phone call should take place soon after the letter is received.

The key staff contact person may vary from setting to setting, but the social worker or other community services contact staff person is often the individual most aware of residents' visual needs. In fact, one of the social worker's major responsibilities is to identify needs and ensure that the appropriate resources (including those from the community) are called upon to meet those needs. In some settings, the nursing staff serves this role and may represent the primary contact. The program administrator is an important contact and should be included in the early discussions, although the details of a new program for vision care often will be determined by other staff. However, regular communication with, and support from, the top administrator can overcome ambivalence from other key staff.

One issue important to management personnel is to what degree their staff will need to be involved. Supervisors and administrators may need to be assured that bringing a vision-care program into their facility will not be time intensive to their staff. Nursing staff, for instance, may be accustomed to doctors seeing patients and expecting a chairside assistant to accompany them during their rounds. This degree of staff support typically is not required in a vision-care program. Nevertheless, a minimum degree of support is needed from the staff. Their involvement typically includes the following: educating patients and their sponsors about the availability of vision-care services on site; making available medical records on the patients; in some settings (for example, nursing homes) facilitating an order from the attending physician requesting vision care; directing or transporting patients to a central site for evaluation; filing reports in the patients' charts; and following up on or initiating treatment recommended by the optometrist (in some settings in conjunction with the patients' attending physicians).

Yet another issue of concern to the agency staff is fees charged for on-site vision care and the need for careful communication regarding this to the patient (in some settings, sponsor approval is required as well). In many agency and institutional settings, patients are insured by a combination of Medicare and Medicaid, and accepting assignment therefore is required. (See Chapter 1.) Nevertheless, patients and sponsors are often quite diligent in their effort to ensure that the Medicare/Medicaid system is not abused. It is encumbent upon the optometrist proposing a vision-care program of this nature to ensure accurate and complete understanding of what fees will be charged and the appropriateness of fees for on-site care (which are likely to be considerably higher than in-office fees for similar levels of care). Some staff anticipate these patient and family concerns and require that they be addressed in advance. A fee schedule will likely be requested and shared with patients and/or sponsors (even in the event that the services provided are on an accept assignment basis).

After due consideration and discussion are given to these issues, a formal agreement should be drafted in order to clarify and document what each party expects of the other. This legal document allows the optometrist to negotiate important issues such as exclusivity of care and to specify other aspects of the on-site visits, such as availability of patient charts, level of staff assistance, and minimum number of patients to be scheduled per visit. In turn, the agency or institution involved may wish to specify the availability of the optometrist, the expected fees to patients (or their insurers), and the expected conduct of both parties to the agreement.

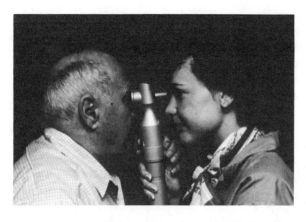

Figure 14.1. Hand-held, Goldmann-type tonometry can be performed with ease and accuracy in any out-of-office setting.

Suggested Instrumentation, Equipment, and Locale

Providing vision care on-site in a non-traditional setting (such as an agency or institution) can be accomplished using a minimum amount of ophthalmic equipment. However, at present, newly available portable versions of in-office instrumentation allow a level of on-site evaluation that formerly was not possible.

Of special note are newly developed, portable versions of lensometers, applanation tonometers (Figure 14.1), biomicroscopes, interferometers (Figure 14.2), and fundus cameras. Private practices that place special emphasis on the provision of on-site care in non-traditional settings often include these types of instrumentation for such vision-care programs. This equipment also has uses in

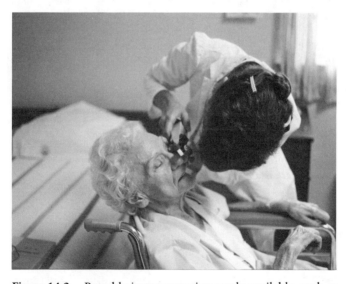

Figure 14.2. Portable instrumentation newly available, such as the Randwal, IRAS interferometer, provide for the provision of even sophisticated testing on-site in any setting.

the traditional office as well, especially for wheelchair-bound patients and other physically challenged patients who cannot easily use traditional office instruments. Table 14.1 lists essential and recommended equipment for use in providing vision care on-site in the non-traditional setting. Optometrists vary according to their preference and use of this equipment and the level of care provided.

Scheduling of appointments should be based on considerations for maximizing patient performance as well as minimizing extraneous distractions during the examination. As a rule, older adults may prefer mid-morning appointments. Medication schedules (as some medications cause drowsiness), social activities (as many older adults prefer not to miss a favorite crafts class or television show), the desire of family members to be present during the examination (and hence the need to consider their schedules), and, when in an institutional setting, staff shift changes are additional considerations.

The exact location chosen for providing care within the agency or institution is to be viewed with flexibility. In the initial phases of proposing and implementing any new program, an appropriate locale should be discussed and decided upon. Appropriate locales may include treatment rooms, conference rooms, class-

Table 14.1 Equipment useful in out-of-office examinations

Essential Equipment	Optional Equipment	Miscellaneous Equipment
Diagnostic kit	Hand-held slit lamp	Tape
Occluder	Worth 4-Dot	Extension cords
BIO	Portable lensometer	3-pronged adapters
Trial lens set	Low-vision devices	Portable lighting
Halberg/Janelli clips	Hardwire (assistive	Measuring tape
Hand-held JCC	listening device)	Rx pads
Trial frames	Frame warmer (air)	Penlight
Acuity charts (distance:	Fundus camera (portable)	PD ruler
10 ft Snellen, Feinbloom	Interferometer (portable)	Extra bulbs/batteries
low-vision, Bailey-Lovie	Tangent screen	Tissues
low contrast; near:		
reduced Snellen,		
Lighthouse near-vision		
card, Duke reading card)		
Frames (traditional styles		
with adjustable nosepads)		
Ophthalmic tools/materials		
(tools, screws, hinges,		
temples)		
Tonometer (hand-held		
Goldmann, tonomat,		
Schiotz)		
Ophthalmic drugs		
Stethoscope/Sphygmomanometer		
Amsler grid/Diamond chart		
Burton lamp		

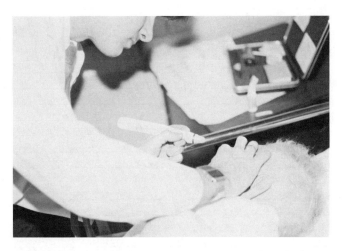

Figure 14.3. Patients who are confined to their beds may undergo a greater degree of testing using miniature, highly portable instruments made possible by new technologies (shown here, Tonopen by Biorad [Norwell, CT]).

rooms, private offices, patient rooms (Figure 14.3), and even large closets. It is desirable to have access to an area that can be closed off from noise and activity, in which lighting can be controlled separately from the remainder of the room used, and in which a sink is reached easily.

Value of Advance Patient Information

One important means of increasing the clinician's efficiency when providing vision care on-site is through the use of patient questionnaires and advance history forms. Whenever possible, a standard set of questions that constitutes the history section of a standard optometric examination should be asked in advance of the scheduled visit (Figure 14.4). This can maximize the clinician's time and allow greater opportunity for other necessary test procedures. Such questionnaires or forms can be completed by patients, by family members, or by staff at the agency or institution involved. Another option is for a designated staff member from the optometrist's office to phone a patient (or a significant other) in order to complete the form in this way. The optometrist must, of course, be prepared to devote some time and attention to augmenting the advance information obtained as a portion of the patient encounter.

Recommended Examination Sequence

As is the case in the examination of an older adult in any setting, emphasis must be given to clear and accurate communication skills throughout the process. Proper communication strategies remain important throughout the examination.

Advance History Form

Patient Name _____

Address _____

_____

Phone _____ Contact Person _____

Who will be present during the exam? _____

Relationship _____

Directions: _____

_____

_____

_____

Primary Physician _____ Phone _____

Last Seen _____ For what purpose? _____

_____

Pharmacy Name _____ Phone _____

Previous Eye Doctor's Name _____ Last seen _____

Nature of Current Vision Problems/Complaint

_____

_____

_____

Insurance Information

What is your primary insurance? (name of company) _____

_____, (address) _____,

_____, (phone) _____

(policy number) _____, (under whose name?) _____

What is your secondary insurance? (name of company) _____

_____, (address) _____,

_____, (phone) _____

(policy number) _____, (under whose name?) _____

Have you met your deductible for this year? _____

How will you be handling your fees? _____

Figure 14.4. Advance history form

Medical History

What prescription medicines are used regularly? _____

_____

What non-prescription medicines are used? _____

_____

What home remedies are used? _____

Are you allergic to any medications including eyedrops? _____
If so, list _____
What health problems are being treated or monitored by your other
doctors? _____

_____

What operations have you had? _____
Have you ever had eye surgery for cataracts? _____ If so, who was
your surgeon? *Right Eye* (doctor) _____ (date) _____
Left Eye (doctor) _____ (date) _____ Any other eye
surgeries? _____
Were you ever told you had: Glaucoma Y/N, Diabetes Y/N, Any Other Eye
Disease (list)? _____

Do you wear glasses? Y/N When? for reading, watching TV
Does anyone in your family have: Glaucoma Y/N (who?) _____
Diabetes Y/N (who?) _____ Any other eye disease?
(list eye problems and relation) _____

Figure 14.5. Advance medical history form

In some settings (for example, nursing homes or adult day-care settings), the risk
of encountering an older adult having cognitive difficulties (including communication disorders) is greater. Additional time is required in communicating with
these patients, and a greater emphasis on obtaining history and other data from
secondary sources is needed (for example, medical charts, significant others, staff
who work regularly with the patients). Nevertheless, a problem-oriented medical
history approach is recommended (Figure 14.5), with greater emphasis on the
social history and functional history aspects.

 In testing visual acuities, the clinician working on-site in a non-traditional
setting should anticipate the need for auxiliary lighting. Clip-on spot lighting is
commercially available to address this need. Portable visual acuity test charts (traditional Snellen and others) are appropriate, as well as low-vision test charts.

Newly developed acuity charts offering varying levels of contrast are useful in these settings (See Chapter 7). In non-communicative patients, techniques such as OKN drum and, more recently, Teller card preferential viewing are appropriate (Marx et al., 1990). It is likely that a 10 foot test distance (or less) will be used, depending on the room characteristics where the exams will take place. In regard to testing near visual acuity, lighting and the use of a test chart which features a wide range of letter sizes are appropriate considerations.

Pupillary testing, gross observation of the eyes and adnexa, and evaluation of motility and binocularity are appropriate tests to next consider in the exam sequence (Figure 14.6). In regard to binocularity, patient symptoms from the history are a significant indicator of the need for indepth testing and/or treatment (see Chapter 10). In addition, the neurologic implications of disorders in these areas cannot be overlooked (see Chapters 2 and 3).

Refraction should proceed using trial frame or Halburg/Janelli clip methods while giving appropriate consideration to increased difference thresholds expected in this population (See Chapter 7). Retinoscopy is of considerable value in many patients and should be used routinely, although some patients have pupillary miosis or media opacities that reduce the usefulness of this test. Radical retinoscopy may serve as a means of overcoming these problems (see Chapter 7). Subjective refraction is best conducted using Halberg/Janelli clips over the patient's habitual correction when possible (otherwise, trial frame methods suffice). The habitual correction can be neutralized using a portable lensometer or

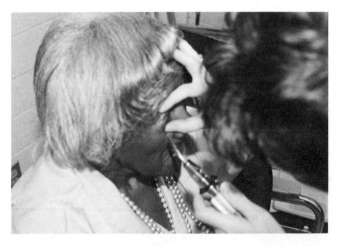

Figure 14.6. The standard diagnostic kit can be used for multiple procedures such as pupil testing, gross observation of the adnexa, Hirschberg testing, as well as refractive analysis and internal health screening.

through hand lens neutralization techniques. Trial lenses and hand-held (or trial frame model) Jackson Cross Cylinders provide a means for accurate cylinder refraction in any setting. The availability of both $\pm$ 0.50 and $\pm$ 1.00 cross cylinders provides for most needs. Vertex distance considerations are more likely to arise in this patient population because of the frequency of high hyperopic prescriptions.

Biomicroscopy and evaluation of the anterior structures of the eye are appropriate tests to follow. In the absence of hand-held, portable slit-lamps, a diagnostic kit or other illumination source used in conjunction with a magnification system (condensing lens or magnifier) provides additional information beyond that obtained from gross observation only. A simple cobalt blue filter can be attached to the end of a transilluminator or penlight to assess tear quality or detect gross corneal staining. Tonometry is essential, and any number of validated portable instruments are available to the optometrist for this aspect of the examination (Chiara et al., 1989).

Binocular indirect ophthalmoscopy should be performed on each patient (except in those rare cases where it is contraindicated because of the risk of angle closure). Information gained through this procedure is invaluable and not otherwise obtainable through any other test means. In addition, medical-legal precedents dictate that the procedure be used routinely in optometric evaluations (Classe, 1989).

Visual field assessment can take place during an on-site evaluation in a number of ways. Confrontation fields can be used in any setting without special equipment. Portable tangent screen fields, Amsler grid charts, and hand-held arc perimetery can be made available as well.

Just as it is difficult or impossible for these patients to obtain vision care in the community, it is equally difficult for them to obtain glasses in the community. Therefore, any on-site optometric evaluation must include services for the repair and ordering of glasses. In many instances, simply reconditioning existing glasses will fulfill the patient's needs. In some cases, emergency repair and frame modification are required. However, any examination in a non-traditional setting should offer selection and ordering of glasses. Ophthalmic optic designs appropriate for spectacle corrections for older adults should be given consideration. (See Chapter 8.)

Optometrists who provide care regularly in these settings may also wish to provide certain special procedures and services on-site. These may include contrast sensitivity testing, glare disability testing, interferometry, ocular photography, and low-vision care. Newly available portable versions of instruments used in providing these services are currently available. Providing care in a non-traditional setting also creates an opportunity for input (formally or informally) on issues of environmental design from the optometrist's background and expertise. In any setting, the optometrist can assess use of lighting, color, and contrast and make recommendations to improve the visual environment for older adults. (See Chapter 12.)

Reporting and Follow-Up Activities

Because of the high incidence of eye health problems in this population, the need to follow-up with patients regularly on subsequent visits often exists. This is facilitated in an arrangement for regularly scheduled visits to an agency or institution as opposed to serving on an "on-call" basis.

Patients examined in non-traditional, out-of-office settings are likely to present special challenges in the area of follow-up and compliance. Therefore, the clinician must invoke additional measures to diligently facilitate understanding and compliance with recommendations made. This most often includes providing documentation in the form of reports to all concerned parties (patients, staff at the agency or institution, other health-care providers, and family or sponsors). Forms can be designed that facilitate reporting with minimum time required from the clinician. In particular, the use of a three-part, carbon copy form (one copy for the patient or their family/sponsor, one for the agency or institution, and one for the clinician) conveniently meets this need in most instances (Figure 14.7). A brief cover letter with a copy of the report can be provided to other health-care providers to augment general information contained in the exam report.

THE LONG-TERM CARE SETTING
Description

With the increase in the older population of the United States, there has been a proportionate increase in the nation's nursing home population. Five percent of the elderly population reside in nursing homes at any given time, although one in four will require the use of a nursing home at some time during their life (Aging America: Trends and Projections, 1985; American Foundation for the Blind, 1986; Blake, 1986). Furthermore, the chances of an older adult entering a nursing home increase with age. Approximately 14% of those 75 years and older reside in nursing homes, while approximately 22% of those 85 years and older are nursing home residents (Whitmore, 1989). Convalescent hospitals provide similar types of care to this same population, with there being greater emphasis on the patient's return to the community after a greater degree of recovery from their illness has been accomplished.

Patient Visual Characteristics and Needs

Nursing home residents have a high incidence of vision disorders and eye health problems (Kornzweig et al., 1957; National Center for Health Statistics, 1977; Whitmore, 1989; Durkin and Newcomb, 1992). The more common ocular disorders in the 65 years and older population are age-related cataracts, age-related macular degeneration, open-angle glaucoma, and diabetic retinopathy (National Society to Prevent Blindness, 1980; Rosenbloom, 1982). Visual handicaps are known to negatively influence quality of life (Gillman et al., 1986), and still vision needs go largely unmet in these settings (Beliveau et al., 1986). Snyder

TO: _____

FROM: Dr. _____

RE: SUMMARY OF VISION EVALUATION

Patient Name: _____ DOB _____
Where evaluation took place: _____
Date evaluation took place: _____

At the request of _____
_____ was evaluated by _____ on
_____, 19 ___ with the following complaints: _____

As a result of this evaluation, the following visual issues were identified:
_____
_____
_____.

Recommendations for treatment are as follows: _____
_____
_____.

Follow-up evaluation is planned for: _____.

Special Instructions for Caregivers

Additional Information/Comments

_____, O.D.
Phone Number: _____

Figure 14.7 Summary of vision evaluation form

et al. showed that 80% of nursing home patients had no record of vision care noted in their charts during an average of the past 5 years (Snyder et al., 1976). In another study, 51 (almost 25%) of 238 residents were identified as being in need of low-vision evaluation (Morse et al., 1988). In short, the optometrist's role in providing care in the nursing home setting is significant (Gorman, 1990; Mancil, 1989).

Existing Protocols

In providing vision care in an institution such as a long-term care facility, the optometrist is operating within the medical model of patient management. Established protocols are based on those in effect in the hospital setting when an attending physician requests a consultation from another doctor. It is important for the optometrist to realize that in this model, one individual is given responsibility to manage the patient in the overall sense. Therefore, it is appropriate and customary to communicate with the nursing home patient's attending physician prior to and after the visit. Furthermore, it is essential to seek the attending physician's authorization prior to initiating treatment of any nature. This avoids unnecessary risks created to the patient's health and well-being when multiple health-care providers initiate care without the benefit of an overall perspective on the patient. That perspective is maintained by the "attending" practitioner. In serving as a consultant to the attending physician, certain reporting protocols need to be followed. This need normally can be met by reports and orders left in the patient's chart for the attending physician's approval. When providing a level of care best defined as consultation, additional communication and reporting protocols must be followed under Medicare guidelines. (See Chapter 1.)

One way to initiate this level of communication is through a phone call made to the attending physician, advising him or her of the planned visual evaluation. This can be accomplished by speaking directly with the attending physician or by communicating with the physician's staff. Often, nursing home staff or family members of the patient can attend to this task (although there is certainly great value in the optometrist communicating directly with the physician concerning the patient). In this way, if the patient has an unstable condition that may impact on the timing of the visual evaluation (for example, is recovering from a recent myocardial infarction), the attending physician has an opportunity to provide input. In the majority of cases, however, the optometrist will be encouraged to move forward with the planned evaluation.

A report on the results of the vision evaluation must be added to the patient's chart in the nursing home. This can be done by simply adding notes in SOAP format (subjective; objective; assessment; plan) to the consultants section of the chart. Copies of the evaluation will need to be maintained by the optometrist. Some optometrists use multicopy, carbon-backed printed forms on site for this purpose, and others mail a report back to the nursing home to be later placed on file.

In most facilities, the director of social work is an essential person to whom examination results should be provided as well. This individual is more likely to be aware of vision-care needs among the residents and to have responsibility for seeing that these needs are met. Furthermore, this individual is generally best able to communicate with the patients' family members or sponsors concerning recommendations that result from visual evaluations.

On-site interactions with nursing and other staff should be based on the optometrist's role as a consultant physician seeing the patient at the attending physician or family's request. In most instances, nursing staff will have minimum or no experience with optometry. Given the fact that the staff members' training most often has taken place in settings which rarely include optometrists, special efforts may be required to educate them about the role of a modern optometrist in a nursing home setting. Professionalism and respect for standard protocols in the facility should be the rule. For example, many staff are taught not to sit on patient's beds (as this is viewed to contribute to the spread of germs from room to room). Furthermore, the head of nursing should be consulted regarding any orders left that will involve nursing staff. With time and experience, more routine protocols for such issues will develop, but especially in the beginning of a new program, greater degrees of communication should be the rule. In-service training should be offered to nursing staff on common procedures that might be ordered (for example, lid scrubs).

THE HOSPITAL SETTING

In today's scheme of health-care, hospitals are reserved for the treatment of acute illnesses. Older adults are more frequently hospitalized than the rest of the population and, in fact, in 1983 the elderly accounted for 29% of all hospital discharges, despite the fact that this group represented only 12% of the population (Aging America: Trends and Projections, 1985). Health policy decisions such as length of stay (LOS) restrictions influence the types of services hospitals are likely to provide (Agency for Health Care Policy and Research, 1991). Routine vision care is not requested often for patients undergoing hospitalization for acute illnesses. In some settings in which optometric services are routinely available, acute care patients are seen for a variety of purposes, ranging from eye health evaluations to replacing lost glasses to vision rehabilitation services.

Optometrists are commonly on staff in hospitals operated by the Department of Veterans Affairs, the Public Health Service, and the various branches of the military. In other hospitals, optometrists in the community may establish hospital privileges and, therefore, may be called on for a variety of needs involving specific patients. These vary from rural hospitals that may rely on optometrists for consultations on emergency patients to rehabilitation hospitals in which a community optometrist may serve as a member of a multidisciplinary or interdisciplinary care team assembled for the patient's overall rehabilitation. The American Optometric Association offers guidelines to optometrists who are interested in establishing hospital privileges (American Optometric Association).

COMMUNITY SERVICE AGENCY SETTING

The Older Americans Act, passed initially in 1965 and later amended, mandates the provision of supportive community resources for older adults. Through the Administration on Aging (AoA), a branch of the Department of Health and Human Services, State Units on Aging and Area Agencies on Aging were created (Ficke, 1985). In addition to these government programs, various religious and private agencies exist to meet the needs of older members of a community. In short, a host of programs exist on the local level to provide community assistance for the elderly. Despite the existence of these programs, however, many needs of the elderly in the community remain unmet.

Examples of community service agency settings in which older adults may be accessed for on-site care include senior centers or nutrition centers, senior clubs, day hospitals, adult day-care centers, and rehabilitation centers. Some of these settings are more likely to have seniors who are highly independent. In such a setting, the optometrist's role is more likely to provide health education and vision screening. Indeed, health promotion activities among the elderly by all health professions are highly valued and are directed toward providing knowledge, skills, and resources that enable them to meet their own health-care goals and objectives (Minkler and Pasick, 1986). In other settings, however, it may be more appropriate to provide comprehensive optometric services on-site (Mancil, 1989).

In each setting, an appropriate contact person must be identified in an effort to access older adults who can benefit from optometric care. This individual may be titled a center director, program administrator, or ombudsman. Meeting with the director of the local Area Agency on Aging generally can provide all the information and contacts needed to instigate a new program. Contact may be initiated through an introductory letter followed by a phone call. In many instances, administrators in these settings are most interested in having a presentation and/or vision screening provided by the optometrist. Some settings will be appropriate for providing more comprehensive care on-site (described elsewhere in this chapter).

THE PRIVATE HOME SETTING

The vast majority of older Americans reside in private homes. However, with advancing age, the chances of an older adult who resides in a private home requiring assistance with activities of daily living increase dramatically. While 2.6% of the population age 65 to 69 years require such assistance, almost 32% of the population over age 85 years require assistance. Almost 71% of the long-term care population reside in the community (DeSylvia and Williams, 1989). Special housing needs are concentrated among the population of those 75 years and older, a reflection of the high incidence of physical disability in this population (Newman, 1985). Furthermore, 30% of the non-institutionalized elderly reside alone (DeSylvia, 1990).

Community-based or home care has been shown to be an alternative to inappropriate or premature institutionalization (Holt, 1986). Furthermore, this alternative for caring for frail, elderly people is more cost effective than institutionalization and, in fact, is preferred by potential program beneficiaries (Nassif, 1986). The success of the home-care option in the future depends on a number of factors, including commitment on the part of health policy makers and the availability of health-care professionals with interest and expertise in this area of health care (Bernstein et al., 1990; Cummings, 1987). Innovative pilot programs demonstrate the success of home care when resources, man-power, and commitment co-exist (Lombardi, 1986; Swanson, 1990; Walters and Nussenblatt, 1989).

The provision of optometric care in the home setting incorporates many of the considerations discussed previously in this chapter. In seeking to access these patients, caregivers must be made aware of the availability of the service through any possible means of communication or marketing. In an existing private practice, patients who receive care in the practice can become a source of referrals. In addition, other optometric and ophthalmologic offices that do not offer the service, as well as all members of the network of resources for older adults, must be informed. Brochures, press releases, and newspaper articles also can be prepared to inform the local aging network and the community at large of the service. In some areas, brokers who market health-care services to nursing homes can assist in placing optometrists in these settings.

Interaction with caregivers and family members is a major aspect of providing home care. Eighty percent of the care provided to frail elderly is provided by families (Rubin, 1985). These individuals represent a major source for information prior to an examination through the use of advance forms and/or phone calls, and these are also likely to be the on-site support persons during the examination. It should be noted that a caregiver's presence in the examination is not always desired. There are instances when the patient will perform better and be more at ease if a caregiver is not present. Once the clinician is made aware of an adverse relationship, steps should be taken to remove the distraction from the examination. In extreme cases of adverse relationships where elder abuse is suspected, some states have mandatory reporting requirements that apply to all professionals (including optometrists) who provide care to an older adult. (See Chapter 7.) In arranging for the appointment, it is helpful to know who will be present, their relationship to the patient, and their goals for the examination (as well as the patient's goals). Consideration for optimum time of day, equipment needed, examination sequence, environmental vision assessment, and reporting parallel those discussed previously.

Methods of reporting examination results for these patients can range from verbal explanation to an alert patient to reporting solely to the caregiver. In cases where numerous community services are being delivered, an entire team of professionals may need to be informed, sometimes in the context of a team meeting. Techniques for facilitating compliance and understanding (discussed elsewhere) take on additional importance in this setting. In such a setting, the possibility that no other professionals may be involved in the patient's care to reinforce recommendations (such as would be the case in a long-term care setting) is strong. Referral for additional evaluation or specialty care may require regular phone follow-up (and documentation of such) to reinforce the seriousness of identified problems. In many situations of home care, circumstances make leaving the home for care virtually impossible. Therefore, the value of an optometrist providing a wide scope of treatments on-site, as regulated by state law, cannot be overstressed. Not only are supplemental diagnostic procedures of greater value when called for (for example, interferometry, retinal evaluation, serial tonometry, and lacrimal dilation and lavage), but the need to manage common eye diseases through the use of therapeutic pharmaceuticals is especially great in this population.

ADDITIONAL SETTINGS FOR THE DELIVERY OF OPTOMETRIC CARE ON-SITE

Optometrists who specialize in low-vision and vision rehabilitation care are frequently called upon to provide care to older adults in rehabilitation centers, most often related to the occurrence of a cerebral vascular accident (CVA). Neuro-optometric evaluation and vision rehabilitation techniques are increasingly valued by the entire rehabilitation team treating these patients (Gianutsos and Ramsey, 1988). (See Chapter 12.) In this very specialized setting, traditional low-vision care can be merged with optometric vision therapy to manage functional vision problems and increase quality of life of these patients. Furthermore, the entire rehabilitation process is enhanced through a better team understanding of the effects of the neurologic insult on vision. Due to the sometimes severe cognitive and physical deficits that result from CVA, much of this optometric care needs to be provided on-site in the rehabilitation center setting.

THE MOBILE CLINIC SETTING

Yet another means of providing vision care in non-traditional settings is through the use of a mobile eye clinic. An increasing number of optometrists who emphasize on-site care as an aspect of their practices operate mobile clinics. Indeed, the mobile vision clinic adds a dimension of versatility in that it can serve patients in any of the settings described previously in this chapter. Additionally, there are optometrists who practice full-time optometry in so-called "non-traditional" settings, thus eliminating the physical confines (and overhead expenses) of a traditional office.

The mobile clinic method of health-care delivery can take place in a number of ways. In one scenario, the clinic is designed for bringing patients on board and providing care within the mobile unit itself. In another, the necessary equipment simply is transported (through the use of whatever vehicle) to the site where the care will be delivered. This latter method is perhaps best suited for accessing bedridden patients in nursing homes, private homes, and rehabilitation facilities.

Establishing the former type of mobile clinic involves additional and unique expenses, and considerable energies must be devoted to custom-design considerations. No such vehicle exists as a standard item, and many considerations exist in the custom design of such a clinic above and beyond the equipment considerations described elsewhere in this chapter. These include size of the vehicle, heating/cooling needs for the clinic compartment, the need for running water, and the need for access by physically challenged patients. Even the overall size of the vehicle takes on practical importance, as small vans are more easily squeezed into small alleys and driveways than larger recreational vehicles, but at the same time, the smaller vehicle is more confining once a patient is aboard. Van conversion suppliers, recreation vehicle dealers, and suppliers of orthopedic supplies can be consulted to make arrangements for items as diverse as wheelchair lifts to air conditioners. Ultimately, optometrists who maintain a mobile vision clinic are almost certainly to be those who heavily emphasize on-site care in a variety of non-traditional settings.

FUTURE TRENDS IN THE NON-TRADITIONAL SETTING

Given rapidly emerging trends in population demographics, the need for delivering optometric care in non-traditional settings may be expected to increase. The development of on-site services for home care, nursing home care, as well as for other settings has been shown to be instrumental in reaching a large and growing underserved population. However, as stated by Berkowitz et al., (1982), "As governments and organizations pursue cost avoidance strategies, individuals will get squeezed into 'solutions' that do not fit their real needs." Two current health-policy trends seem to epitomize this observation: the present health-care policy emphasis on cost containment, as well as the concurrent and paradoxical failure to realize that maintaining independence in the community (through the provision of a variety of community-based services) is more cost effective than other options. These issues represent perhaps the greatest obstacles to the provision of optometric care in non-traditional settings. Despite such formidable barriers, however, optometrists are better prepared educationally, better equipped technically, and better dispersed geographically than ever to meet this need.

REFERENCES

1. Agency for Health Care Policy and Research. *Delivering Essential Health Care Services in Rural Areas: An Analysis of Alternative Models.* U.S. Department of Health and Human Services, AHCPR pub. No. 91–0017.
2. *Aging America: Trends and Projections.* (1985–1986 Edition). U.S. Department of Health and Human Services [PF3377(1085)].
3. American Foundation for the Blind. *Recommendations from the 1981 Mini-White House Conference on Vision and Aging.* 15 West 16th Street, New York, NY 10011.

4. American Optometric Association, Hospital Privileges Committee, 243 North Lindbergh Blvd., St. Louis, MO 63141.
5. Beliveau, M., A. Yeadon, S. Aston. *Innovative Curriculum Development Research: To Develop In-service Training Curriculum for Providers of Long-term Care to Elderly Blind/Visually Impaired*. Final Report. National Institute for Handicapped Research, No. G008535147.
6. Berkowitz, M., M. Horning, S. McDonnell, J. Rubin, J.D. Worrall. An Economic Evaluation of the Beneficiary Rehabilitation Program. In: Rubin, J. (ed.). *Alternative in Rehabilitating the Handicapped*. New York: Human Sciences Press, 1982.
7. Bernstein, L.H., P.E. Hankwitz, J. Portnow. "Home Care of the Elderly Diabetic Patient." *Clin. Geriatr. Med.* 6 (1990): 943–957.
8. Blake, R. "Disabled Older Persons: A Demographic Analysis." *J. Rehabil.* (October/November/December, 1981): 19–27.
9. Chiara, G.F., L.P. Semes, J.W. Potter, G.R. Cutter, W.R. Tucker. "Portable Tonometers: A Clinical Comparison of Applanation and Indentation Devices." *J. Am. Optom. Assoc.* 60 (1989): 105–110.
10. Classe, J.G. "A Review of 50 Malpractice Claims." *J. Am. Optom. Assoc.* 60 (1989): 694–706.
11. Cummings, J.E. "Innovations in Homecare." *Generations* 12 (1987): 61–64.
12. DeSylvia, D.A. "The Older Patient: Part I." *High Performance Optometry*. 4 (1990): 1–5.
13. DeSylvia, D.A., A.K. Williams. Health and Housing Continuum. In: *Optometric Gerontology: A Resource Manual for Educators*. Rockville, MD: Association of Schools and Colleges of Optometry. 1989, pp. 5.1–5.13.
14. Durkin, J.R., and Newcomb, R.D. Optometry in nursing homes. *J. Am. Optom. Assoc.* 63 (1992): 102–105.
15. Ficke, S.C. *An Orientation to the Older Americans Act* (Revised Edition). Washington, D.C.: National Association of State Units on Aging, 1985.
16. Fozard, J.L., S.J. Popkin. "Optimizing Adult Development: Ends and Means of an Applied Psychology of Aging." *Am. Pyschol.* 33 (1978): 975–989.
17. Gianutsos, R., and G. Ramsey. "Enabling Rehabilitation Optometrists to Help Survivors of Acquired Brain Injury." *J. Vis. Rehabil.* 2 (1988): 37–58.
18. Gillman, A.E., A. Simmel, E.P. Simon. "Visual Handicap in the Aged: Self-Reported Visual Disability and the Quality of Life of Residents of Public Housing for the Elderly." *J. Vis. Impair. Blind*. February (1986): 588–590.
19. Gorman, N.S. "Nursing Home Practice." *Optom. Econ.* (1990): 18–21.
20. Holt, S.W. "The Role of Home Care in Long Term Care." *Generations* 11 (1986): 9–12.
21. Kornzweig, A.L., M. Feldstein, J. Schneider. "The Eye in Old Age IV. Ocular Survey of Over One Thousand Aged Persons with Special Reference to Normal and Disturbed Visual Function." *Am. J. Ophthalmol.* 44 (1957): 29–37.
22. Lombardi, T. "Nursing Home Without Walls." *Generations* 11 (1986): 21–23.
23. Mancil, G.L. "Delivery of Optometric Care in Non-traditional Settings: The Long-Term Care Facility (symposium). *Optom. Vis. Sci.* 66 (1989): 9–11.
24. Mancil, G.L. "Eye Care Delivery in Nontraditional Settings. In: Aston, S.J., DeSylvia, D.A., Mancil, G.L. (eds.). *Optometric Gerontology: A Resource Manual for Educators*. Rockville, MD: Association of Schools and Colleges of Optometry. 1989, pp. 16.1–16.12.
25. Marx, M.S., Werner, P., Cohen-Mansfield, J., and Hartmann, E.E. Visual Acuity Estimates in Noncommunicative Elderly Persons. *Invest. Ophthalmol. Vis. Sci.* 31 (1990): 593–596.

26. Minkler, M., and R.J. Pasick. Health Promotion and the Elderly: A Critical Perspective on the Past and Future. In: Dychtwald K. (ed.). *Wellness and Health Promotion for the Elderly*. Rockville, MD: Aspen Publications, 1986.
27. Morse, A.R., W.O. O'Connell, J. Joseph, H. Finkelstein. "Assessing Vision in Nursing Home Residents." *J. Vis. Rehabil.* 2 (1988): 5–14.
28. Nassif, J.Z. "There's Still No Place Like Home." *Generations* 11 (1986): 5–8.
29. National Center for Health Statistics. *The National Nursing Home Survey, 1977 Summary for the United States*. Vital and Health Statistics Series 13, No. 14. Hyattsville, MD: 1979.
30. National Society to Prevent Blindness. *Vision Problems in the U.S.* New York, 1980.
31. Newman, S.J. "The Shape of Things to Come." *Generations* 9 (1985): 14–17.
32. Rosenbloom, A. "Care of Elderly People with Low Vision." *J. Vis. Impair. Blind.* June (1982): 209–212.
33. Rubin, R.J. Private Versus Public Responsibilities for Long-Term Care. In: Dunlap, B.D. (ed.). *New Federalism and Long-Term Care of the Elderly*. Millwood, VA: Center for Health Affairs, 1985.
34. Snyder, L.H., J. Pyrek, K.C. Smith. "Vision and Mental Function of the Elderly." *Gerontologist* 16 (1976): 491–495.
35. Swanson, M.W. "Optometric Care of the Homebound and Institutionalized Older Adult." *Optom. Vis. Sci.* 67 (1990): 323–328.
36. Walters D.L., and H.L. Nussenblatt. "Team Approach to Home Health Care Delivery: Optometry as the Primary Vision Care Provider." *Optom. Vis. Sci.* 66 (1989): 17–19.
37. Whitmore, W.G. "Eye Disease in a Geriatric Nursing Home Population." *Ophthalmology* 96 (1989): 393–398.

15

Low-Vision Care in a Clinical Setting

Samuel M. Genensky
Steven H. Zarit

To insure good communication and a clear understanding of terms, the authors have carefully defined the visual groupings of subsets referred to in this chapter. No claim is made as to the merit of these definitions relative to alternatives offered by other researchers. However, these definitions are rational, self-consistent, and operational:

- *Fully sighted.* People are fully sighted if they are not visually impaired.
- *Functionally blind.* People are functionally blind if they are either totally blind or if they have, at most, light projection.
- *Legally blind.* People are legally blind if the best-corrected visual acuity in their better eye does not exceed 20/200, or if the maximum diameter of their visual field does not exceed 20°, even though the best-corrected visual acuity in their better eye exceeds 20/200.
- *Light perception.* People have light perception if, with their better eye, they can only see light but are unable to determine the direction from which it is coming.
- *Light projection.* People have light projection if, with their better eye, they can only see light and determine the direction from which it is coming.
- *Partially sighted.* People are partially sighted if the best-corrected visual acuity in their better eye does not exceed 20/70 but is better than light projection, or if the maximum diameter of their visual field does not exceed 30°, even though the best-corrected visual acuity in their better eye exceeds 20/70.
- *Partially sighted and legally blind.* People are partially sighted and legally blind if they are legally blind but not functionally blind.
- *Partially sighted and not legally blind.* People are partially sighted and not legally blind if they are visually impaired but not legally blind.
- *Totally blind.* People are totally blind if they cannot visually detect light with either eye.

- *Visual enhancement devices.* Various visual devices permit partially sighted people to perform tasks that otherwise would be beyond their visual capability or that they could handle only with great difficulty. Examples of visual enhancement devices are telescopic spectacles that permit partially sighted people to view objects at a distance, microscopic spectacles that allow them to view objects at very close range, and closed-circuit television systems that permit them to read ordinary ink-printed material, write with a pen or pencil, and carry on other tasks that require precise eye-hand coordination.
- *Visual enhancement techniques.* Visual enhancement techniques may or may not involve the use of visual devices, but they permit partially sighted people to handle one or more tasks using their residual vision (for example, pouring dark-colored liquids into light-colored glasses in order to be able to distinguish more clearly the surface of the liquids in the glasses and hence avoid underfilling or overfilling those containers).
- *Visual substitution devices.* Visual substitution devices call for the use of one or more senses other than sight (for example, talking watches or calculators, or the Opticon, a device that uses an electro-optical probe to scan printed material letter by letter and presents a raised image of each scanned letter to an index finger resting on a cradle or in a slot).
- *Visual substitution techniques.* Visual substitution techniques require the use of one or more senses other than sight (for example, the non-visual procedures that are needed to properly use a white cane or dial a telephone without viewing the dial.)
- *Visually impaired.* People are visually impaired if they are either functionally blind or partially sighted.

THE POPULATION

Since this book is primarily concerned with older people, the reader undoubtedly will be interested in the population breakdown for individuals who are at least 65 years old. Table 15.1 gives estimates of the partially sighted, partially sighted but not legally blind, legally blind, legally blind but not functionally blind, and functionally blind populations in the United States for 1990. It also shows estimates of the age distribution for each of these populations.

These estimates were made by first using (1) information obtained by the National Institute for Neurological Diseases and Blindness (NINDB) and by its successor, the National Eye Institute (NEI), in the course of a 1962–1971 population data collection and analysis study known as the Model Reporting Area (MRA) study and (2) estimates of the 1970 legally blind, as well as partially sighted and not legally blind, populations made by a committee of the National Academies of Sciences and Engineering. Subsequently, the change in age distribution that occurred in the United States population from 1966 to 1990 was taken into account.

From Table 15.1 it can be seen that 1,336,400, or 57.8%, of the partially sighted population is estimated to be at least 65 years old. Likewise, 1,071,500, or 57.8%, of the partially sighted but not legally blind population is in that age range; 335,800, or 55.8%, of the legally blind population; 264,900, or 57.8%, of the legally blind but not functionally blind population; and 70,900, or 49.5%, of the functionally blind population.

There is a very large difference between the number of people at least 65 years old who are legally blind but not functionally blind and those who are functionally blind. This difference can be explained in part by the fact that, with the exception of diabetic retinopathy, the other three major causes of severe visual loss among older people rarely lead to functional blindness either because of the inherent nature of the ocular pathology or because surgical and medical techniques exist that, in most cases, either check the progression toward functional blindness or, with the help of appropriate visual devices, nearly restore lost eyesight.

Common Visual Disorders in the Older Population

An erroneous myth prevails that individuals who are both partially sighted and legally blind should learn vision substitution methods and techniques to cope with daily needs, because most of them eventually will become blind or will at best be left with only light perception. Fortunately, as the previous section pointed out, medical evidence clearly indicates that most people who are both partially sighted and legally blind will continue to retain vision that is better than functional blindness throughout the remainder of their lives and, hence, in most cases, will continue to benefit from visual enhancement techniques and devices. A study by one of the authors (Genensky, 1978) has shown that even under the most pessimistic assumptions concerning the visual future of people who are both partially sighted and legally blind, a partially sighted child aged 5 years would have less than 12 chances in 100 of becoming functionally blind before age 65. If

Table 15.1 Summary of national data on various components of the visually impaired population, 1990

Age (yrs)	PS	PS-LB	LB	LB-FB	FB
0–4	6,200	5,000	2,000	1,200	800
5–19	117,200	94,000	35,400	23,200	12,200
20–44	390,600	313,200	106,500	77,400	29,100
45–64	463,600	371,700	122,200	91,900	30,300
65–74	394,700	316,500	101,700	78,200	23,500
75–84	483,300	387,500	120,900	95,800	25,100
85 +	458,400	367,500	113,200	90,900	22,300
Total	2,314,000	1,855,400	601,900	458,600	143,300

Abbreviations: PS, partially sighted; PS-LB, partially sighted but not legally blind; LB, legally blind; LB-FB, legally blind but not functionally blind; FB, functionally blind.

the data were available to permit the use of more realistic assumptions, it is probable that the chances of the child's becoming functionally blind over the 60-year span would turn out to be less than 5 in 100. The probability of an older partially sighted and legally blind individual's losing total sight is very likely greater than that for a child, but it is still small enough not to invalidate the assertion previously made concerning the likelihood of a partially sighted person's becoming functionally blind.

The four most commonly encountered visual diseases that afflict older people are age-related maculopathy, diabetic retinopathy, glaucoma, and cataracts. They account for more than 75% of severe visual impairment among older people in the United States. For a description of these eye diseases, see Chapter 4. The following section concerns these four major causes of visual loss as they bear on the visual care of the low-vision patient.

Age-Related Maculopathy

Age-related maculopathy patients tend to respond well, visually speaking, to a variety of visual devices that can help them see details up close, as well as far away. As to the acceptance of visual devices, this depends heavily upon patient motivation, self-image, and the presence or absence of other sensory disorders and physical or mental disorder.

Diabetic Retinopathy

There are two major forms of diabetic retinopathy: background retinopathy and proliferative retinopathy. All retinopathy begins as background retinopathy, and most patients do not develop the proliferative type. People with proliferative retinopathy make up between 3% and 10% of all diabetics. Individuals with proliferative retinopathy often encounter large, sometimes reversible fluctuations in the quality of their eyesight. One day they may be seeing well enough to drive a car or at least take a walk by themselves, and the next day they may be functionally blind (sometimes temporarily and sometimes permanently). Although individuals with proliferative retinopathy usually retain valuable eyesight over many years, some individuals suffer significant nonreversible losses rather suddenly. Vision-care professionals should help these people use all their remaining eyesight as long as they have it. However, such people also should be advised to acquaint themselves with various visual substitution techniques and devices so that if they become irreversibly functionally blind, they will have useful information about what can be done for them and what they can do for themselves.

Partly because of the potential effects of diabetes itself, and partly because of the fluctuations in vision, people with diabetic retinopathy, as well as members of their immediate families, frequently benefit from counseling. In addition, diabetics often find participation in patient support groups very beneficial.

Glaucoma

Glaucoma patients frequently have difficulty seeing at night and are bothered by glare during both the day and night. Impairment of night vision usually is the result of partial loss of rod, or peripheral, vision. Furthermore, in the early stages of the disease, many people with glaucoma have good central vision, even though an examination of their visual fields indicates that they have substantial scotomas in an annular or partially annular region about the macula.

Cataracts

Some ophthalmologists hesitate to remove a cataract if the patient is severely visually impaired by way of age related maculopathy in the affected eye, even if the patient has no other ocular diseases. They argue that (1) the removal of the cataract will not restore the patient's vision; (2) the patient will very likely remain legally blind; and, hence, (3) cataract surgery is contraindicated. The authors believe that this argument is sometimes fallacious. For example, in some instances, the cataract is very dense and either pervades a large portion of the lens or obscures a critical portion of it. If this is the case, and if the patient has no other ocular or systemic disorders that make surgery inadvisable, it appears reasonable to seriously consider removing the cataractous lens. New, low-vision techniques and visual devices frequently will permit the patient who has undergone successful cataract surgery and who has age-related maculopathy to advance from functional blindness to partial sightedness and to make better use of remaining eyesight.

PHILOSOPHY OF LOW-VISION CARE AT THE CENTER FOR THE PARTIALLY SIGHTED

One example of a low-vision care facility providing comprehensive rehabilitation services is The Center for the Partially Sighted in Santa Monica, California. The Center, established in 1978, has demonstrated that it is possible to provide partially sighted people of all ages with a set of services that are tailored to meet their special needs and that permit them to use all their remaining sensory capabilities, including their residual vision, to gain, regain, or maintain their visual independence.

At the Center, the needs of each patient are assessed, and a determination is made as to which of the following services might prove beneficial to the patient: low-vision optometric care; psychological counseling; orientation and mobility instruction; and direction to educational, vocational, social, and recreational services not offered at the Center. All services are given on an out-patient basis. Every attempt is made to help patients understand the difference between partial sightedness and functional blindness; the value of residual vision and how that vision can be used to perform tasks that are important to the patient; and how all sensory capabilities, including residual vision, can be used to enter, reenter, or remain within the framework of fully sighted society. This program provides partially sighted people with visual devices and teaches independent living skills that can reduce their medium and long-range dependence on scarce tax dollars.

LOW-VISION OPTOMETRIC CARE

A low-vision optometric examination differs from a general ophthalmologic examination in that it concentrates on determining what patients can do with their remaining eyesight rather than on determining the nature and extent of patients' ocular diseases and how best to treat them medically or surgically.

Low-vision optometric examinations should be designed to determine the patients' functional visual capabilities. Based on the results of these examinations and information gleaned from patients concerning their personal objectives and significant vision-related environmental problems, optometrists should determine which visual devices, if any, will help the patients perform one or more of these problematic tasks with comparative ease. Before purchasing these devices, patients should be encouraged to borrow and work with one or more appropriate loaner devices. A loaner program permits patients to try the devices in their homes or work environments and enables them to make more informed decisions about which devices to purchase for long-term use. Patients should be trained in the use of the devices, including the loaner devices, before they take them home. Thorough training is essential for patients to use visual devices effectively and avoid the devices being relegated to the bureau drawer.

About two to four months after the initial low-vision examination, a follow-up call or visit should be made to patients at their homes or work places by, for example, a case coordinator, social worker, or independent living skills instructor. These contacts enable staff members to determine how the patients are getting on with the devices prescribed for their use and to ascertain whether a recheck or additional visual device training is necessary. At this time, these professionals also can discuss inexpensive modifications that would make the visited environment safer or more visually comfortable.

PSYCHOLOGICAL ASPECTS OF AGING AND LOW VISION

To successfully work with older patients with low vision, the clinician needs technical skills, such as those for the measurement of remaining vision or prescribing appropriate visual devices. However, the difference between a good or poor outcome will depend on the interactions between the patient and clinician. Under the best of circumstances patients can be difficult, but especially following the loss of vision, they may be irritable, contrary, or distractible, or they may not even hear what the clinician has to say. Some patients will not accept the clinician's conclusions about their condition, or they may reject the visual device or other assistance offered. In the face of all evidence, they even may maintain that all they need is a new pair of glasses to correct their vision loss.

Many older people approach low-vision services enthusiastically and learn to use devices quickly and effectively. However, some have a great deal of difficulty adapting, even when their vision loss is not severe. Clinicians who expect that patients will be rational or will know what is best for them will be continually frustrated in low-vision work. The challenge is to learn effective ways of interacting with many difficult patients to increase their positive responses to optometric services. Just as the eye-care specialist relies on the scientific foundations of practice, there are appropriate procedures for managing doctor-patient interactions, and the practitioner can increase the number of people who can benefit from low-vision optometric services.

To work effectively with older patients, optometrists experienced in low-vision practice must be able to evaluate the possible causes of a poor response to services and what remedies can be tried. One potential cause is the effects of aging on behavioral capacity to respond. A second area, which applies to patients of any age, involves problems in compliance with treatment. These two areas will be reviewed, and the program of psychological services at The Center for the Partially Sighted, which has been developed to address these concerns, will be described.

Psychological Changes with Age

The most central question in dealing with older patients is the extent to which aging can be expected to interfere with successful adaptation to a vision loss. The predominant belief is that aging is associated with decline. There are certainly people who have suffered irreversible physical and mental declines that interfere with their response to low-vision services. However, the course of aging is highly variable. Some older people function at or near levels typical of the young, whereas others experience only mild, relatively benign psychological changes. Major decrements in functioning typically result from illnesses rather than aging per se. Nonetheless, many people confuse the effects of age and illness and view all older people as having major psychological impairments.

An example of the way old age and disease are confused is senile dementia. Senility involving severe decrements of memory and personality is considered by many people to be synonymous with old age. However, only 5% to 7% of people over 65 years have the type of progressive mental deterioration that could properly be termed senile (Mortimer, 1988). Furthermore, senile dementia is brought about by degenerative diseases of the brain, the most common being Alzheimer's disease and multi-infarct dementia. (See Chapter 2.) Just as older people are more prone to other chronic and degenerative conditions, the prevalence of dementia increases at advanced ages, but it is not a universal part of the aging process.

Individuals with senile dementia will be recognizable by their extreme forgetfulness. The dementia patient literally may be unable to remember from one minute to the next. This is different from the average older person, who — like everyone else — will forget occasionally. A person who is anxious or depressed may be more distractible, and it is important not to mistake forgetfulness in this person for the more permanent, persistent type found in dementia.

Working with dementia patients usually involves enlisting the cooperation of family members or other people involved in their care. Because of their extreme forgetfulness, the patients need to be reminded to follow any procedures that the clinician might recommend. Furthermore, problems they have with reading may involve comprehension as well as vision. Although the gains dementia patients can make from low-vision services are small, it is worthwhile at least to evaluate their response to visual devices.

In the absence of the catastrophic decrements caused by an illness creating dementia, the psychological changes associated with aging are relatively mild. Some practical suggestions can help the practitioner adjust for age-related differences in three areas of functioning: (1) learning and memory, (2) cautiousness, and (3) hearing.

The older person generally will need more time to learn new information, especially when it is novel or unusual. When information is given at too fast a pace, learning can be disrupted seriously. Distractions also may interfere with learning to a greater extent for older people than for younger ones. Problems in learning often are magnified by hearing and vision losses. Once information is learned, however, the older person will remember effectively, perhaps as well as when the person was younger (Howard, 1991; Craik, 1977). Steps the clinician can take to enhance learning include pacing the presentation of information or instructions more slowly, cutting down distractions, and writing or typing instructions in large print with bold letters so the patient can review them later.

Another dimension of behavior with practical relevance is cautiousness. In general, older people have been found to make more cautious responses in a number of situations. For instance, they are less likely to guess when taking tests, even when they are fairly sure they know the answer (Botwinick, 1978). This reluctance to guess carries over to other situations. In an auditory examination, for example, older people failed to report hearing tones that were faint but had previously been determined to be within their range of hearing (Rees and Botwinick, 1971). As a result, they gave the impression of having far more hearing loss than was actually present. Cautiousness may have a similar effect on the vision examination. Encouraging older patients to guess can overcome this inhibition.

Hearing loss is fairly common among older people and may be a major reason for communication problems (Fozard, 1990). The hearing-impaired person can, at times, be mistaken as senile or confused, although with proper methods of communication, the effects of the hearing loss can be minimized. Some ways of working with patients with hearing loss include speaking slowly, distinctly, and in complete sentences; using a room with good acoustics; and eliminating background noises. It is not necessary for people to shout to be heard. Although many hearing-impaired people are helped by hearing devices, some have conditions that cannot be corrected. New developments in hearing device technology are increasing the number of people who can benefit while decreasing limitations such as the difficulty of filtering out background noise. As with vision devices, adaptation to hearing devices may take time and training.

Perhaps the most important factor that emerges from studies of normal aging is that older people as a group are more variable or different from one another than are younger people. On any given test of abilities, some older people will score as well as the young, whereas others will do more poorly (Zarit and Zarit, 1987). Even for reaction time, where the most consistent differences between old and young have been reported, some older people can respond as fast as younger individuals; for others, the slowing is minimal. It therefore is difficult to make predictions about the "average" older person. More so than at any other age, averages are misleading. One older person will have difficulty with memory; another will be rigid; and still another will be lively, flexible, and have a good memory.

A major implication for working with older patients is to evaluate each person individually and not make assumptions based on chronologic age. People's current behaviors and attitudes can be understood in the context of values and habits they had in the past, as well as their current circumstances. Rather than look upon an elder as someone for whom nothing can be done, the vision-care practitioner can consider the role vision has played in the person's life and how that individual has adapted to change in the past. Although adaptation may be slower than for younger patients, the practitioner who takes time with older people will obtain good results.

Common Problems in Adaptation and Compliance

The aging person who has experienced recent losses in vision represents a major challenge for the vision-care practitioner. As with any major life stress, adaptation to visual loss is a difficult process. Often the person's emotional reaction will be intense or self-defeating and will interfere with appropriate adaptational responses. The key to a successful outcome is for the clinician to understand that the patient's emotional response is an integrated part of the eye problem and has to be dealt with as part of the rehabilitative process. By understanding the basis of self-defeating or irrational behaviors, clinicians can assist patients to make better choices about visual devices and other low-vision assistance.

Many older patients have a poor initial response to low-vision devices. They may reject them without trying them, use them briefly and then give up, or use the devices in ways that do not produce maximum benefit. Perhaps as many as one of every two older patients has a poor first response to low-vision devices.

These patients often are described as "unmotivated." The vision care specialist may believe that if only the patient wanted to get help, the response to treatment would be adequate. However, lack of motivation is too general a concept for understanding patients. A few patients derive benefits from their vision loss, such as having someone take care of them or being eligible for disability, and they are not interested in increasing their own independence. Most partially sighted people, however, truly want to use their vision again. Furthermore, patients who are difficult or noncompliant rarely believe they are the cause of the problem. Instead, they regard the treatment as inadequate for their condition. Even when patients are aware they are noncompliant, they may not be able to understand why.

The low-vision specialist must identify the specific reason for noncompliance of a given patient. This means gathering information from several sources, including the patient's verbal reports about the eye problems and observations of how the patient uses visual devices. Possible reasons for noncompliance include the patients' beliefs about their visual condition and about the use of visual devices, as well as behavioral problems that prevent adequate adaptation to visual devices. Once the basis of noncompliance has been identified, interventions can be made to improve the response to treatment. Such interventions may involve testing self-defeating beliefs, involving patients in managing their own problems better, and breaking down complex visual tasks, such as reading, into a series of simpler steps. These interventions have been found useful for dealing with a variety of emotional problems (Teri, 1991; Beck et al. 1979; Lewinsohn et al. 1978). Several common problems and ways of managing them will be described.

One of the most straightforward and frustrating obstacles to compliance is when patients believe that what they need is a new, stronger pair of spectacles, and they do not understand why the optometrist has shown them more cumbersome devices such as magnifiers or telescopes. When they first come to a low-vision service, patients have varying degrees of information about their condition. Some may not understand what their condition means for visual functioning. Although the low-vision specialist can give a careful explanation and answer the patient's questions, that does not always mean the patient will understand.

When a patient does not respond to a brief explanation, it is important to go into more detail. The clinician can discuss why new glasses would not correct the condition — for example, the clinician can state that glasses correct for errors in refraction, whereas the patient's condition involves damage to the retina. Using the analogy that the eye is like a camera sometimes helps. It should then be determined if the patient believes the explanation. If so, the patient then can be encouraged to try visual devices again, with the instruction to find out if there is anything that makes even a small difference. By emphasizing to the patient the importance of determining if there is a "small difference," the clinician guards against creating other unrealistic expectations, such as being able to see as well as in the past. However, if patients do not respond to these efforts to explain the nature of the vision problem or continue to insist that they just want a new pair of glasses, they can be encouraged to continue their search. However, it must be stressed that these patients are welcome to come back if they decide to try the other devices available. For some patients, keeping open the possibility of returning at a later date may be the best that can be done.

A related belief that interferes with adjustment is that it is too embarrassing or demeaning to use visual devices. Some patients think the devices will call too much attention to them or will cause others to pity them or think of them as strange. Through questioning a patient, the optometrist can determine the specific reason why devices are embarrassing and the situations in which the patient would be uncomfortable. It sometimes may be sufficient to explain that most partially sighted persons are a bit ill at ease when they first use their devices. They generally find that other people respect them rather than pity them. One patient, for example, said he initially would not use his device (a hand-held telescope for distance viewing), but he subsequently found that when he did use it in social situations, it provided a helpful way to initiate conversations with strangers. He evaluated the change in his attitude this way: life had handed him a lemon (his visual problem), but he was trying to turn it into lemonade. Sometimes giving patients examples such as this one helps, but occasionally the best tactic is to introduce them to other partially sighted people who are using devices. Hearing firsthand from someone who has a similar problem that the gains from using devices far outweigh any minor embarrassments can make the most difference.

Other beliefs that interfere with compliance involve pessimism and hopelessness about what the device can do. Some patients believe they cannot be happy unless the devices restore their vision to what it used to be. Using what Beck et al. (1979) call "all-or-nothing" thinking, these patients maintain there is no reason to use low-vision devices, because their vision is not restored totally. They will make statements such as, "It's not the same," or "It's just no good," and they will actively frustrate efforts by the clinician to determine how much use they potentially might get from a given device. They also may be disturbed by some aspects of how they see with the device. For instance, some patients complain about the reduced visual field they have when using magnifiers. Others complain about how they have to use the devices; for example, a reading portion might be too awkward or uncomfortable, or they may have to read more slowly than in the past.

There are several ways in which patients can be helped to question these pessimistic attitudes. First, the clinician can explain to them that it takes time to get used to a device. Improvement is gradual and does not occur all at once. This is particularly the case with someone who maintains that the devices are too awkward or uncomfortable, or who reports reading too slowly or tiring too easily. The clinician also can ask patients about other situations in which they faced changes to determine how they generally adapt to new circumstances. One woman who did not like the way she had to read with microscopic spectacles remembered that she did not like Talking Books either when she first received them, but now she uses them all the time. Once she gave this example, she was able to understand that she often responds negatively to changes. At that point, she was able to accept the microscopic spectacles that were being suggested to her.

A particularly difficult type of patient is the "help rejector." This person says "Help me," but then refuses anything that is offered. The help rejector maintains that nothing makes a difference, even when objective testing of visual functioning with devices indicates differently. Once someone with this negative belief has been identified, the clinician needs to present the devices in a paradoxical way, for example: "This is a device that helps a lot of people, but I am not sure you can use it. Tell me if it makes a difference." This approach upsets the patient's usual negative response. Another strategy is to ask the patient what amount or percent of improvement he or she would consider significant. Many people with all-or-nothing thinking will scale down their expectations when forced to be more specific. The extent to which devices can help them fulfill their expectations then can be discussed.

With some oppositional and negative patients, the best approach is to give them a choice between different visual devices. They may not always choose the device that gives them the most benefit, but their choice will reflect other, intangible factors, such as which device fits best into their life-style.

One final reason for a poor response to low-vision devices is a patient's never having been a good reader. Adequate magnification of print is possible, but the patient cannot put together the simplest words or sentences. These patients differ from those with just negative expectations in that their reading skills are just not adequate to meet the increased challenge of reading with magnification. An approach using the method of "successive approximations" may be beneficial to these patient (Rimm and Masters, 1978). Successive approximations involves breaking a task down into small, manageable components. A person can master a skill by starting at the simple level and gradually increasing the complexity level. Most of the problems with poor readers appear to be in figuring out individual words quickly. To build up this ability, they can begin with simple words or pairs of words. When their speed begins to pick up, they can move to sentences and, eventually, to printed material. The goals often can be modest, since patients' goals may involve reading a label or letter, not a complicated test.

Psychological Services for Low-Vision Patients

A viable psychology program should have five components: assessment, individual and family psychotherapy, patient groups, consultation, and peer counselors. Assessments should be made when patients are referred by an optometrist or by other health or rehabilitation professionals or paraprofessionals. The assessment seeks to determine if the person has a significant psychological problem interfering with rehabilitation and what type of intervention would be best. Depending on the assessment, the patient may be referred for individual or family psychotherapy, he or she could be recommended to a patient support group, or there could be a consultation between the psychologist and other clinical personnel on better ways of interacting with the patient.

People judged to be in need of psychotherapy are those who manifest severe adjustment reactions. Some examples are severely depressed, anxious, angry, or worried individuals or those having pronounced interpersonal difficulties. In many instances, the problems preceded the vision loss but may have been exacerbated by it. Individual or family therapy that may be time limited should be offered; or, if the patient lives too far away to travel regularly for assistance, referrals should be made to mental health professionals in their own communities.

When the symptoms of distress are not severe, or if the person is isolated socially, a patient group often is useful. Such a group should emphasize the exchange of information among patients and developing positive self-images. Much of the benefit will come from observing and learning from the successes of other patients. For instance, people may observe others using visual devices successfully or learn strategies from compensating for their visual loss, such as how they might identify people in a social situation. Finding out they are not alone in having a vision problem is often very helpful in itself for older patients.

Groups also may revolve around specific medical diagnoses that cause vision loss along with other physical problems. Typically, these groups are time-limited and provide introductions to other rehabilitative services as well as the peer support mentioned above. Often, information about the core medical problem is discussed, and visually accessible informational materials are distributed. Examples of such groups at the Center include the Diabetes Education and Support Group and the HIV and Vision Loss Support Group.

A consultation with the optometric staff should occur for each patient who is referred for psychological assessment. The consultation should involve conveying the findings of the assessment and working out strategies for interacting with the patient. Many of the referrals will involve patients who do not have prominent psychiatric symptoms such as depression or anxiety, but whose attitudes or behaviors interfere with successful adaptation, as described earlier. In collaboration with the low-vision staff, the psychologist will use the findings of the assessment to formulate new approaches for working with the patient in question.

Because of the benefits patients can derive from talking to someone else with a similar vision problem, a peer counseling program is recommended. Volunteers for the program might be former patients who have gone through a special training program in communications skills. Their role might be to greet new patients and answer any questions they might have while waiting for their examination. They should not respond to technical questions about vision; they should tell the patient to ask the low-vision specialist these questions. Instead, they should talk about the different services available and how they have been able to adjust to their vision problem. New patients will frequently welcome the opportunity to ask questions of a peer and often will be surprised and pleased to meet someone else with a vision problem.

Summary

Although aging has some effects on mental processing, most older people have the capacity to adapt to changes, including learning to use visual devices. Many patients, however, make a poor initial response to low-vision devices. The clinician's task is to identify the reasons for this poor response and give the patient information that counters the negative beliefs. Patients' compliance and understanding can be increased considerably by working with them in this way.

ENVIRONMENTAL ADAPTATION

As can be gleaned from the prior sections of this chapter, we believe that comprehensive low-vision care is much more than a low-vision examination, the prescription of visual devices as a result of such an examination, and training in the proper use of those devices. This chapter has demonstrated the relevance of competent psychological counseling to comprehensive low-vision care. This section will discuss orientation and mobility; home visits; independent living skills; and information that can and should be conveyed to the older partially sighted patient during those visits, as well as at comprehensive centers.

Orientation and Mobility

In general, emphasis should be placed on teaching patients how to move about safely and independently using visual enhancement techniques (that is, all their remaining sensory capabilities, including their residual vision, augmented when necessary with appropriate visual devices). Thus, patients should be taught, for example, how to use a monocular, binoculars, or telescopic spectacles to perform distance tasks such as determining the status of a traffic signal, the number or name of a bus, the name of a street, a street address or office number, or a name on an office door in a public building. However, the mere acquisition of a monocular or other distance-viewing device does not guarantee that it will be used or used properly. Patients need training in the use of the devices, and the training preferably should take place daily in a context in which the patient can be expected to use the devices.

There are circumstances in which some partially sighted people should be encouraged to carry and display a cane, even though visual parameters such as best-corrected distance visual acuity and size and shape of visual fields would not indicate a need for such a device. For example, people who have both macular degeneration and very slow reaction rates to visual and other sensory information should be encouraged to carry and display a cane when moving on a crowded street or passing through automobile traffic in order to inform others that they have a visual problem.

Some partially sighted people should be taught to use a cane properly to move from place to place. For example, people who have very restricted visual fields, regardless of what their best-corrected visual acuities might be, should be encouraged to obtain thorough training in the proper use of a cane. This follows from the fact that these people cannot visually comprehend enough of a complicated traffic situation fast enough to avoid being injured or perhaps being the cause of injury to others. Many people with retinitis pigmentosa or with advanced glaucoma fall into this category. Partially sighted people who experience fluctuations in vision that at times leave them functionally blind (as is sometimes the case among people having very advanced cases of diabetic retinopathy) also need instruction on how to use a cane properly during periods in which they are effectively functionally blind.

Home Visits

Whenever possible, it is strongly recommended that older adults receive a follow-up visit to their homes. Follow-up visits are the best assurance that patients have successfully transferred the information and training received at the agency to their homes. The visit should last no longer than 90 minutes and be conducted by a professional who is trained to conduct a multifaceted evaluation such as the following.

1. *Safety Check.* Common hazards such as loose rugs, unmarked stairs, cluttered pathways, and electrical or telephone cords that obstruct pathways should be noted and practical alternatives suggested.
2. *Basic Markings.* Stove dials, appliances, and telephones should be marked with large print numbers and/or orange fluorescent high marks. Appliances and such become more accessible to the visually impaired person, utilization is increased, and safety is enhanced.
3. *Lighting.* Assessment of glare sources as well as an investigation of general and task-specific lighting should be conducted. Recommendations should be made to minimize glare and enhance in-home lighting.
4. *Low-Vision Device Check.* Use of prescribed low-vision devices should be checked to ensure proper utilization and patient satisfaction. Individuals who require more training or who voice dissatisfaction with their low-vision devices should be encouraged to return for more training and/or optometric assistance.

Often, low-vision patients don't mention the everyday problems they encounter at home because they believe nothing can be done about them. They simply do without. They very often are amazed during the home visit when these "unsolvable" problems are solved quickly and easily with a wide variety of solutions (Genensky, 1979, 1980, 1981; Genensky et al., 1979).

Independent Living Skills

Independent living skills (ILS) training is designed to restore, strengthen, and help maintain the safe and independent functioning of visually impaired persons within the home. Areas of training include identification and organization (for example, labeling medications), personal management (for example, money management), cooking skills, communication skills (for example, telephone use) and leisure activity (using high-tech CDs, VCRs). Instruction is generally provided in two formats:

Class Instruction usually is geared to someone who has many problems functioning within the home. The class is limited to a maximum of eight students, meets once a week for two hours, and has a structured, sequenced curriculum in which all instruction is "hands-on." Class participants receive the added benefit of peer interaction and support, thus decreasing the feeling of being the only one with vision-related problems.

Individual In-home Training consists of two to five home visits focused on problem areas identified by the patient. Usually younger persons (under 50), people who work or attend school, or people who have a few specific problem areas prefer this shorter training program.

IMPORTANT AND USEFUL INFORMATION FOR THE PARTIALLY SIGHTED

What follows illustrates the kinds of information and advice that teacher counselors of the blind and rehabilitation counselors of the blind should give to their partially sighted clients, whether they are or are not legally blind. General information about services available to the visually impaired is useful. For example, local services may include special transportation services or discounted taxi fares, and state services may include identification cards available from the State Department of Motor Vehicles, which are similar in appearance to drivers' licenses and which can be used for identification or check-cashing purposes.

Probably the best known national program is the Talking Book Program. For people who enjoy reading and who cannot read long articles or books for long enough periods of time or rapidly enough to make it practical, the Library of Congress provides a service that may prove useful. The Talking Book Program provides free recordings or tape cassettes of a large number of current and classical books and periodicals for handicapped people who are not able to read printed material. The Talking Book Program provides record players and tape recorders for use with its records and tapes, and it also services this equipment — all at no charge to the user. Talking Books and Talking Book machines (record players and tape recorders) are distributed by the Library of Congress through a system of regional and branch libraries. Although this program is admirable and has enriched the lives of tens of thousands of legally blind and physically handicapped people for more than 40 years, the selection of materials available is limited. Thus, it would appear that the partially sighted person who is a serious reader and who can use visual devices for reading also will want to use the devices to maintain reading independence and avoid curtailing the selection of reading material.

In addition to the information already described, patients should receive specific advice concerning things they should or should not do to make their adaptation to partial sight smoother and perhaps more efficient. Table 15.2 gives specific examples illustrating the scope, degree, or kind of advice and information that most partially sighted older people might benefit from having.

A comprehensive program of supportive rehabilitative services is essential to achieve success with selected low-vision patients. It is strongly recommended that vision-care specialists who do not have such supportive services available through their own offices or clinics seek them in their communities for those patients who might benefit.

Table 15.2 Aids to daily living guidelines for the partially sighted

1. Keep all room doors totally open or totally closed to minimize the dangers of inadvertently walking into the vertical edge of a door.
2. Use dishes and glasses that contrast in color with the tablecloth or table (that is, white or light dishes on a dark cloth or table, or dark dishes on a light cloth or table). When pouring liquids, pour dark liquids into light cups or mugs and light liquids into dark cups or mugs. For example, pour coffee into a white cup and milk into a dark mug. This use of the color-contrast technique will help to avoid underfilling as well as overfilling the container.
3. Tack down or otherwise inhibit the motion of a scatter rug. This will reduce the possibility of falling because of rug slippage.
4. Avoid placing lamps and other sources of artificial light in places or positions that result in people having to look at bare lightbulbs or at reflections of those bulbs coming from reflectors that may be associated with them. Bare lightbulbs or light coming from such reflectors can be annoying even to fully sighted persons. For many partially sighted people, it can be physically painful or blinding in the sense that other objects in the visual field that otherwise would be visible are fully or nearly completely obscured by the light generated by the bulbs or off the reflectors.
5. When reading or writing, make sure the lighting sources illuminate the printed work or the writing paper and not the eyes of the person trying to read or write.
6. Arrange clothing according to color or put clothes together in matched sets. In the former case, for example, clearly labeled dividers can be placed on clothes racks to distinguish one color set from another. Many partially sighted people have good color vision, but many others have difficulty distinguishing among low- or medium-saturation colors, especially in the presence of incandescent lighting.
7. Use brightly colored reflecting tape to mark dial settings on stoves, washers, dryers, and other appliances to indicate critical settings. Partially sighted people frequently have great difficulty reading these dials and need this additional visual boost.
8. Do not reach across burners on a gas or electric stove. Partially sighted people often have difficulty determining visually whether or not a gas burner is lit or an electric element is heated, particularly when the color or gray value of the flame or heated coil is not in high contrast with the color or gray value of the portion of the stove immediately adjacent to it. For safety's sake, try to confine cooking to the gas burners or electric elements closest to the front of the stove. By doing this, there will be less chance of inadvertently reaching across a lit burner or hot electrical element.
9. Avoid the use of glass-top coffee tables or other low glass-top furniture to prevent severe leg bruises caused by bumping into the virtually invisible glass.
10. Clearly mark sliding glass doors with colorful decals or other clearly visible markings to reduce the chance of serious injury from glass door-human collision.
11. Mark the leading edge of all interior and exterior steps with a stripe of paint or a strip of nonskid material that runs the width of the step. The strip should be 5 cm wide on both the runner and the riser and have a color and gray value that stands out in high contrast to the color and gray value of the rest of the step. (A coating of clear resin mixed with clear transparent aggregate protects painted stripes and provides some traction.) Steps marked in this way can be seen by at least 95% of all partially sighted people. Furthermore, marking steps in this way is also useful to fully sighted older people, many of whom have a great fear of falling or tripping on stairs (Genensky, 1979, 1980, 1981).

Table 15.2 continued

12. Place knives, forks, and other sharp objects with their points downward in drainers and dishwasher silverware baskets. This will avoid the problem of inadvertently grasping the blade of the knife or the prongs of a fork.

13. Never move the face close to an object to view it more clearly until the object has been checked carefully and cautiously with the hands to determine whether it has any pointed or sharp edges that could injure eyes. Similarly, never move an object close to the face to see it more clearly until it has been inspected with the hands.

14. If a steel needle or a common pin is missing and its approximate location is known, a small, strong magnet can be used to "sweep" the area and find the missing needle or pin. If the sharp object is in the area and the magnet is close enough to the surface — say, about 1 cm to 3 cm — the needle or pin will be attracted to the magnet. To determine that the needle or pin has in fact been picked up by the magnet, move fingers carefully over or near the magnet. Never bring the magnet close to the eyes; if the needle or pin is present, it could cause serious injury.

15. When sweeping or washing a floor or vacuuming a rug, mentally divide the floor or rug into squares or other convenient shapes enclosing about 9 to 16 square feet. First, thoroughly sweep (wash, or vacuum) a square in one corner of the room; then do the same to the square to the immediate right (or left) of it and to each successive square in the row until the end of the row is reached. Follow the same procedure across each row, and continue doing this until the last row has been completed. In this way if the dirt or dust on the floor or rug cannot be seen, one still can be reasonably sure a good job of cleaning was done. A still better procedure requires that the successive squares overlap somewhat with their closest neighbors.

16. Carefully order the paper money in a wallet or billfold either in increasing or decreasing order of value. For those who still would have difficulty telling one bill from another even with the aid of a visual device that they carry about with them, a money-folding convention used by the totally blind may prove useful. The convention calls for leaving one-dollar bills unfolded, five-dollar bills folded in half lengthwise, 10-dollar bills folded in half widthwise, and 20-dollar bills folded in half widthwise and then folded in half again widthwise. You also may find it convenient to separate bills of various denominations from one another by ordinary paper clips. Thus, the one-dollar bills are all clipped together, the five-dollar bills are all clipped together, and so on, and the clipped bills are arranged in the billfold either in increasing or decreasing order. Imaginative use of the paper clips would make it possible to differentiate the various denominations from one another without having to see them visually. For example, a single paper clip at the longest side of the bills indicates that they are one-dollar bills, a single paper clip at the shorter side of the bills indicates that they are five-dollar bills, two paper clips at the long side of the bills indicates that they are ten-dollar bills, and so on.

17. If one has trouble seeing the numbers on a telephone dial, a special enlarged telephone dial cover that has enlarged numbers and letters can be used. One also may be able to learn to dial strictly by touch. For many people, this is not hard to do with a bit of practice. For example, placing the nonthumb fingers of the right hand in the first four holes of the dial immediately tells you where the numbers 1,2,3 and 4 are located and that the number 5 is below and slightly to the left of your index finger. Placing the same fingers in the last four holes of the dial immediately tells

Table 15.2 continued

you where the numbers 7, 8, 9, and 0 are located and that the number 6 is above and slightly to the left of your index finger. Using this finger map, the right index finger can be trained to dial as rapidly as you please. For many individuals, "dialing" with push buttons is much easier than dialing with the circular dial. With the right hand, the index finger can be placed on the button labeled 1, the big finger on the button labeled 2, and the ring finger on the button labeled 3. The same fingers on the second row of the push buttons cover 4,5, and 6, respectively, and on the third row they cover 7,8, and 9, respectively. On the fourth row they cover the asterisk, the 0, and the number sign, respectively. For those who prefer to use the push button telephone with a display of enlarged numbers and letters, a plastic cover having these properties is also available.

18. To avoid losing contact with friends, for example, on the street or at a large gathering, one should ask fully sighted friends to say hello and to tell their names when they first see them. One should explain that because of impaired vision, they are no longer recognized, even if they are standing very close. By doing this, both partially sighted people and their friends are put at ease. The former no longer wonder who passed by, who is approaching them, or who is standing in front of them, and the latter are no longer at a loss as to how to cope with their friend's visual impairment in this regard. Furthermore, friends tend to respect people who have accepted their partial sightedness and have, as it were, taken command of their visual loss. Thus, both parties are more at ease. As a result, they frequently find it easier to talk to one another about the visual problem and, perhaps, further ease any tension that might still exist because of the reduction in vision.

19. When it is necessary to approach the entrance of a bus and ask the driver a question, such as what is the number of this bus, it is best to also let the driver know that you cannot see well. For example, say to the driver, "Excuse me. I don't see very well. Could you please tell me if this is the number 38 bus?" By doing this, the driver is alerted to the existence of the visual problem and the chances of responses like "Can't you read?" or "You blind or something?" will be reduced. Both of these responses are uncalled for, but the driver is human and is subject to making "dumb statements." This same technique would be helpful in asking people for directions or assistance in determining the name of a street or number of a building. It is best to help others assist a partially sighted person, and in so doing, avoid confrontations.

20. One should not let an ego or vanity interfere with using vision and visual devices. Experience has shown that fully sighted people soon get used to the use of visual devices, and they accept their presence and use as perfectly normal. In addition, they frequently develop a greater admiration and respect for the partially sighted person because that person has accepted his or her visual status; uses the devices; and, as a consequence, participates more effectively in fully sighted society. Also, as noted in Item 18, when one uses devices, fully sighted friends and family are put at ease. The anxiety they sometimes experience is eased because they want to help and do not know what to do.

REFERENCES

1. Beck, A., D. Rush, D. Shaw, and G. Emery. *Cognitive Therapy of Depression.* New York: Guildford Press, 1979.

2. Botwinick, J. *Aging and Behavior,* 2nd ed. New York: Springer Publishing, 1978.
3. Craik, F.I.M. Age Differences in Human Memory. In: *Handbook of the Psychology of Aging,* J.E. Birren and K.W. Schaie (eds.). New York: Van Nostrand Reinhold, 1977.
4. Fozard, J.L. Vision and Hearing in Aging. In: *Handbook of the Psychology of Aging,* 3rd ed. J.E. Birren and K.W. Schaie (eds.). (pp. 150–168). New York: Academic Press, 1990.
5. Genensky, S.M. "Data Concerning the Partially Sighted and the Functionally Blind." *J. Vis. Impair. Blind.* 72, no. 5 (1978):177–180.
6. Genensky, S.M. "Architectural Barriers to Partially Sighted Persons." *Report (National Center for a Barrier Free Environment)* 5, no. 2 (1979):8.
7. Genensky, S.M. "Architectural Barriers to the Partially Sighted-And Solutions." *Architectural Record* (May 1980):65–67.
8. Genensky, S.M. "Design Sensitivity and the Partially Sighted." *Building Operation Management* (June 1981):50–54.
9. Genensky, S.M., S.H. Berry, T.H. Bikson, and T.K. Bikson. *Visual Environmental Adaptation Problems of the Partially Sighted: Final Report (CPS-100-HEW).* Santa Monica, CA: Santa Monica Hospital Medical Center for the Partially Sighted, January 1979.
10. Howard, D.V. Implicit Memory: An Expanding Picture of Cognitive Aging. In: *Annual Review of Gerontology and Geriatrics,* v. 11, K.W. Schaie and M.P. Lawton (eds.). New York: Springer, 1991, pp. 1–22.
11. Lewinsohn, P.M., R.F. Munoz, M.S. Youngren, and A.M. Zeiss. *Control Your Depression.* Englewood Cliffs, N.J.; Prentice-Hall, 1978.
12. Mortimer, J.A. "Epidemiology of Dementia — International Comparisons." In: J. Brody and G. Maddox (eds.). *Epidemiology of Aging.* New York: Springer, 1988.
13. Rees, J., and J. Botwinick. "Detection and Decision Factors in Auditory Behavior of the Elderly.: *J. Gerontol.* 26 (1971):133–136.
14. Rimm, D.C., and J.C. Masters. *Behavior Therapy: Techniques and Empirical Findings,* 2nd ed. New York: Academic Press, 1978.
15. Teri, L. Behavioral Assessment and Treatment of Depression in Older Adults. In: P.A. Wisocki (ed.). *Handbook of Clinical Behavior Therapy with the Elderly Client.* New York: Plenum, 1991, pp. 225–244.
16. Zarit, J.M., and S.H. Zarit. Molar Aging: Physiology and Psychology of Normal Aging. In: L.L. Carstensen and B.A. Edelstein (eds.). *Handbook of Clinical Gerontology.* New York: Pergamon, 1987, pp. 18–30.

SUGGESTED READINGS

1. "Argon Laser Photocoagulation for Senile Macular Degeneration." *Arch. Ophthalmol.* 100 (June 1982): 912–918.
2. Bernstein, C. "Altering SMD Victims in Time." Sight-Saving: *J. Blindness Prevention* 51, no. 2 (1982): 16–20.
3. Birren, J.E., and J. Botwinick. "Age Differences in Finger, Jaw, and Foot Reaction Time to Auditory Stimuli." *J. Gerontol.* 10 (1955): 429–432.
4. Botwinick, J. Intellectual Abilities. In: J.E. Birren and K.W. Schaie (eds.). *Handbook of the Psychology of Aging.* New York: Van Nostrand Reinhold, 1977.
5. Chown, S.M. "Age and the Rigidities." *J. Gerontol.* 16 (1961): 353–362.
6. Coughlin, W.R., and A. Patz. "Diabetic Retinopathy." *Diabetes Forecast,* 1978.
7. Hassinger, M.J., J.M. Zarit, and S.H. Zarit. "A Comparison of Clinical Characteristics of Multi-infarct and Alzheimer's Dementia Patients." Paper presented at the meeting of the Western Psychological Association, Sacramento, CA 1982.

8. National Institutes of Health, U.S. Department of Health, Education, and Welfare. *Model Reporting Area for Blindness Statistics.* Washington, D.C.: U.S. Government Printing Office, 1962–1970.
9. NIA Task Force. "Senility Reconsidered." *J.A.M.A.* 244, no. 3 (1980): 259–263.
10. Rosenbloom, A.A. "Care of Elderly People with Low Vision." *J. Vis. Impair. Blind.* (June 1982): 209–212.
11. Schaie, K.W., and G. Labouvie-Vief. "Generational Versus Ontogenetic Components of Change in Adult Cognitive Behavior: A Fourteen Year Cross-Sequential Study." *Dev. Psychol.* 10 (1974): 305–320.
12. "SMD: Clearing up the Picture." *Eye Care Digest* 1, no. 1 (1982): 4.
13. Zarit, S.H. *Aging and Mental Disorders.* New York: Free Press, 1980.
14. Zarit, S.H. "Affective Correlates of Self-reports about Memory of Older People." *Int. J. Behav. Geriatrics* 1 (1982): 24–34.
15. Zarit, S.H., and J.M. Zarit. "Families Under Stress." *Psychotherapy: Theory, Research and Practice* 19 (1982): 461–471.

ACKNOWLEDGMENT

The authors wish to gratefully acknowledge the assistance of Phyllis Amaral, Ph.D, Javier Gomez, M.A., and Pamela Thompson, Ph.D. in completing this manuscript.

Index

Note: Page numbers in italics indicate figures; page numbers followed by t indicate tables.